Cultures of the Abdomen

Cultures of the Abdomen

Diet, Digestion, and Fat in the Modern World

Edited by

Christopher E. Forth
and
Ana Carden-Coyne

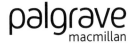

CULTURES OF THE ABDOMEN
© Christopher E. Forth and Ana Carden-Coyne, 2005.

First published in 2005 by
PALGRAVE MACMILLAN™
175 Fifth Avenue, New York, N.Y. 10010 and
Houndmills, Basingstoke, Hampshire, England RG21 6XS
Companies and representatives throughout the world.

PALGRAVE MACMILLAN is the global academic imprint of the Palgrave Macmillan division of St. Martin's Press, LLC and of Palgrave Macmillan Ltd. Macmillan® is a registered trademark in the United States, United Kingdom and other countries. Palgrave is a registered trademark in the European Union and other countries.

ISBN 1–4039–6521–8

Library of Congress Cataloging-in-Publication Data

Cultures of the abdomen : diet, digestion, and fat in the modern world / edited by Christopher E. Forth and Ana Carden-Coyne.
  p.cm.
Includes bibliographical references and index.
ISBN 1–4039–6521–8 (hc : alk. Paper)
  1. Abdomen—Social aspects. 2. Abdomen—History. 3. Food habits.
4. Fat. 5. Obesity. I. Forth, Christopher E. II. Carden-Coyne, Ana.

GT498.A24C85 2004
306.4′613—dc22   2004050508

A catalogue record for this book is available from the British Library.

Design by Newgen Imaging Systems (P) Ltd., Chennai, India.

First edition: January 2005

10 9 8 7 6 5 4 3 2 1

Printed in the United States of America.

Contents

Notes on Contributors

Ken Albala teaches early modern European history at the University of the Pacific in Stockton, California, where he is also department chair. Among regular history courses, he also teaches A Global History of Food and A History of Medicine. His first book, *Eating Right in the Renaissance*, was published by the University of California Press in 2001, and his second, *Food in Early Modern Europe*, was published by the Greenwood Press in 2003. He is also series editor for Greenwood's "Food Culture Around the World" series. He is currently starting a history of dining in the late Renaissance, to be published by the University of Illinois Press.

Ana Carden-Coyne is Lecturer in the Cultural History of Modern War at the Centre for the Cultural History of Modern War, University of Manchester. She has published articles on bodybuilding, war memorials, and the cultural history of medicine, and is currently working on a monograph, *Revenge of the Body: Classicism, Modernism and the First World War.*

Lucia Dacome is a Research Fellow at The Wellcome Trust Centre for the History of Medicine at University College London working on early modern European medicine. She has written on the history of nutrition, anatomy, and resurrection.

Christopher E. Forth is Reader in History at the Australian National University, where he teaches courses in the cultural history of gender, sexuality, and the body. He is the author of *Zarathustra in Paris: The Nietzsche Vogue in France, 1891-1918* and *The Dreyfus Affair and the Crisis of French Manhood*, as well as coeditor (with Ivan Crozier) of *Body Parts: Critical Explorations in Corporeality*. His current project is a history of the male body in the Western world (under contract with Palgrave).

Jay Geller is Senior Lecturer of Modern Jewish Culture at Vanderbilt Divinity School and the Vanderbilt University Department of Religious Studies. He has published numerous articles on Freud's Jewish identity and on the relationship between antisemitism and modern European Jewish identity formation. More recently, his work has focused on the Shoah and film. Currently completing a manuscript that includes chapters on Levin Varnahgen, Heine, Nordau, Schreber, Kafka (inter alia) as well as on Freud, he had earlier co-edited *Reading Freud's Reading* and a special issue of *American Imago* on "Postmemories of the Holocaust."

Sander L. Gilman is Distinguished Professor of the Liberal Arts and Medicine at the University of Illinois in Chicago and the director of the Humanities Laboratory. A cultural and literary historian, he is the author or editor of over sixty books. His recent books include *The Fortunes of the Humanities: Teaching the Humanities in the New Millennium* (2000), *New Germany in the New Europe* (edited with Todd Herzog, 2000), and *Fat Boys: A Slim Book* (2004).

Joyce L. Huff is Visiting Assistant Professor of English at St. Mary's College of Maryland. Her scholarship brings together disability studies and fat acceptance. Her essay, "A 'Horror of Corpulence': Interrogating Bantingism and Mid-Nineteenth-Century Fat-phobia," appeared in the anthology *Bodies Out of Bounds: Fatness and Transgression*, published by the University of California Press in 2001. She is currently working on a book on representations of corpulence in Victorian Britain.

Fredrik Albritton Jonsson is a doctoral student at the University of Chicago. His dissertation deals with the sciences of internal colonization in the Scottish Highlands, 1760-1820. He is the author of "Enlightened Hands," in Christopher E. Forth and Ivan Crozier, eds., *Body Parts: Critical Explorations in Corporeality*.

Ronald L. LeBlanc is Professor of Russian and Humanities at the University of New Hampshire and Research Associate at the Davis Center for Russian and Eurasian Studies at Harvard University. The author of a book on Russian picaresque fiction (*The Russianization of Gil Blas*, 1986), he is currently at work on a book-length manuscript, "Slavic Sins of the Flesh: Food, Sex, and Carnal Appetite in 19th-Century Russian Fiction," which examines how a number of Russian writers express male sexual desire through food imagery and eating metaphors.

Alison Moore is Lecturer in late modern European history in the Department of History, University of Sydney. Her general interests include the cultural and political history of modern France, histories of sexuality, psychoanalytic theory, and more specifically, the history of European consumerism and of discourses of sexual perversion. She is currently writing a book about concepts of excretion in the cultural history of nineteenth-century Europe.

George Rousseau has just retired from the Regius Professorship of English at King's College Aberdeen in Scotland and as Professor of the Humanities at De Montfort University in England. Based in Oxford, he is currently an Honorary Professor in the Faculty of Modern History at Oxford University. He recently published, with Roy Porter, *Gout: The Patrician Malady* (Yale University Press, 2000) and *Framing and Imagining Disease in Cultural History* (Palgrave, 2003). His essays, entitled *Nerves, Spirits and Fibres: Essays on literature and Sensibility* is due from Palgrave in 2004.

Peter N. Stearns is Provost and Professor of History at George Mason University (U.S.), and editor of the Journal of Social History. His research interests focus on the history of human behavior, with an eye to explaining present patterns through historical change and continuity, and world history. His many books include *Fat History: Bodies and Beauty in the Modern West* (1997; rev. ed. 2002) and, recently, *Anxious Parents: A History of Modern Childrearing in America* (2003).

Anne C. Vila is Associate Professor in the Department of French and Italian at the University of Wisconsin-Madison. She is the author of *Enlightenment and Pathology: Sensibility in the Literature and Medicine of Eighteenth-Century France* (Johns Hopkins University Press, 1998). She is currently completing a book entitled *Thinking Bodies: Literature, Medicine, and the Cult of the Intellectual in France, 1700-1840*.

Introduction ✌

THE BELLY AND BEYOND

BODY, SELF, AND CULTURE IN ANCIENT AND MODERN TIMES

Ana Carden-Coyne and Christopher E. Forth

We live in a world obsessed with abdomens, where the "belly," "tummy," or "gut" are objects of vigilance and, quite frequently, sources of anxiety. If in modern Western societies post-Cartesian thought has often disqualified the body in favor of the mind, in everyday life the belly continues to bear considerable cultural weight. Embracing as it does much of the digestive system, physiologically the belly is the primary site of *incorporation*, where food is directly assimilated into the body, where it is literally made into flesh. This deceptively simple point is complicated by the many ways in which eating, digestion, and excretion have been understood, both as objects of medical and scientific knowledge as well as targets of personal bodily reform. After all, at the same time that it does the work of digestion, the belly is also considered the metaphorical location of appetite itself. Far from dying out, these concerns have persisted throughout the early modern period and well into the nineteenth and twentieth centuries, and have included along the way anxieties about proper chewing, constipation, nutrition, exercise, and weight loss. Although historians of food and nutrition sometimes address these issues in simple health terms, in most cases it is not only physical health that is on the line; rather, insofar as health and well-being are often conceptualized through moral frameworks, personal character too seems jeopardized by poor diet and faulty habits.

Whether referring to size, shape, tone, or internal processes, the abdomen remains an integral aspect of our sense of self as well as a favored site of self-fashioning. The constitution of the self through experience, medicine, and ideology are therefore critical factors brought to light by the myriad cultures of the abdomen. Until recently, scholars have been conspicuously silent about these aspects of corporeal experience, ostensibly confirming the rather lowly status the abdomen has endured in the Western intellectual tradition. For the most part, historians of medicine have not examined dietetics very carefully, perhaps, as Steven Shapin speculates, because the content of dietetic expertise has changed so little from ancient times through to the early modern period. For scholars "who conceive of the history of medicine as the history of its novel ideas," the apparent common sense and continuity of dietetic knowledge has proven singularly unattractive.[1] The situation is not much different among cultural historians, whose relative silence may spring in part from the abstract manner in which "the body" is conceptualised as a discursive construct rather than as a lived, fleshy experience. While it is not our historical intention to recapture "real" bodies behind their cultural representations, attention can be directed to a wider range of bodily experiences, however mediated those experiences are, in order to provide a more comprehensive account of how the body has been lived in different contexts. Indeed, outside of the history of cuisine and nutrition, the past decade has registered a growing academic interest in many aspects of abdominal experience, including diet, constipation, excretion, and fat, less as physical "facts" than as aspects of personal embodiment that illuminate broader issues of society, politics, culture, and morality.[2] This significant development has implications for how we approach the embodied self in the past and present. For instance, it has been recently suggested that historians have some way to go in understanding the history of the body beyond its discursive constructions and institutionalized rhetoric. We should, rather, consider the constitution of the self within the realm of agency and experience, and with a degree of empathy.[3] The abdomen is such a site of personal, medical and cultural deliberation that this dynamic has profound consequences for the writing of history.

I

We should not confuse the blind spots of historiography with the complexity of the historical record, for throughout history men and women have been reminded of the importance of attending to their own abdomens. Ranking rather low in the hierarchy of senses proposed by the ancient Greeks, the stomach and intestines have often been denigrated as the organs closest to man's animal nature, despite Plato's admission that it was the duration of the digestive process that provided people with leisure time for philosophizing.[4] As Steven Shapin reveals in an important recent essay, however, the belly has played a special role in the philosophical and scientific search for truth, mainly insofar as it exempts itself from the pursuit altogether. This age-old trope of the ascetic scholar denying his appetites in order to access the truth is, as Shapin points out, a sleight-of-hand concealing an inescapable fact: that these are "embodied people *portraying* their disembodiment and that of the knowledge they produce or the documentary records of such portrayals."[5] Since classical antiquity, physicians have cited the centrality of digestive and excretory processes in maintaining health and morality, and thus the proper functioning of body and mind. Medical writers from Hippocrates, Galen, and Soranus, to Celsus (writing in Latin) located three main streams to their approach: regimen (*dieta*, which included diet as an important element), drugs (*pharmaka*, which included food), and surgery. By Roman times, this was combined with emetics and bathing.[6] Clearly, our modern understanding of dietetics has come from the Graeco-Roman concept of *dieta*, which in its original usage connected food and nourishment to a way of life and a quality of existence.

While the Epicureans saw "the pleasure of the belly" as the origin of all good, Hippocratic sources and moral philosophers limited this perception by entwining moderate eating, drinking, and exercise habits with the social morality of *sophrosyne* (soundness of mind, balance). As well, the rhetoric of "a sound mind in a sound body" had profound implications for the democracy: quite literally, the well-being of the healthy and fit body reflected the state of the moral and political corpus. Hence, the ancients regarded appetite not just as located in the belly but, more crucially, as an indicator of the social status and moral worth of a person. It is with this awareness that the Hippocratic texts advised "fleshy people" to walk faster.[7] Embroiled in the complex construction of ancient selfhood, the stomach was sometimes seen as possessing a will of its own. The Roman moralist Cato observed: "It is a hard matter, my fellow citizens, to argue with the belly, since it has no ears."[8] Although the belly seemed not to be a good listener, Romans nevertheless talked (and wrote) about diet, digestion, and fat as disorders of the self. The Roman shame of *incontinentia* (lack of self-control) compacted the stomach into a moral code about sexual and bodily license. The god Priapus, with his massive, erect, but impotent penis, was a symbol not just of ugly and excessive fleshiness but the folly of *incontinentia*.[9]

The self-consciousness with which this minor god compared his body to that of other gods enacted a warning to Roman citizens about the public and private consequences of immoderation. Bodily appearance wrapped self-identity in wider civic and religious ideologies. Moralists in the Graeco-Roman tradition had a profound influence upon Christian ethics, turning the bodily and civic disorder associated with excess into specific transgressions of gluttony, avarice, envy, lust, pride, sloth, and wrath. Under Christian law, unrestrained appetites became the deadliest of sins.[10] Recent research has shown that St. Paul was preoccupied with what he called "belly worship." In Paul's rhetoric, the belly had become a kind of false god. Christian moral philosophers turned the stomach into the paradigmatic organ through which a Christian life could be measured.[11] Control of earthly desires and appetites was directly linked to holiness and the promise of paradise in the hereafter.

The belly was, then, not simply the source of appetite for food, but the seat of all appetites, whether physical, alimentary, or sexual. The belly and sexuality were interlinked, even interchangeable in ancient thought. Romans regarded prostitutes as given over to indulgence, not only for their sexual cravings, but because they ate too much. Since payment for sexual services often included a meal, this complaint reveals just how restrained the Romans were prepared to be. The worse excess, however, was homosexuality, especially as the receiver (*kinaidos* in Greek, *cinaedus* in Latin), shamefully (*aidos*) relinquished his power by "acting like a woman," that is, inviting and enjoying penetration. Taking in the penis was the function of the female vessel. Like the uterus, the stomach was an animate being, aware of its own lack and in search of fill. When ancient writers confused the uterus with the belly, stomach and sexual desire were intimately bound to each other, and to the feminine.[12] Since the days of Homer's Sirens, women had seduced men with drunken feasts and sexual promises, luring them to their peril. Resistance to desires was bound to a rite of passage from boyhood to manhood. Whereas women (and all other noncitizens) were thought to be unbounded like water and dirt, the masculinity of restraint characterized ideas about citizenship.[13] The perfection of manliness was molded onto civic virtue. Although drives and appetites made up one-third of the human soul (reason and action the other two-thirds), they were also the most unruly and required containment. Hence Plato banished homosexuals from the utopia of the Republic. In Roman times, sex and food were easily associated with female abandon and *luxuria*. This latter Roman category grouped together a range of excesses, especially genital and digestive. By the eleventh century, the theologian Peter Damien had condensed *luxuria* into a neologism, the sin of *sodomia*.[14] Moreover, Christian teachings about the body and sin spread throughout the Western world, creating new forms of self-awareness.[15] Sins such as gluttony and sodomy enabled Christianity to construct the identity of a person, based upon the crimes they committed. Enter the Sodomite and the Glutton. Arguably, the history of sin and the identity of the sinner can be seen within the history of the abdomen.

Christians, just like pagans, were indeed frequent sinners. Appetites and consumption, especially in relation to food and drink, were actually revered in the lifestyles of wealthy Christians. In the late antique period, the Greek Christian writer Clement felt compelled to critique the luxurious habits of wealthy Christians residing in the plentiful environs of Alexandria. Clement cleverly used warnings about overeating, imbibing, and poor digestion as a way of promoting a simple and healthy life. In the late third century, the pagan philosopher Porphyry wrote *On Abstinence*, locating the dining table as a hub for menacing spirits to tempt the living with meat. Not only was meat a symbol of sexual congress, but it was also a corrupt and foul pollutant that produced what Peter Brown refers to as "raucous hiccups and unruly farts."[16] Pagans and Christians, however, were motivated by different spiritual convictions. Although Porphyry's pledge to vegetarianism reflected wider and increasingly influential notions of abstinence, both sexual and dietary, Christians came to value absolute denial: virginity, celibacy, and asceticism. Individual sins could be seen as direct assaults on the body of Christ.[17] The Eucharist put this belief into daily practice. Ingesting the bread and wine was like ingesting the body of Christ, "since bodies become what they consume."[18] This communion between Christ and participants conceptualized Christian unity as devout respect for Christ's body. By the early medieval teachings, the physical acts of eating and drinking were consolidated as metaphorical and spiritual concepts, entwining the self with God. Influential in Anglo-Saxon culture, this shift was reflected in Old English verse and prose.[19] Animalistic associations with feasting, for instance, were reinforced by Christian ideas about fasting, abstinence, and purity.

By the early modern period, belief in the humoral system as governor of both digestive and sexual health was challenged not just by the spread of syphilis, but also by concomitant ideas about the soul and new medical thinking. Diet and digestion affected mood, mentality and soul, so that gluttony was "unholy" in both physiological and moral ways. Like the alimentary canal, the path to godliness was seen as "blinde," "dirty," and "winding."[20] Spiritual understandings of digestion and eating, although dominant since the Renaissance, slowly gave way to more profound associations with personality and self-identity, productions steeped in the shifts and changes wrought by early modernity and the struggles within the gender order. The abdomen bore some of the weight of these changes. It was no coincidence that by asserting her role as monarch in a time of threat and instability, Queen Elizabeth identified herself as possessing "the body of a weak and feeble woman, but [having] the heart *and stomach* of a King."[21] This was Elizabeth's famous speech at Tilbury in 1588, rallying her forces to defend England against the invading Spanish Armada. Locked within the secrets of the stomach were the characteristics of manly fortitude and courage needed to face the enemy in battle. Hence, Elizabeth located the stomach as a gendered body part, but one bound to the identity and self-perception of a female king.

The "interiority" of the self was thus a rather corporeal affair. In this period, as Michael Schoenfeldt concludes, the stomach "played a central role in the development of political individuation and the articulation of devotional inwardness."[22] At the same time, the German healer and mystic Paracelsus contrived the stomach as a chemical laboratory, and helped to establish the genre of the "regimen[t]," an advice manual on both personal and social order. The painful disfigured syphilitic body, for example, came to resemble the excessive actions of the Stuart monarchs.[23] Looseness too was a physical as well as moral quality, and evidence of laxity in one area could be evidence for its presence in others. This was true whether this "looseness" was noted on the outside (as in fat or flabby flesh) or on the inside of the body. The uncontrollable flow of diarrhea, for instance, suggested a looseness that spoke volumes about a more general laxity, leading John Locke to note that people who are "very loose have seldom strong thoughts, or strong bodies."[24]

By the modern era, the belly continued to be closely connected with matters of character, gender, health, and sexuality. Eighteenth- and nineteenth-century physicians attached great significance to mental and genital functions, especially in the developing child, pointing to what Vernon Rosario had dubbed a "cerebrogenital axis" connecting the body's most developed organ to what many considered its most primitive ones. By the same token, physicians also pointed out the primacy of digestion in the bodily economy, sometimes claiming that the stomach and the brain are in fact the most important organs. In her recent study of sensibility in the eighteenth century, Anne C. Vila has revealed the widespread insistence upon what amounts to a "cerebrodigestive" axis that often eclipsed the genital function altogether, at least among men of letters.[25] Nineteenth-century commentators made similar claims, and one need only glance at Sidney Whiting's fanciful book, *Memoirs of a Stomach*, to see the close and ongoing association of the belly with "Mr Brain."[26] Such ideas echo the statement made by Victor Hugo around the same time: "The serpent is in man. It is the intestine. The belly is a heavy burden; it disturbs the equilibrium between the soul and the body... it is the mother of vices. The Colon is King."[27] This emphasis on the pivotal role of digestion in the moral complexion of the person persisted well into the twentieth century. "Someone once thought it was good to define a man as a brain served by organs," observed a French physician in 1908. His retort to this idea is telling: "He should have said the opposite: it is the organs of vegetative life whose functioning dominates the rest."[28] At the beginning of the twentieth century, the abdomen sustained its vital role in the constitution of the self, shaping what it meant to be a modern person.

II

For centuries, then, the digestive and appetitive dimensions of the abdomen have been inextricable from our concepts of the embodied self. They continue to be the target of what Michel Foucault describes as "techniques of the self," by which he means "those intentional and voluntary actions by which men not only set themselves rules of conduct, but also seek to transform themselves, to change themselves in their singular being, and to make their life into an *oeuvre* that carries certain aesthetic values and meets certain stylistic criteria."[29] The culture or shaping of the abdomen may be understood in this light, for these techniques call for bodily reforms that aim as much at internal processes as at external appearances. In the twentieth century, the development and diversification of body and health industries has enabled social customs to become cultural obsessions, inflecting a range of anxieties about late modernity and individualism. In 1934, the health reformer F. A. Hornibrook proposed a system that promised to "cultivate those parts of the body that, owing to man's posture and to his civilized habits, are the most neglected parts of his body, albeit the most important, viz., the muscles of the abdomen and the organs of digestion and excretion."[30] Pursuing what Hornibrook called "the culture of the abdomen" promised nothing less than the recuperation of the modern person, in body and mind, from the many traps of modern, "civilized" life. Techniques of the self, then, have clearly persisted in our modern ways of approaching our food, our appetites, and our bodies. The steps we take to feed, manage and sculpt our bellies have been intimately connected with who we are and what we wish to be.

As the following chapters indicate, attention to the size, shape, and processes of the abdomen is at once widespread and diverse in modern society.

Although we no longer judge disease as the result of a "false" way of life, in the way the ancient Greeks and early Christians did, the origins of modern selfhood may well be located in a premodern tradition of linking the experience of individual embodiment with a range of collective identities. These preoccupations have undergone transformations over time, and every period and national culture features a range of prescriptions and beliefs about how the stomach should be managed. In other words, the way in which we cultivate our bellies reveals a great deal about our culture generally. We can go beyond Hornibrook to discover that there is not one but many "cultures of the abdomen," revealing different yet related ways of crafting the self through the administration of the belly in many of its manifestations.

Cultures of the Abdomen demonstrates that a consideration of the belly requires rethinking a number of current themes in the cultural history of the body. Acknowledging that the digestive process has long been conceptualized as playing an integral role in the proper functioning of the body highlights the ways in which digestion and elimination are interlaced with mental life, sexuality, and the nervous system. This was not simply a concern of medical specialists, but was taken for granted by most people as a given of physical health. We thus need to revise our understanding of how desire and personality are inflected by bodily states and processes. Despite the proliferation of contemporary scholarship examining how medicalized discourses of sexuality structure personal identity, historically speaking, it is also clear that the abdomen has always competed with the genitals as the recognized seat of appetites, whether we understand "appetite" to mean desire for food, sex, or some other sensual experience.

Moreover we need to reassess the relationship between fat and gender identity. That "fat is a feminist issue" has become a truism in both activist and academic circles since Susie Orbach made that observation in 1979, exciting subsequent generations of interest in this vexed question.[31] Today, the disastrous effects that beauty imperatives toward slenderness have had on the bodies and minds of girls and women are notorious and undeniable. Yet in light of recent scholarship on masculinity and men's bodies, we need to revise our commonly held beliefs about the relationship between dietary habits and gender identities, both historically and in our own time. As several essays in this book suggest, fat has for centuries been an issue for men as well as women: indeed, insofar as they can imply sedentariness, luxury, and the abdication of self-control, fat male bodies have continually raised doubts about the "masculine" capacity to conquer appetites, brave hardships, and remain "active" in physical, sexual, and moral terms.[32] By carefully interrogating changes in cultural attitudes toward male and female bodies, we may better understand how both are subjected to, and actively engage with, norms of health, beauty, and gender while remaining attentive to the obvious specificities that distinguish each case.

Cultures of the Abdomen is divided thematically so as to address a spectrum of concerns pertaining to the abdomen, from diet, digestion, and excretion to physical culture and weight loss. Part I explores how dietetic, digestive, and excretory imagery has been used in the modern period to construct perceptions of social class and gender identity, whether among the English leisured classes in the eighteenth century (Jonsson), the laboring classes of the nineteenth (Huff), or American men in the twentieth (Carden-Coyne). It also examines how excrement, that infamous by-product of digestion, related to European enthusiasm for hard eating chocolate in the modern era (Moore). Part II considers the role of dietetic and alimentary issues in the works of eminent cultural figures like Voltaire (Vila), Samuel Taylor Coleridge (Rousseau), Ludwig Feuerbach (Geller), and Leo Tolstoy (LeBlanc), revealing the prominence these writers accorded issues of diet, whether as factors in sustaining health and morality or, in the case of Feuerbach, as a means of denigrating Jews. Part III focuses exclusively on the problem of fat in the modern world, identifying its medical roots in the seventeenth century (Albala), its steady advance among the eighteenth-century English elite (Dacome), its entwinement with images of effeminacy in fin-de-siècle France (Forth), its unique role in the depiction of portly detectives in German, English, and American crime fiction (Gilman), and its special place in the history of American diet and culture to the present day (Stearns). This collection thus marks an important development in the cultural history of the body while suggesting areas where further research may be directed and new questions might be asked.

Notes

1. Steven Shapin, "Trusting George Cheyne: Scientific Expertise, Common Sense, and Moral Authority in Early Eighteenth-Century Dietetic Medicine," *Bulletin of the History of Medicine* 77 (2003), 268.
2. Michael C. Schoenfeldt, *Bodies and Selves in Early Modern England: Physiology and Inwardness in Spenser, Shakespeare, Herbert, and Milton* (Cambridge: Cambridge University Press, 1999); John Coveney, *Food, Morals and Meaning: The Pleasure and Anxiety of Eating* (London: Routledge, 2000); James C. Whorton, *Inner Hygiene: Constipation and the Pursuit of Health in Modern Society* (Oxford: Oxford University Press, 2000); Jana Evans Braziel and Kathleen LeBesco, eds., *Bodies Out of Bounds: Fatness and Transgression* (Berkeley: University of California Press, 2001); Ken Albala, *Eating Right in the Renaissance*

(Berkeley: University of California Press, 2002); Karl Olav Sandnes, *Belly and the Body in the Pauline Epistles* (Cambridge: Cambridge University Press, 2002).

3. Bertrand Taithe and Mark Jenner, "The Historiographical Body," in *Medicine in the Twentieth Century*, John Pickstone and Roger Cooter, eds. (New York: Harwood Publishing, 2000), 187–200.

4. Plato, *Timaeus*, in *The Dialogues of Plato, Volume Two*, B. Jowett, trans. (New York: Random House, 1937), 49, 51. See also Carolyn Korsmeyer, *Making Sense of Taste: Food and Philosophy* (Ithaca: Cornell University Press, 1999).

5. Steven Shapin, "The Philosopher and the Chicken: On the Dietetics of Disembodied Knowledge," in *Science Incarnate: Historical Embodiments of Natural Knowledge*, Christopher Lawrence and Steven Shapin, eds. (Chicago: University of Chicago Press, 1998), 23.

6. Elizabeth Craik, "Diet, Diaita and Dietetics," in *The Greek World*, Anton Powell, ed. (London: Routledge, 1995), 389–391.

7. Hippocrates, "Regimens in Health," in *Greek Medicine: From the Heroic to the Hellenistic Age*, James Longrigg, ed. (London: Duckworth, 1998), 112.

8. Marcus Porcius Cato, quoted in Plutarch, *Lives*.

9. Maurice Oleander, "Misshapen Priapus," in *Antiquities*, Nicole Loraux, Gregory Nagy and Laura Slatkin, eds. (New York: New Press, 2001), 283–291.

10. Craik, "Diet, Diaita and Dietetics," 401.

11. Sandnes, *Belly and Body*.

12. Thomas Laqueur, *Making Sex: Body and Gender from the Greeks to Freud* (Cambridge: Harvard University Press, 1990), 27.

13. Anne Carson, "Putting Her in Her Place: Women, Dirt, and Desire," in *Before Sexuality: The Construction of Erotic Experience in the Ancient Greek World*, David Halperin, John Winkler, and Froma Zeitlin, eds. (Princeton: Princeton University Press, 1990), 135–69.

14. Mark D. Jordan, *The Invention of Sodomy in Christian Theology* (Chicago: University of Chicago Press, 1997), 29–44.

15. Robin Lane Fox, *Pagans and Christians* (London: Penguin, 1986), 23.

16. Peter Brown, *The Body and Society: Men, Women and Sexual Renunciation in Early Christianity* (New York: Columbia University Press, 1988), 182.

17. Frank Bottomley, *Attitudes to the Body in Western Christendom* (London: Lepus, 1979), 34–36.

18. See I Corinthians, X, 20f. Cited in Bottomley, *Attitudes*, 35.

19. Hugh Magennis, *Anglo-Saxon Appetites: Food and Drink and their Consumption in Old English and Related Literature* (Dublin: Four Courts Press, 1999).

20. Michael Schoenfeldt, "Fables of the Belly in Early Modern England," in *The Body in Parts: Fantasies of Corporeality in Early Modern England*, David Hillman and Carla Mazzio, eds. (New York: Routledge, 1997), 253.

21. Carole Levin, *The Heart and Stomach of a King: Elizabeth I and the Politics of Sex and Power* (University Park: University of Pennsylvania Press, 1994).

22. Schoenfeldt, "Fables of the Belly," 258

23. Margaret Healy, *Fictions of Disease in Early Modern England: Bodies, Plagues and Politics* (Basingstoke: Palgrave, 2001).

24. John Locke, *Some Thoughts Concerning Education*, in *The Educational Writings of John Locke*, John William Adamson, ed. (Cambridge: Cambridge University Press, 1922), 23.

25. Vernon A. Rosario, *The Erotic Imagination: French Histories of Perversity* (New York: Oxford University Press, 1997), 25; Anne C. Vila, *Enlightenment and Pathology: Sensibility in the Literature and Medicine of Eighteenth-Century France* (Baltimore: Johns Hopkins University Press, 1998), 97–100.

26. Sidney Whiting, *Memoirs of a Stomach, Written by Himself, That all who Eat May Read* (London: W. E. Painter, 1853).

27. Victor Hugo, quoted in Michaela Sullivan-Fowler, "Doubtful Theories, Drastic Therapies: Autointoxication and Faddism in the Late Nineteenth and Early Twentieth Centuries," *Journal of the History of Medicine and Allied Sciences,* 50 (July 1995), 364–90.

28. Dr. F. Aumont, *L'Estomac des gens du monde: Neurasthénie digestive* (Paris: n.p., 1908), 26.

29. Michel Foucault, *The Use of Pleasure*, Robert Hurley, trans. (New York: Vintage, 1985), 10–11.

30. F. A. Hornibrook, *Cultures of the Abdomen: The Cure of Obesity and Constipation* (Garden City, NY: Doubleday, Doran & Co., 1934), 5.

31. Susie Orbach, *Fat is a Feminist Issue* (Feltham: Hamlyn Paperbacks, 1979). See also Naomi Wolf, *The Beauty Myth* (London: Chatto & Windus, 1990), and Susan Bordo, *Unbearable Weight: Feminism, Western Culture, and the Body* (Berkeley: University of California Press, 1993).

32. See the essays by Dacome, Forth, and Gilman, Chapters 10–12 in this volume, as well as Sander L. Gilman, *Fat Boys: A Slim Book* (Lincoln, NE: University of Nebraska Press, 2004).

Part I ❧

DIET, DIGESTION, EXCRETION

Chapter 1 ∽

THE PHYSIOLOGY
OF HYPOCHONDRIA IN
EIGHTEENTH-CENTURY BRITAIN

Fredrik Albritton Jonsson

During the eighteenth century, the stomachs of the British upper ranks threatened to turn on their owners and devour them from the inside. These fears of gastric rebellion in the polite interior were articulated in a series of medical manuals on hypochondria between the 1720s and the early 1800s. Physicians like George Cheyne, Bernard Mandeville, Robert Whytt, and William Smith jostled to capture a slice of the market. What came first—the cannibal stomach or the book-peddling physician—is quite impossible to say. Both were parasites of a churning consumer economy. Yet, the precise meaning of this peculiar disease remains elusive. One line of interpretation, promoted by John Mullan, stresses the literary and philosophical character of hypochondria in the period. Another angle, supplied by Roy Porter, emphasizes its wider social meaning, as a locus for anxieties tied to the moral and medical effects of consumption.[1] My essay offers a third perspective on the boom and bust of this disease, giving particular weight to the social distinctions encoded in the physiology of hypochondria.

These physicians portrayed the genteel stomach as a dangerously unreliable organ, prone to catastrophic disruptions. Such pathological sensitivies were traced back to the dual position of the stomach in the symbolic hierarchy of the organs, at the same time a site of debasing labor and refined consumption. This blurring of functions in turn made the elite stomach the symbolic stage for wider anxieties about the bodily causes of disorder.

Here, the vision of a corrupt and enfeebled elite threatened by mindless convulsions was performed by organs and vital fluids in a gastric drama, which illuminated the precarious foundation of genteel authority in the uncertain mastery of the private body.

Cashing In

Hypochondria is a disease with a long tradition and many variations. Only in the nineteenth century did it acquire the overriding meaning of a morbid preoccupation with imaginary diseases. Until the eighteenth century, physicians knew it as a somatic disease of the humors, more specifically, the result of an excess of black bile produced by the liver. This excess defined the melancholic temperament, equally predisposed to madness and learning. In seventeenth-century England, works like Thomas Burton's *Anatomy of Melancholy* (1621) identified humoral hypochondria as a form of religious melancholy. For some, the condition shaded into the pathology of excessive intellectual activity termed "the disease of the learned." Sedentary reading habits among savants were said to damage their health, by "stooping and squeezing the Belly against the Books, which hinder[ed] the free Descent of the Diaphragma, and consequently the Circulation of the Humours."[2] Significantly, hypochondria also figured as the male version of hysteria, centered on the abdominal region rather than the uterus, but with similar symptoms of derangement and debility.[3]

However, in the early eighteenth century, hypochondria changed bodies. The association with the physiology of the humors gave way to a neurological incarnation of the disease, made possible by the exploration of the function of the nervous system conducted by Thomas Willis (1621–1675) and others.[4] In the wake of this research, physicians relocated hypochondria in the peculiar exchanges of the digestive process, where aliments, digestive juices, nervous fluids, and blood mixed in vital ferment. The parallel with hysteria also underwent a significant mutation, since this malady lost its narrow association with the mobility of the womb and came to signify instead the general weakness of female nerves and animal spirits. Both diseases were seen as the result of pathological sensitivity, typical of a specific kind of constitution distinguished by lax and delicate fibers, rendering women hysterical and men effeminate (in sharp contrast with the robust nerves and strong vascular system characteristic of the male and female victims of gout).[5]

The enterprising doctor could now begin to cash in on contemporary anxieties concerning the vicious affinities between nervous sensibility and excessive consumption. Here was a disease born out of a luxurious diet rather than solitary intellect.[6] In his seminal work *The English Malady* from 1733, the fashionable Scottish physician George Cheyne (1671–1743) deemed a heavy diet, saturated with consumer goods like tea, coffee, snuff, chocolate, and sugar, especially pernicious. For Robert Whytt (1714–1766), another major Scottish authority in medicine, the consumption of luxury played a double role, at the same time constituting a predisposing cause and a characteristic symptom of the disease. He defined the latter in terms of a "strong desire for rare or uncommon sorts of food, or for things that can afford no nourishment." When such alimentary urges were combined with an idle lifestyle void of exercise and a weak nervous constitution, disaster threatened. For this reason, Cheyne saw nervous disorder as the special province of "the Rich, the Lazy, the Luxurious, and the Unactive," namely, "those who fare daintily and live voluptously, those who are furnished with the rarest Delicacies, the richest Foods, and the most generous Wines."[7]

Fashionable Pathologies

The introduction of the concept of nervous pathology allowed physicians to medicalize the contemporary status symbol of sensibility. For the established elite as well as the upwardly mobile sort, sensibility emerged as a new form of cultural capital from the middle decades of the eighteenth century. Such sensibility justified moral and aesthetic judgments in the name of nervous superiority. Exquisite nerves not only magnified the power of the senses, but also increased the strength of the imagination and the moral sentiments. This superiority was properly demonstrated in bodily performances like embraces, tears, swooning, and olfactory sensitivity. The conceit of sensibility broadened the corporeal basis of the elite, offering the authority of nervous refinement as an alternative to aristocratic birth and blood. Indeed, it formed a cultural and literary code, elaborated in numerous genres, from Edmund Burke's aesthetics of the sublime and Adam Smith's *Theory of Moral Sentiments* to James Macpherson's poems of Ossian. These models of sensibility could be assimilated and performed by anyone with sufficient attention to its gestures and language as well as the education, income, and leisure to sustain such social theatrics.[8]

Through the link with sensibility, hypochondria became a pathology in vogue, the mark of genteel consumers everywhere, beset by the horrors of a sedentary and indulgent style of life. The medicalization of sensibility rested on the implicit or explicit assumption that nervous refinement conferred pathological sensitivity. John Hill (1716–1775) declared: "those who have the nervous system in the highest perfection, are the most liable to have it disordered: for that greatest perfection infers the greatest tenderness and delicacy."[9] Cheyne's diagnosis in *The English Malady* carefully equated such sensitivity with a broadly patrician status. To create a broad but genteel pool of patients, he proclaimed that the nation was in the grip of a nervous epidemic with a third of the population suffering from such disorders. In this way, he could insist on the aristocratic orientation of weak nerves while leaving the condition accessible to social climbers of all kinds (contradicting his own claim that the middling sort possessed immunity from such disorders by virtue of its moderate desires).

Cheyne's diagnosis implied that physicians were the indispensable managers and therapists of hypochondriac modernity, offering the sole escape from the corruption of luxury consumption. This new centrality of the doctor to modernity found a striking expression in the personal and professional alliance between Cheyne and the sentimental novelist and printer Samuel Richardson. The latter embraced his doctor's medical views not only for the purpose of personal therapy but also to shape the language of character and sympathy in his literary works. Indeed, because the popularity of Cheyne's work preceded the first successful sentimental novels, we should define his therapeutic success not as an appropriation of literary fashion, but as a prolegomenon to the latter. Medicine ushered in literature in the case of the doctor–patient relation between Cheyne and Richardson.[10]

The genre of the hypochondria manual crucially reinforced and expanded the reach of the individual physician over the market of potential patients. Addressed directly to the patient in the vernacular, the accessible character of these texts at the same time diffused the disease as far as print could take it and advertised the reputation of particular remedies and doctors across the country. Ostensibly composed to safely diagnose and cure the disease, the hypochondria manual in fact defined it as a protean malady characterized by a nearly infinite variety of symptoms, so that any number of ailments could be colonized by the empire of hypochondria. To stack the odds further in their favor, the physicians gave hypochondria a close set of pathological relatives, ranging from consumption, dyspepsia, and atonic gout to the incubus and the vapors, each one of them said to emanate from the nervous stomach and its digestive problems.

The manuals portrayed the progress of the disease as relatively slow rather than virulent and lethal, insisting on the need for costly medical attention by skilled physicians, without guarantees of definite recovery. Cheyne emphasized from the outset of his book that many of his patients should not expect a return to full health: "The noble organs may be spoilt or irretrievably obstructed." Such a chronic condition obviously facilitated the link between hypochondria and social status in as much as it promised the reader a long life as a distinguished patient. Accordingly, Clark Lawlor and Akihito Suzuki have characterized Cheyne's "English malady" along with tuberculosis and gout as peculiarly fertile in producing forms of identity and status, contrasting this class of "diseases of the Self" with more quickly lethal pathologies like cholera, plague, and syphilis.[11]

The physicians of hypochondria entrenched the chronic character of the disease by prescribing as remedies the same luxuries they also identified as causes of the disease. William Cullen recommended tea and coffee whereas Whytt favored brandy and "spiceries." Even Cheyne was willing to relativize his austere regimen according to the size of the belly (perhaps a result of his own struggles with obesity): "The great Rule of Eating and Drinking for Health is to adjust the Quality and Quantity of our Food to our digestive Powers." Another fashionable cure—opium or laudanum—tended to aggravate gastric complaints more than heal them. Such flattering restoratives helped guarantee the status of hypochondria as an exclusive condition caused and perpetuated by luxury.[12]

Slippery Organs

The successful spread of hypochondria required intimidation as much as flattery to capture the attention of potential patients. This helps explain why doctors gave the malady such a peculiarly subversive character. Gastric physiology was interpreted in a language rich with social and moral resonance, drawing on metaphors of rank, convulsion, and sympathy. Unsurprisingly, the uncanny aspect of hypochondria was rooted in the inversion of contemporary images of corporeal order. Physicians in eighteenth-century Britain conceived of the body as an intricate and nearly self-regulating balance of solids and fluids—an animal economy—designed by God to operate in accordance with the laws of nature and the proper regimen prescribed by respectable doctors. This ideal of partial homeostasis was reinforced by other images of orderly design, patterns believed to permeate the wider universe, repeated in a myriad of natural, aerial, rural, political, and vegetable economies. Within such a chain of economies, enlightened doctors claimed exclusive knowledge of the natural rules of health, making them the sole authority capable of managing and recuperating the ideal bodily equilibrium of solids and fluids.[13]

The internal equilibrium of the body was founded on the structure of the animal economy as a miniature polity, expressed in the ranking of organs and fluids as noble or base. In descending order, the organs of the brain, heart, stomach, and intestines formed a hierarchy, bound together into a harmonious polity by the involuntary operations of the nervous system. The hierarchical logic applied also to physiological processes like digestion. In his *Dissertation upon the Nerve* (1768), William Smith portrayed the extraction of nutrition from aliments as a sequence of selective refinement, permitting a limited, upward mobility for the most subtle and valuable particles. In this way, chyle was extricated from food while indigestible matter exited through the anus. The chyle in turn entered the circulation of the blood, which after further refinement in turn yielded the precious nervous fluid. Thus, the bodily juices formed a hierarchy of their own, parallel to that of the organs.[14]

It was this harmonious polity of organs and fluids that hypochondria threatened to subvert. Physicians defined the disease as a perversion of the animal economy, pitting the lower organs of the body against the higher ones, even turning the hierarchy upside-down, so that the base stomach dominated the noble brain. In Robert James's (1703-1776) gruesome tableau from his mid-1740s *Medicinal Dictionary*:

> When thick and viscid Humours are, by the Spasms of the Lower Belly, copiously convey'd to the superior Parts and Head, where they circulate slowly in the Vessels of the Brain; the animal Functions are destroyed; the Senses languish; the Force of the Memory, and Brightness of the Genius, are impair'd.... [It is a] spasmodico-flatulent Disorder of the *Primae Viae*, of the Stomach and Intestines, arising from an Inversion or Perversion of their Peristaltic Motion, and by mutual Consent of the Parts, throwing the whole nervous System into irregular Motions, and disturbing the whole Oeconomy of the Functions.[15]

In the healthy organism, the digestive process of the stomach labored obediently to provide nutrition for the nobler organs above it. Yet the greater the sensitivity of the nervous system, the higher the risk of disruptions in the internal hierarchy of the organs. The digestive process constituted the weak link in the system of consumption and waste management, which maintained the circulation of vital fluids within the animal economy. Physicians like William Smith and Robert Whytt insisted that the stomach and intestines occupied a privileged position in the nervous system, enjoying a more direct connection than the other organs with the brain. In *A View of the Nervous Temperament*, Thomas Trotter (1760–1832) went even further. Not only did he attribute to the stomach "the most complex properties" of any organ in the body, but he also asserted that the "centre of sympathy" the stomach formed between "our corporeal and mental parts" possessed "more exquisite qualifications than the brain itself."[16]

Ultimately, the subversive force of hypochondria derived from the ambiguous status of the stomach implicit in these medical writings, simultaneously an organ of production and consumption. While eighteenth-century doctors did not frame the problem in those abstract terms, the gist of the contradiction—how to maintain the elite stomach at work under the pressures of luxury and excessive refinement—was perfectly clear to them. On the one hand, the digestive system performed the lowest yet most necessary form of labor to supply the nobler parts of the body with nutrition. On the other hand, physicians endowed the stomach with such an exceptional degree of nervous sensibility that it must necessarily be perpetually unsettled among patricians since it constituted the physical receptacle of all their alimentary indulgences. When hypochondria struck, these two powers combined perversely to give the stomach a riotous authority over the body. It polluted the blood with noxious chyle and the acid of gastric juices. It reversed the peristaltic movements of the intestines, clogging them with indigestible food, and swelling the constipated body with miasmatic gases. Worst of all, it exercised an insidious influence on the other organs through the nervous system, striking the heart with palpitations, the eyes with dimness, and the brain with melancholy.

Such convulsions reflected a social contradiction within eighteenth-century physiology as much as a deliberate marketing strategy. The ambiguity exposed in the genteel stomach was ultimately generated by the fundamental patrician value prescribing a strict distinction between refined consumers and base labor. Digestive processes turned out to be conceptually slippery and therefore pathological because they blurred this boundary. Quite possibly, the ambiguity may have upset physicians as much as patients. In fact, the distasteful consequence of mixing social categories in the stomach was perhaps particularly acute to the upwardly mobile physicians of hypochondria, who, after all, were professionally sensitized to the medical hazards of their own habits of consumption. In other words, the profit motive of the doctor did not necessarily give him immunity from the disease. George Cheyne may have been quite earnest in proclaiming himself a hypochondriac.[17]

The link between physiology and patrician values surfaced with unusual clarity in the thought of the Edinburgh physician Robert Whytt. In the same period that his fellow Scots David Hume and Adam Smith developed their notion of moral sympathy to account for the normative bonds of civil society, Whytt pioneered the concept of organic sympathy to explain the dissemination of nervous pathologies among his patients. At one level, the concept explained how nervous disorder spread within the individual body. By means of sympathy, a diseased organ could generate similar or new symptoms in other body parts through the conduit of the nervous system. At a second level, Whytt postulated that the same organic sympathy could be transmitted between the animal economies of different persons, "whence various motions and morbid symptoms are often transferred, from one to another, without any corporeal contact or infection." The simple observation of nervous actions in others, especially in the form of facial expressions, might induce spontaneous nervous imitation in the observer. Whytt's catalogue of contagious motions ranged from the innocuous (yawning), uncouth and unpleasant (vomiting, sore eyes), to the frightening (bagpipe music) and dangerous (epileptic and hysteric fits). Organic sympathy appeared best suited to convey grossly physical and collective actions, which violated the ideal of individual self-restraint embodied in polite etiquette. Most spectacularly, Whytt announced that nervous spasms had the power to overtake entire crowds, leading to collective convulsions.[18]

This catalogue of spasms undermined not only polite etiquette but also the theory of moral sense and spectatorial sympathy underpinning Scottish moral philosophy by suggesting that sympathy might account for plebeian enthusiasm as much as genteel solidarity. Although Whytt never made the tension between organic and moral sympathy explicit, he invoked both forms in his *Essay on the Vital and Involuntary Motions of Animals*. Curiously, he selected (female) hysteria to represent the most violent type of organic sympathy, reporting a recurring phenomenon of collective spasms among hysteric women in Edinburgh: "it has frequently happened, in the Royal Infirmary here, that women have been seized with hysteric fits from seeing others attacked with them." He found further support in observations made by the eminent physician Boerhaave on convulsions among female workhouse wards in the Dutch town of Harleem.[19]

An effort to resolve the tension between the two kinds of sympathy was not undertaken until several decades later, outside the realm of medical literature, in the philosophy of Adam Smith's disciple Dugald Stewart (1753–1828). As part of a larger project exploring the elements of the human mind, Stewart proposed to subsume organic and moral sympathy under a higher principle he termed the law of sympathetic imitation. This law was rooted in the "mimical powers connected with our bodily frame," which "in certain... circumstances" were produced "with little intervention of our will, from a sympathy between the bodily organizations of different individuals." Besides Smithian moral sympathy, the range of nervous imitation in Stewart's work extended to the phenomena catalogued by Whytt as well as to more elaborate actions which incorporated elements of training and skill, such as the acquisition of speech among children, the physiognomy of mimics and the dexterous acrobatics of popular entertainments. Stewart put special emphasis on the uses of the law of sympathetic imitation to account for collective behavior, including "the contagious nature of convulsions, of hysteric disorders, of panics, and of all the different kinds of enthusiasm." He also limited the explanatory reach of his model by admitting that other "powerful causes" could also be at work in generating some of these phenomena, like the sway of the imagination over crowd passions.[20]

Yet, despite his fascination with convulsions and enthusiasm, Stewart's commitment to a Baconian science of the human mind (cemented by a secure position as an Edinburgh professor in moral philosophy) distracted him from Whytt's medical conception of organic sympathy as the sinister vehicle of disease. The delicate and easily disturbed animal economy imagined by Cheyne and Whytt was swept aside by Stewart's urgent insistence on the social utility of the law of sympathetic imitation. As a cautious progressive intimidated by the counter-revolutionary forces dominating Britain in the 1790s, Stewart chose to couch his hopes for reform in the development of a unified set of human sciences. One vital element in this project involved the exploration of the "mimical powers," which Stewart believed underpinned sympathetic imitation. Such knowledge would allow this bodily force to be domesticated and oriented toward practical moral and economic uses. Observing that the proclivity to imitate was the most spontaneous and effective among children, in part because of the greater flexibility of their "muscular system," he suggested that the management of the "mimical powers" should begin as early as possible. Unable to conceal his enthusiasm, he described the practices of Count Rumford's House of Industry in Munich, where he claimed to have witnessed how the youngest children learnt their trade by playfully mimicking the operations of the older children. By interpreting the exploitation of child labor in terms of his law of sympathetic imitation, Stewart held up the possibility of a social order where pleasurable imitation served as a foundation of manufacturing production and a guarantee against plebeian unrest. Separated from Whytt and Cheyne by an age of revolution, Stewart searched in the body for the sources of social stability rather than upheaval and convulsion.[21]

Regurgitating the Imagination

Unfortunately, we do not yet have a clear understanding of how hypochondria was experienced by the majority of its victims. Some testimony can be found among the savants and literati who succumbed to it, such as James Boswell and Samuel Richardson. However, very little is known about how the manuals on hypochondria were interpreted and appropriated by the general reader. Questions about the wider circulation and influence of these texts will have to await further research.

Here I will limit myself to some final comments about the changing perception of hypochondria toward the end of the eighteenth century. At this point, physicians were forced increasingly to concede that consumer goods had penetrated into new, low-end markets. Such a popularization of old luxuries in turn undermined the definition of hypochondria as a genteel disease. Some medical writers sought to profit from the expanding demand, turning out catchpenny pamphlets and universal potions like Dr. Hodson's Aromatic Nervine Tea, but the market for elite sufferers appears to have been faltering.[22] A dramatic reevaluation of sensibility probably also damaged the fashionable character of hypochondria. During the French Revolution and the Napoleonic Wars, the language of nerves was smeared with the taint of radical politics. In the face of the French threat, the British elite heeded a call for cultural and corporeal regeneration, embracing a new ideal of robust and martial manhood, antithetical to the high-strung sympathies of the man of feeling. The ennobling element of pathological sensibility seems to have survived mainly in the related figures of the romantic genius and the ethereal victim of tuberculosis (consumption). This shift also crucially displaced the locus of sensitivity upward in the body away from the stomach to the lungs and the mind.[23]

In the decline of gastric hypochondria, a decisive turning point may have come in 1807, when the Newcastle physician (and former surgeon's mate in the Royal Navy, trained at Edinburgh) Thomas Trotter proclaimed that the spread of nervous diseases now amounted to a national emergency, involving two-thirds of the entire population. While singling out bankers, investors, and shopkeepers as the worst affected victims, his enormous tally by necessity also included large groups of laborers. In the highly charged atmosphere of the Napoleonic Wars, Trotter intended his book as a wake-up call to a nation enfeebled by "its vast wealth, so diffused among all ranks of people." If the population could not be redeemed from the debilitating influence of "refined modes of life and luxurious habits" and returned to a fundamental "simplicity of living and manners," a plague of nervous disorders "must inevitably sap our physical strength of constitution [and] make us an easy conquest to our invaders." This announcement of a nervous epidemic may have served to rob hypochondria of much of its aristocratic frisson, consequently killing the fashionable status of the disease among the upwardly mobile. For the same reason, the sheer scope of Trotter's threat probably helped make his work the final best seller in the genre of the hypochondria manual.[24]

The downward mobility of hypochondria in turn began to transform the etiology of the disease. As nervous disorders spread outward from the genteel interior and descended to the lower ranks, Trotter hesitated between psychological and physiological explanations of the condition. Certainly, the stress on non-somatic causes had some precedent in earlier theories of the disease, conceived long before Trotter proclaimed that hypochondria had struck the plebeian orders. Robert Whytt's *Observations* for example listed violent passions of the mind as one of the "particular occasional causes" of hypochondria and hysteria. However, Trotter's etiology gave unprecedented weight to the claim that hypochondria, despite the clear importance of bodily causes, ultimately derived from a certain "disposition of mind." His own perception of the pervasive spread of the disease apparently tempted him to identify it with forces of culture and history rather than a privileged order of bodies. Perhaps we could say that the social resonance encoded in the physiology of the animal economy became increasingly irrelevant when the disease lost its genteel status. The more vulgar the victim, the less acute the conflict between noble and base organs. How could a plebeian really suffer from possessing a plebeian stomach? This would explain why Trotter announced in the Dedication of his book that he did not see any need to illustrate his argument by recourse to anatomy and physiology (he merely referred his "young readers" to "Dr Whytt on nervous disorders"). Certainly, we should not take him entirely at his word. *A View of the Nervous Temperament* still discussed the operation of nerves and digestion in great detail. A careless reader would find little to distinguish his work from earlier literature in the genre. The usual suspects of diet, sedentary life, and excessive nervous sensibility all figured prominently in the narrative. Yet at several points, Trotter abandoned physiological explanation and turned instead to the record of history and culture. The strongest statement of this kind came in a discussion of the reign of Terror during the French Revolution, when he insisted that the violence and fury unleashed by the Jacobins had shocked the French nation so profoundly that "all diseases, usually called nervous, low spirits, or hypochondriacism, [had] quickly disappeared." To Trotter, this provided binding proof that these nervous disorders were "so nearly connected with the tenor of the mind, that great commotions in the moral world, may both induce and remove them."[25]

In the same spirit, Trotter looked to the course of British history to explain the national proliferation of nervous disorders in his own time. He singled out the South Sea Bubble of 1720 as a pivotal event when the anxieties engendered by financial chaos and sudden reversals of fortune had caused a very large number of cases of "hypochondriacism and low spirits." The disaster marked the beginning of a permanent epidemic to Trotter, who believed that the precarious financial cycles of the City had come to dominate British society from this moment onward. He denounced the London Stock Exchange as the "the puddle of corruption" that had "filled the nation with degenerate fears, apprehension, and hypochondriacism."[26] Trotter's contempt for financial markets should be seen in the light of his primitivist critique of modernity. Once man had departed from the savage state, forsaking "a mode of life that had been presented to him by nature," existence had lost its original simplicity, uniformity, and stability. Instead, man found himself transformed into a "creature of art," governed by a dangerous proliferation of "new passions and desires," not the least of which were stocks and bubbles. Elsewhere, in his *Essay on Drunkenness*, Trotter laid the blame squarely at consumer desire: "In the present stage of society, human kind are almost taken out of the hands of Nature; and a custom called fashion . . . now rules everything." Trotter's fellow propagandist for medical reform Thomas Beddoes (1760–1808) agreed, proclaiming that the wants of consumption were boundless in scope: "Before one set of desires is well gratified, new ones are kindled by the infinity of bright temptations, which ingenuity is daily displaying in the view of taste."[27]

By stressing this link between desire and the imagination, Trotter and Beddoes envisioned a consumer disease unlimited by simple bodily constraints. Even the threat of the predatory stomach appeared rather innocuous in comparison with the apparently infinite scope of this new danger. The convulsions of the mind threatened the body with lethal exhaustion as imaginary wants forced the nervous system into a state of continuous excitement: "[T]he body is not merely worn down by the perturbations of the mind. It is directly attacked," Beddoes exclaimed. The ultimate source of nervous disorder then, lay in the unnatural proliferation of fickle and transient desires fostered by a mind steeped in artifice. In this way, the proliferation of nervous disorders forced hypochondria to ascend upward in the body, out of the bowels and into the imagination.[28]

Notes

For helpful comments on earlier drafts of this chapter, I wish to thank James Delbourgo, James Elwick, Margaret Jacob, Alison Winter, John Brewer, and the editors of this anthology.

1. John Mullan, *Sentiment and Sociability: The Language of Feeling in the Eighteenth Century* (Oxford: Clarendon Press, 1988); Roy Porter, "Addicted to Modernity: Nervousness in the Early Consumer Society," in *Culture in History; Production, Consumption and Values in Historical Perspective,* Joseph Melling and Jonathan Barry, eds. (Exeter: University of Exeter Press, 1992); Idem. "*Consumption*: Disease of the consumer society?" in *Consumption and the World of Goods,* John Brewer and Roy Porter, eds. (London: Routledge, 1993). Also, Karin Johannisson, *Kroppens tunna skal; sex essäer om kropp, historia och kultur* (Stockholm: Norstedts/Pan, 1997), 105–34.

2. Bernard Mandeville, *A Treatise of the Hypochondriack and Hysterick Diseases* (London, 1730, second edition [first 1711], reprint New York: Delmar, 1976), 216.

3. Roy Porter, *Mind Forg'd Manacles: A History of Madness in England from the Restoration to the Regency* (Cambridge: Harvard University Press, 1987), 62–81. M. J. Lieburgh, *The Disease of the Learned: A Chapter from the History of Melancholy and Hypochondria* (Rotterdam, 1990); Adrian Johns, *The Nature of the Book: Print and Knowledge in the Making* (Chicago: University of Chicago press, 1998), Chapter Six; Ilza Veith, *Hysteria: The History of a Disease* (Northvale, NJ: Jason Aronson, 1993).

4. Robert G. Frank, Jr., "Thomas Willis and his Circle," in *The Languages of Psyche; Mind and Body in Enlightenment Thought,* G. S. Rousseau, ed. (Berkeley, University of California Press, 1990); G. S. Rousseau, "Nerves, Spirits, and Fibres: Towards Defining the Origin of Sensibility," in *Studies in the Eighteenth Century III,* R. F. Brissenden and J. C. Eade, eds, (Toronto: University of Toronto Press, 1973).

5. Porter, *Mind-forg'd Manacles,* 48–49; Mandeville, *A Treatise,* 239–49.

6. John Sekora in *Luxury: The Concept in Western Thought, Eden to Smollett* (Baltimore: Johns Hopkins University Press, 1977); Christopher Berry, *The Idea of Luxury* (Cambridge: Cambridge University Press, 1994); Maxine Berg and Helen Clifford, *Consumers and Luxury: Consumer Culture in Europe, 1650–1850* (Manchester: Manchester University Press, 1998); Roy Porter, "The Patient in England, c. 1660–c. 1800," in *Medicine in Society: Historical Essays,* Andrew Wear, ed. (Cambridge University Press, 1992), 108.

7. George Cheyne, *The English Malady: or, a Treatise of Nervous Diseases of all Kinds, as Spleen, Vapours, Lowness of Spirits, Hypochondriacal, and Hysterical Distempers* (First edition 1733, reprint: New York: Scholars' Facsimiles, 1976) 21, 34; Whytt, *Observations,* 98, 111. I hope to analyze elsewhere the process by which Cheyne's gastric hypochondria marginalized Bernard Mandeville's earlier and alternative diagnosis focused on managerial anxieties over property and capital rather than diet and luxury.

8. John Brewer, "Sensibility," in *The New Cambridge History of English Romantic Literature*, James Chandler, ed. (Cambridge: Cambridge University Press, forthcoming).

9. John Hill, *The Construction of the Nerves, and Causes of Nervous Disorders; with A Regimen and Medicines which have proved successful* (London: 1758), 14. For "genteel" and "patrician," see Amanda Vickery, *The Gentleman's Daughter: Women's Lives in Georgian England* (New Haven: Yale University Press, 1998), 13; E. P. Thompson, "Patricians and Plebeians," in Idem., *Customs in Common: Studies in Traditional Popular Culture* (New York: New Press, 1993).

10. Cheyne, *The English Malady*, ii; C. A. Moore, "The English Malady," in *Backgrounds of English Literature 1700–1760* (Minneapolis: 1953), 179; G. J. Barker-Benfield, *The Culture of Sensibility: Sex and Society in Eighteenth-Century Britain* (Chicago: University of Chicago Press, 1992), 7–15; Juliet McMaster, "The Body inside the Skin: The Medical Model of Character in the Eighteenth-Century Novel," *Eighteenth-Century Fiction*, 4:4 (1992), 277–300.

11. Cheyne, *The English Malady*, vi; Roy Porter, "Laymen, Doctors and Medical Knowledge in the Eighteenth-Century: The Evidence of the Gentleman's Magazine," in *Patients and Practitioners*, Roy Porter, ed. (Cambridge: Cambridge University Press, 1985), 283–314; Wayne Wild, "Doctor-Patient Correspondence in Eighteenth-Century Britain: A Change in Rhetoric and Relationship," Timothy Erwin, ed., *Studies in Eighteenth Century Culture* (29): 47–64; Clark Lawlor and Akihito Suzuki, "The Diseases of the Self: Representing Consumption, 1700–1830," in *Bulletin of the History of Medicine* 74:3 (2000), 458.

12. William Cullen, *First Lines of the Practice of Physic, for the Use of Students in the University of Edinburgh* (Edinburgh, 1783), vol. 3, 134; Whytt, *An Essay on the Vital and Involuntary Motions of Animals*, in the *Works of Robert Whytt* (Edinburgh, 1768), 49; Idem., *Observations*, 128; Cheyne is quoted in Roy Porter, "Consumption: Disease of the Consumer Society?," 64; Anita Guerrini, *Obesity and Depression in the Enlightenment: The Life and Times of George Cheyne* (Norman: University of Oklahoma Press, 2000).

13. Cheyne, *The English Malady*, 21; Emma C. Spary, "Political, Natural and Bodily Economies," in *Cultures of Natural History,* Nicholas Jardine, James A. Secord, and E. C. Spary, eds. (Cambridge: Cambridge University Press, 1996), 178–196.

14. William Smith, *A Dissertation upon the Nerve* (London: W. Owen, 1768), 49–59 (also 192); Whytt, *An Essay on the Vital and other Involuntary Motions of Animals*, 51; See also Herman Boerhaave's *Institutiones Medicae* (1708), discussed in Anne C. Vila, *Enlightenment and Pathology: Sensibility in the Literature and Medicine of Eighteenth-Century France* (Baltimore: Johns Hopkins University Press, 1998), 18; Cheyne, *The English Malady*, vi.

15. Robert James, *A Medicinal Dictionary*, 4 vols (London: 1743–45), vol. 2, "Hypochondriacus Morbus."

16. William Smith, *A Dissertation upon the Nerve*, 208–209; Whytt, *Observations on the Nature, Causes, and Cure of those Disorders which have been Commonly Called*

Nervous, Hypochondriac, or Hysteric, 127; Thomas Trotter, *A View of The Nervous Temperament* (London: Longman, 1807; reprint, New York: Arno, 1976), 203.

17. Cheyne, "The Case of the Author," in *The English Malady*. For a recent interpretation of work and leisure in the period, see Sarah Jordan, *The Anxieties of Idleness: Idleness in Eighteenth-Century British Literature and Culture* (Lewisburg, PA: Bucknell University Press, 2003).

18. Whytt, *Observations on the Nature, Causes, and Cure of those Disorders which have been Commonly Called Nervous, Hypochondriac, or Hysteric*, 217–220, quotes from 219 to 220; Idem., *An Essay on the Vital and Involuntary Motions of Animals*, 134. For "special sympathy" in Whytt, see Christopher Lawrence, "Medicine as Culture: Edinburgh and the Scottish Enlightenment," Doctoral Dissertation, University of London, 1984, 137–138, 149–155; Idem., "The Nervous System and Society in the Scottish Enlightenment," in *Natural Order: Historical Studies of Scientific Culture,* Barry Barnes and Steven Shapin, eds. (London: Sage, 1979).

19. Whytt, *An Essay on the Vital and Involuntary Motions of Animals*, 151; Idem., *Observations on the Nature, Causes, and Cure of those Disorders which have been Commonly Called Nervous, Hypochondriac, or Hysteric*, 217–218.

20. Dugald Stewart, "Law of Sympathetic Imitation," in *Elements of the Philosophy of the Human Mind*, in *The Collected Works of Dugald Stewart,* William Hamilton, ed. (Edinburgh: Thomas Constable, 1854), vol. 4, 117–118, 129, 136, 147–148, 155; J. B. Morrell, "Theophobica Gallica: Natural Philosophy, Religion, and Politics in Edinburgh 1789–1815," in *Notes Received by the Royal Society*, London: 26 (1971): 43–63; Stefan Collini, Donald Winch, and John Burrow, *That Noble Science of Politics: A Study in Nineteenth-Century Intellectual History* (Cambridge: Cambridge University Press, 1983), 32.

21. Stewart, *Elements of the Philosophy of the Human Mind,* vol. 4, 120–121.

22. James Hodson, *Nature's Assistant to the Restoration of Health* (London, 1794, thirteenth edition). Other examples include James Graham, *The Guardian of Health* (Newcastle upon Tyne, 1790); William Perfect, *Cases of Insanity, the Epilepsy, Hypochondriacal Affection, Hysteric Passion, and Nervous Disorders, Successfully Treated* (Rochester, 1785); James Rymer, *A Tract upon Indigestion and the Hypochondriac Disease, with the method of cure, and a new remedy or medicine recommended* (London, 1785); William Brodum, *To the nervous, consumptive, and those of debilitated constitutions, and with full evidence of astonishing efficacy in numberless trials of the Restorative Nervous Cordial, invented and prepared by W. Brodum* (London, 1797).

23. Linda Colley, *Britons: Forging the Nation, 1707–1837* (London: Pimlico, 1994); Chris Jones, *Radical Sensibility: Literature and Ideas in the 1790s* (London: Routledge, 1993); Clark Lawlor and Akihito Suzuki, "The Diseases of the Self." On Victorian constipation, see James C. Whorton, *Inner Hygiene: Constipation and the Pursuit of Health in Modern Society* (Oxford: Oxford University Press, 2000).

24. Trotter, *A View of the Nervous Temperament*, viii, xi–xii, xviii, 71–73; Peter Melville Logan, *Nerves and Narratives: A Cultural History of Hysteria in Nineteenth-Century British Prose* (Berkeley: University of California Press, 1997), 16.

25. Whytt, *Observations on the Nature, Causes, and Cure of those Disorders which have been Commonly Called Nervous, Hypochondriac, or Hysteric,* 188. Trotter, *A View of the Nervous Temperament,* xi, 155–156, 195, 203–208.

26. Trotter, *A View of the Nervous Temperament,* 147, 156–157.

27. Ibid., 26–27, 30–31. See also Roy Porter, *Doctor of Society: Thomas Beddoes and the Sick Trade in Late-Enlightenment England* (London: Routledge, 1992); Trotter, *An Essay, Medical, Philosophical and Chemical, on Drunkenness and Its Effects on the Human Body* (London, 1804), 153, quoted in Porter, "Addicted to Modernity," 87. Thomas Beddoes, *Hygëia,* (Bristol: J. Mills, 1802–1803), vol. 1, essay two, 72. Compare with Adam Smith, *The Theory of Moral Sentiments,* D. D. Raphael et al, eds. (Oxford: Oxford University Press, 1976), 184: "The capacity of [the genteel consumer's] stomach bears no proportion to the immensity of his desires...."

28. Beddoes, *Hygëia,* vol. 1, essay two, 72; Roy Porter, *Doctor of Society*; Brian Dolan, "Conservative Politicians, Radical Philosophy and the Aerial Remedy for the Disease of Civilization," *History of the Human Sciences,* 15:2 (2002), 35–54. For the rise of non-somatic Victorian hypochondria, see Janet Oppenheim, *Shattered Nerves; Doctors, Patients, and Depression in Victorian England* (Oxford: Oxford University Press, 1991), 142–143.

Chapter 2 ∽

CORPOREAL ECONOMIES

WORK AND WASTE IN NINETEENTH-CENTURY CONSTRUCTIONS OF ALIMENTATION

Joyce L. Huff

In British and American culture today, the goal of dietary regimen is generally the elimination of body fat. But the science that underpins the regulation of our dietary intake, with the accompanying stigma that it attaches to fat, was not initially created in response to any real or imagined need to reduce the waistlines of the "well-fed classes."[1] This science had its roots in the 1860s, when medical officers appointed by the British government sought to eliminate the problem of malnutrition and the diseases it fostered among the poor of England. The public relief system by which food was distributed to the unemployed was badly in need of reform, but, as paupers were maintained at government expense, policymakers were working under economic constraints imposed from above. The problem in institutional diet reform was, as prison inspector Sir William Guy argued, how to feed the inmates of institutions without "overburdening" the public with the cost.[2]

Doctors who, like Guy, were in charge of overseeing facilities for the care of the under classes, turned to science in order to discover the dietary regimen that would "yield the largest amount of nourishment at the least cost."[3] These men believed that to reform pauper diet they needed to understand, not only the nutritional elements in food, but also the way in which actual bodies would make use of the food supplied by the government. While, at first, this meant the study of digestion, gradually, digestion itself was contextualized within an overall system of alimentation. Because reformers focused on the working of the body itself, the result was the creation of an epistemological model for framing the body in terms of nutritional requirements and an accompanying disciplinary regime for materializing that body.

The science of alimentation that emerged from the investigations of these dietary reformers placed a high priority on balancing nutrition with cost-effectiveness. Reformers employed a way of talking about the workings of the body as continuous with other forms of labor within the overall economic system of the nation. Thus, the nineteenth century saw the development of a vocabulary for discussing corporeal processes, and specifically those processes by which the body made use of the nutrients in food, in economic terms. This discourse stigmatized fat, and its spread beyond institutions and into the middle-class home helped to foster our current obsession with thinness.

In the 1860s, dietary reformers hoped that a new, scientifically based method would replace the haphazard and inefficient manner by which food was purchased for and distributed to the lower classes. This hope was grounded in utilitarian ideologies. The utilitarian goal was to maximize pleasure and minimize pain, and they believed that this could be achieved through scientific understanding. Mathematics and statistics held the key: if human life could be reduced to that which was measurable, then it would be theoretically possible to calculate precisely what factors were necessary to the maintenance of a harmonious society and to develop a system for managing these factors in order to alleviate the majority of human suffering.[4] When faced with conflicting public pressures—which paradoxically demanded that governing bodies spend as little as possible on the feeding of those individuals who "work not, neither do they spin"[5] while nevertheless insisting that inmates of institutions be treated humanely—utilitarian reformers naturally turned to science for the answer. In order to obey two contradictory mandates, to be both frugal and humane, institutional overseers felt the need to construct a science of alimentation.

The body that emerges from the pages of pamphlets and addresses on dietary reform is a laboring body, valued according to the efficiency with which it uses resources to accomplish tasks. Its worth can be gauged by measuring the amount of work and waste it produces in relation to the amount of the resources it consumes. It is also docile and can be adjusted in order to increase the proficient utilization of materials. And it can be described in paired terms borrowed from economic discourses, such as supply and demand, investment and return, debt and repayment, and excess and waste.

This body also serves as a site for articulating economic concerns; the corporeal economy enacts anxieties about the distribution of economic resources and the circulation of consumer goods in the national economy, naturalizing a view of the existing economic conditions based on capitalism, colonization and the exploitation of natural resources, and attendant assumptions about the gendering of labor.

This model of the body did not allow for a positive view of the corpulent subject. When dietary reformers talked about the body in terms of work and waste, they interpreted corpulence as a signifier of the latter; a fat pauper was the living symbol of government waste. In an 1850 address to the College of Physicians, Dr. Thomas King Chambers called for the medical profession to systematize its approach to the study and management of middle-class fat, as part of the general standardization of medical knowledge that occurred in the nineteenth century. In the following decades, when physiologists and practitioners began their quest to do just that, they turned to the existing alimentary sciences, those constructed for the management of pauper diets, and thus they generalized the stigma that these sciences attached to corpulence.

The Economics of Diet and Digestion in the Nineteenth Century

It is hardly surprising that in the 1860s one of the leading voices in the development of an economic vocabulary for discussing alimentation, Edward Smith, was an inspector in the employ of the Poor Law Board. After the passage of the New Poor Law in 1834, the need to balance cost and nutrition in workhouses became imperative. The New Poor Law was a controversial piece of utilitarian reform legislation that sought to standardize and streamline methods of providing relief to the poor. It was intended to make the distribution of resources to the poor more efficient and cost-effective, while also providing incentive for paupers to reenter the workforce.

Underlying this secondary goal was the assumption that the poor would prefer to live at the expense of the state than to work for their bread. As Smith asserts, "[I]t has always been desired that the arrangements of a workhouse should not be such as would entice able-bodied men to abandon employment."[6] Hunger provided the capitalist system with a primary form of economic incentive. Writing in 1829, just five years before the passage of the New Poor Law, surgeon William Wadd stated that "[a]ccording to an "old English adage, 'It is the stomach makes the legs amble, and not the legs the stomach.' "[7] This sentiment was echoed in an 1861 article that appeared in *Cornhill Magazine,* which proclaims, "Civilization rests on hunger . . . The recurring and unfailing stimulus which the stomach supplies, lies at the root of all those energetic efforts by which men gradually rise from ignorance to knowledge,"[8] and again in an 1864 article in *The Lancet,* which reads, "It is but fair that we see we do not make a full stomach a premium for idleness."[9]

Because of the equation of hunger with economic incentive, after the passing of the New Poor Law, workhouses served a punitive as well as a humanitarian function. To avoid luring poor laborers away from paid employment, the New Poor Law instituted a "deterrent policy," which stated that a workhouse should provide a subsistence level living at a standard lower than that of the lowest-paid worker in the area. It also established that the government would only extend aid to an able-bodied pauper to fulfill scientifically determined physical "needs"; it would not gratify a potential worker's desires.

When Smith began a humanitarian campaign to reform the uneven and inadequate dietary standards in poorhouses, he needed to demonstrate to his superiors, and to the public, that the dietary regimens that he proposed would meet the needs of inmates without fulfilling their desires. The New Poor Law thus demanded a new type of dietary expert, one who could defend decisions about inmate diet on supposedly objective scientific grounds and one who, according to an 1864 article in *The Lancet,* would embody "a combination of the patient social observer, the chemist, the physiologist and the cook."[10] The health inspector became this expert, and by the mid century, discussion of dietary reform was dominated by the search for a "precise scientific method" that would allow institutional managers to provide maximum nutrition for minimal cost.[11]

From the first, however, dietary reformers believed that nutritional knowledge required more than just a familiarity with the nutrients found in food itself. Although they examined various foodstuffs, their goal was not simply to find foods that could provide adequate nutrition at a low cost, for, it was argued, it did not matter how nutritious foods were if they could not be easily digested. Digestion itself had to be investigated.

In the early nineteenth century, dietary reformers concentrated on the digestive process itself and performed experiments to determine the ease with which various foods were broken down. A soldier, wounded in the Napoleonic wars, provided a unique opportunity for study; according to Smith, there was "an artificial hole in his stomach, through which food could be introduced and withdrawn." By the 1860s, however, the focus of research had shifted away from a narrow concentration on the breaking down of foodstuffs within the digestive system and toward a more holistic understanding of the roles played by nutrients within the corporeal economy as a whole. Smith critiques earlier experiments because they "only showed the rapidity of the process."[12] A food that is readily digested, he reasoned, may or may not perform actual work within the body as a whole and, if it does not, then the labor of digesting it would be wasted effort. Smith argues that knowledge about the ease with which foodstuffs are broken down is irrelevant without a broader knowledge of the use to which the nutrients themselves are put within the body.

To truly understand nutrition, according to Smith, reformers needed to determine "the physical requirements of the persons to be fed." But, more than this, Smith emphasized the need to study the workings of the body itself, in order to determine "the conditions under which the inmates should be placed to enable them to make the best use of the food supplied."[13] Paupers themselves were to become part of the standardization and streamlining process, by becoming efficient eaters. Under Smith and men like him, the management of working-class diet depended on the concept of conspicuous production, the inverse of consumer display. As the public did not want to see the poor as consumers, the food they ate had to be figured as part of the process of labor. That is, nutritional scientists needed to demonstrate that food was performing a sort of nutritional labor. It should be noted that, by the 1860s, nutritional labor was not the same as the work produced by individuals; at that time, it was considered inhumane to make paupers work in order to receive food from charitable institutions. Rather, food itself needed to perform work within the body.

Balancing the Corporeal Budget

The utilitarian reformers contextualized digestion within the larger framework of the use of nutrients within the body. The corporeal model that they adopted was a dynamic one in which the living body was the result of a series of chemical processes, rather than simply existing as an object in and of itself. In 1861, surgeon James Hinton explained that "to think rightly of organic bodies, they should be regarded rather from the point of view of their action than of their substance; rather as processes than as things." That is, the Victorian body is not imagined as a separate entity upon which chemical processes act, "a passive mechanism wielded by forces from without." Rather, the body is "active in itself"; it is "constituted by" its chemical processes. Like a flame, Hinton asserts, it gives the effect of stability, but is in fact, continually recreating itself. "For what is such a flame?" he asks.

"Definite as is its form, it is not a 'substance' but a state of burning...In this, it is wonderfully like ourselves—I mean like the bodies in which we dwell. They also are permanent conditions merely, impressed on ever changing materials."[14] Thus, the body in Victorian biomedical discourses is not static, but neither is it radically dynamic. Although bodies themselves are not represented as fixed structures, a sort of structuring is imposed upon them through the idea of the permanent condition.

The flame metaphor could only be carried so far though, because it failed to account for the fact that corporeal processes broke down over time. In 1863, scholar Francis Bond pointed out that the permanent condition is not so very permanent after all: "The human body is continually wearing away; as truly, though perhaps not so evidently, burning away as if it were a bushel of coals in a domestic grate."[15] Although this metaphor reconstructs the body as a thing that is acted upon, Bond nonetheless views the body as far from a stable substance. Rather, he sees it as in a state of continual change, bounded by cycles of physical renewal that inevitably became less and less efficient over time.

The body's renewal was imagined almost entirely in terms of circulating liquids and gases; solid tissues were formed from blood and returned to blood. The circulatory system thus played as important a role in nutritional science as the digestive one did. According to physician Thomas King Chambers, digestion was defined as the conversion of nutrients into "healthy blood," first through the conversion of food to chyme, then a second "cooking" in the stomach, and finally absorption into the blood vessels.[16] From blood, the nutrients are formed into tissues. As Bond adds, the process then is reversed; "chemical and physiological forces...reconvert those tissues into the simpler forms in which, when they have served their part, they are eliminated from the system."[17]

In his catalog for the 1859 South Kensington Food Exhibition, Edwin Lankester asserts that this continual renewal is cyclical. Within the space of six weeks, Lankester explains, all of the tissues of the body are gradually dismantled, excreted and reconstructed afresh. "[W]e may be said," he explains, "to moult or cast away our old body and get a new one every forty days."[18] The creation of knowledge about the body in the mid-nineteenth century thus did not objectify the body as a fixed, bounded, knowable entity, as scientific knowledge is often assumed to do. Rather, in many ways, it anticipated current theories of corporeal performativity, by representing the body as the perceived effect of a series of reiterated actions.[19] However, if the body, like the flame, was wholly constituted by chemical reactions, then it could be rendered knowable by understanding the nature of chemical processes. The underlying assumption here was that chemical reactions were not random phenomena; to understand what went on within the body, one would only have to learn the rules that governed it.

Of course, Edward Smith and his followers were not interested in constructing knowledge for its own sake. As the science of nutrition was circumscribed within the domain of public health, the goals of nutritional scientists were underwritten by the desires of practicing physicians and policymakers. The discourse of nutrition was dominated by the need to develop efficient ways of maintaining bodies in institutions, and this called for a science of nutrition that would insert the body into an overall economic model. In his article, "Bodily Work and Waste," Francis Bond explicates a biomedical theory of corporeal work that facilitates this insertion. Bond divides bodily work into voluntary and involuntary labor; mechanical, and mental work involve volition, while the vital functions that resist decay and the calorific ones that maintain heat are involuntary.[20] Because Bond constructs such involuntary functions as forms of labor, life itself becomes a signifier of the "work" accomplished by the body. Informed by contemporary understandings of the physical sciences, and particularly of thermodynamics, Bond defined work in terms of its visible and therefore quantifiable byproduct—waste. "Exhibitions of force," he explains, "mechanical, electrical, or thermal, alike involve the disintegration, or, in other words, the waste of some form of matter for their production."[21]

Work, Bond explains, is "equivalent" to "waste of bodily substance." Bond proposed therefore that it was through measuring tissue waste that one might measure "the wear and tear of the body" and thus trace the "evolution of force of which that wear and tear is the exponent." Since the tissues that produced force were thought to be formed mainly from nitrogen, the amount of nitrogen found in a grain of urea "represents a certain amount of work done." Bond cites the work of a Dr. Haughton, who had constructed a series of formulas for quantifying ratios of "bodily work to bodily waste." In theory, in order to replace lost tissue, a man (Haughton studied only male subjects) would need to consume an amount of nitrogen equivalent to that which he excreted each day. If manual or mental labor is figured into the equation, it is theoretically possible to calculate the exact amount of nitrogen one would need to consume daily in order to maintain the body in health. With two hours of "hard study" and 200 foot-tons of manual labor daily, for example, a 150 pound man would produce precisely 463.38 grains of urea and require the equivalent amount of nitrogen in his diet to replenish it.[22] These formulas have a practical application, Bond feels, in determining the quantity of food to be included in cost-effective dietaries for laboring men.

Because the dynamic body was continually engaged in renewal, the supply of structural materials had to be continually maintained.[23] But one could not be constantly eating. The process of tissue replacement was thus imagined in terms of waste and replenishment, or, in Bond's economic terminology, as a "debtor and creditor account." A debt is incurred as tissues are used up in the process of producing work and this corporeal deficit must be repaid, in the form of nutrients. In order to maintain the body and prevent corporeal dissolution, a person must continually balance his or her account, or "little bill" as Bond called it, repaying the body for work completed.[24] If one failed to pay the bill, the body would become, in Smith's terms, "impoverished."[25] The body was thus imaged as a credit-based economy, in which individuals paid for services only after they were rendered.

If the body were not properly paid, however, it could not continue to perform its work, including the "vital work" of maintaining life. Accordingly, Bond argues that, if energy were not expended to keep it alive, the body would quickly become "subject to the ordinary chemical laws of inert material."[26] Living is seen as a positive act, as resisting the body's continual impulse toward deterioration. Thus, according to Hinton:

> The most striking circumstance…connected with starvation, is the tendency to decomposition and putridity, alike in the blood and all the organs which the absence of food occasions. The system, left unnourished, not only wastes away, and is consumed; its vitality also fails, and putrid emanations cover the surface. This fact furnishes further evidence that part of the office of the food is to feed the life of the organism.[27]

In this view, nutrition becomes the science of maintaining life; one resists the body's natural tendency to dissolution by remaking it periodically.

Hinton debunks the common notion of life as an object and death as its absence; life, according to him, is not "something existing apart from the other physical powers, and capable of being added to, or withdrawn from, an organism, without any other immediate change."[28] Instead, life and death, as he describes them, are both the sedimented effects of corporeal processes. The life of the body thus dissipates when the processes that create it cease to be reiterated: "The body first breaks down as a machine, and then only dies as a body. After its individual or active life has ceased, by derangement of the requisite adjustments, the life that pervades every part gradually wears out and ceases for want of support and renewal." And, when life dissipates, the processes of decay are "unresisted," producing the effect of death.[29]

The Colonizing Stomach

The nineteenth-century construction of alimentation as the incorporation of outside elements into the body's very structure meant that alimentary processes were easily expressed through imperialist metaphors. Indeed, the language of subjugation and conquest is everywhere in nineteenth-century discourses on eating. Hinton, for example, states, "The living frame is a machine for placing under our control, and at our use, the powers of nature"[30] and "[T]he advancing army of animal existence bears in its train a commissariat which turns to best account the resources of all lands."[31] As Hinton describes it, in the assimilation of food, the body brings nature under its sway; through digestion and chemical interaction, nutrients become "instruments" of man's "will."[32] These metaphors naturalized the colonial enterprise and, with it, fears of reverse colonization by writing them on the body.

Such metaphors are very abstract, however; they avoid any specific discussion of the British exploitation and consumption of foreign resources or of the economic incentives behind empire-building and, instead, construct a generic man, who conquers "Nature," without regards to national boundaries. Nature is depicted as willing to subject "herself" to human rule. She "opens her hand," proclaims Hinton,

> and pours forth to man the treasures of every land and every sea, because she would give him a wide and vigorous life, participant of all variety. For him the cornfields wave their golden grain . . . [P]leasant apple, plum, or peach solicit his ready hand. Beneath his foot lie stored the starch of the potato, the gluten of the turnip, the sugar of the beet . . . Let the various life of all the world throb in the world's ruler.[33]

The use of such metaphors to describe universal human biological processes obscures the specific socio-historical conditions that positioned Britain as the "world's ruler" and gave British citizens access to the produce of "every land and every sea."

In Hinton's description, the relationship of the world to its ruler is imagined, not simply in colonizing, but in patriarchal terms, and thus it serves as an example of the ways in which biomedical theories could serve to naturalize economic assumptions about the gendered division of labor, as well as those about colonization. The language of gendered labor is clear in Hinton's description of the digestive process, in which the "various substances which are blended in the mother's breast" are "scattered" throughout nature and when "man" eats, his body converts these substances back into a liquid form "almost exactly" analogous to "his first food."[34] He quotes "an eloquent author," the anonymous author of "The Human Body and its Connection with Man," who claims that "nature, the mighty mother, offers herself breastwise to all her little natures; she swells in landscape and undulating hill with mammary tenderness; each creation is a dug held forth to a younger creature."[35] Here, female labor is represented as reproductive; a feminine nature works to reproduce the conditions of production for a male laborer/conqueror. The gendered dichotomy serves to naturalize the dominance of the hierarchical opposition of man and nature and vice versa.

The idea that the body needed to be renewed in order to maintain life and the fact that the materials with which it was renewed had to come from outside of it made the nineteenth-century body vulnerable to the world. If food really became part of the body—if in fact, a solid and stable body was simply the perceived effect of a reiterated chain of nutritional processes—then it was impossible to imagine the relationship between the body and world simply in terms of domination. It is important to note that the discourse employed here was a rhetoric of colonization, not of slavery; food was incorporated into the overall structure of the body, just as colonies became part of the empire. It was generally acknowledged that the body adapted itself to the elements of which it was composed. Even Hinton recognizes this "adjustment."[36] The nutrients taken into the body, for example, were popularly thought to transmit certain qualities to it from the world outside. In the early nineteenth century, Wadd remarked on the prevalence of the folk belief that "animal food communicates [the animal's] qualities, with its nourishment."[37]

While doctors might disparage such simplistic associations, they nonetheless had to acknowledge that the dynamic body was open to the world it ingested. To maintain life, as Hinton asserts, food "must be redolent of sunshine, and permeated with light; it must have drunk in the virtue of the airs of heaven. For all these our food must transfer to us—to glow within our veins and animate our nerves."[38] Hinton assumes, however, an ordered and benevolent universe, in which nature affects the body in predictable, if not regular, ways: "The invisible forces which regulate the grand rhythm of the universal order, sweep through it, and draw forth each its own melody. The living body should thrill with every thrill of the wide earth, as the aspen leaf trembles in the tremulous air."[39] Embodied within the romantic rhetoric here is a desire for some connection to the natural world. Through its digestion and incorporation into the body, food becomes the mediator between an alienated, industrialized population and a romanticized nature.

However, if the body's openness to the world could provide an occasion for elegiac celebrations, it could also be a cause of anxiety. The nineteenth-century body, in dynamic interaction with the world, was also vulnerable to what Mary Douglas has described as "symbolic pollution," or "matter out of place."[40] Symbolic pollution is anything that violates the integrity of a perceived whole. The maintenance of the dominant order depends upon the continual reiteration of the boundaries that divide and categorize the world and our experience of it. Symbolic pollution is actively threatening to the dominant order, because it breaks this reiterative chain.

The incorporation of foreign material into the structure of the body paralleled the process of colonization and raised similar fears regarding potential changes to a symbolic whole that could be brought about by the introduction of foreign parts. Just as the Victorians feared the loss of cultural identity attendant upon the adoption of colonial customs and importation of colonial goods, they also felt anxiety about the loss of corporeal identity that might accompany the introduction of new elements into the body. Wadd, for example, noted a popular fear that French styles of cooking would undermine English temperaments; he reports that one of his correspondents worries that French cooking "will degenerate our countrymen, and that the next generation will be the pale-faced puny sons of compound *Entremets*, instead of the lusty offspring of beef and pudding."[41] When the dietary reformers reframed nutritional sciences in terms that favored efficiency, fat was redefined as a foreign element. The writings of dietary reformers thus characterize fat as matter out of place; it is a parasite, rather than a worker, in the corporeal economy.

"Gipsies" and Parasites

In the hands of reformers and policymakers, the science of maintaining life became the science of maintaining life efficiently. To perfect the body's efficiency, it was necessary to understand the nature of the debts it incurred in the process of daily living and to make payment in kind. All foods did not have the same currency value in the corporeal economy. To determine the values of different nutrients, nineteenth-century scientists looked to the writings of German chemist Baron Justus von Liebig, a rival of Louis Pasteur. Liebig's theories would underpin the stigmatization of fat in opposition to "healthy flesh," by dividing the nutritional elements in food into workers and parasites.

By the 1860s, physicians working with Liebig's theories recognized a variety of nutritional building-blocks. Each form of nourishment had a metaphorical part to play in the corporeal economy. Among these, the nitrogeneous or "tissue-forming" matter was thought to supply the actual material of the body. These were the "working" elements that Bond had identified, the ones that replaced wasted flesh. All bodily tissues, except for adipose ones, were thought to be formed from nitrogenous matter. But nitrogen was considered to be a very volatile element. "Of all known bodies [or elements]," Hinton explains, nitrogen "is that which most strongly tends to the gaseous state, and constitutes accordingly, the most unstable compounds. The activity, or proneness to change, of animal bodies, seems to depend chiefly on the presence of nitrogen within them, and its inveterate tendency to escape, and to become free again."[42] While the escape of nitrogen gave the muscles force and motion, its volatile nature made the body unstable. Physician George Wilson fancifully expresses nitrogen's role in the corporeal economy when he compares it to a tamed "gipsy": "Like a half-reclaimed gipsy [*sic*] from the wild, it is ever seeking to be free again; and not content with its own freedom, is ever tempting others, not of gipsy blood, to escape thralldom."[43]

Wilson grounds his metaphor in assumptions about gypsies from both socioeconomic and aesthetic discourses, in which the gypsy appears as part noble savage, part migrant laborer, who may be compelled to work for a time, but will always return to nature, and thus, threatens to destabilize the workforce. This metaphor more completely expresses the dominant mid-nineteenth century understanding of alimentation than others employed at the time, which figured the elements as servants or even slaves and thus reiterated a fiction of control over the body and its processes. As Wilson theorizes, if nutrients are servants, they are "immediate servants" only.[44] Furthermore, this explanation emphasizes the essential dualism of mind and body. This is because the aesthetic resonances of the gypsy from literature and art invoked associations of the essential otherness of body chemistry, its divorce from the brain. The gypsy is both romanticized as a free spirit and viewed with suspicion as a potential criminal element, corrupting others "not of gipsy blood." The metaphor thus reifies an essentially hostile relationship between body and "self," worker and employer.

But nitrogen was not the only important element found in food. Among others, nineteenth-century nutritional science recognized carbonaceous or "heat-producing" ones, which were thought to supply the body with the heat it needed to continue the process of renewal. This category consisted entirely of fatty foods and foods that could be converted to fats, such as starches and sugars.[45] According to Chambers, carbonaceous matter is intended to be the "fuel for the respiration." It is through respiration, Chambers explains, that the body produces the heat it needs to maintain life. "The intention of [dietary] fat," he thus asserts, "is to sustain the animal heat by combustion," and adds, quoting Galen, that it performs its duties "in the same way as oil supplies the flame of a lamp."[46]

A body functioning efficiently would, in theory, burn carbonaceous matter as it was taken in. Adipose tissue is only formed when, according to Chambers, "the materials be digested in a greater quantity than is sufficient to supply carbon to the respiration."[47] As Galen says, it is when the "flame" of life is "less powerful, less required" that "fat is laid by as in a treasure-house."[48] Thus, while nitrogenous food could be compared to payment for work accomplished, carbonaceous food was seen as an investment. Chambers explains that when starch and sugar are converted to fat, the digestive system will "return us our own with usuary [*sic*]."[49] These metaphors would seem to place a high value on fat; it is a "treasure" and a monetary "return." But fat was considered a poor investment; it did not retain its worth in storage, but was only valued if its potential for combustion was realized.

Although adipose tissue, like muscular tissue, could be broken down and consumed, a study of its properties seemed to reveal to medical doctors that this was not its main purpose. While muscles were "quickly decomposing" and "force-exerting" akin to gun-cotton when nitrogen is added, adipose tissue, without the nitrogen, was "slow-changing" cotton, and thus, not intended primarily to be broken down and used.[50] The retention of a certain amount of fat appeared to be necessary provide the body with a layer of protection necessary both to retain heat and to pad the joints and organs. But, beyond this, carbonaceous matter stored in the body was simply extra matter—matter out of place—that did not contribute in any way to the corporeal economy. Like the able-bodied pauper in nineteenth-century economic discourses, it appears as something that has to be supported by more "productive" members of the economy.

If flesh-forming substances were "gypsies," fat-forming ones, unless burned off as fuel, became, as self-proclaimed diet expert William Banting's 1863 pamphlet labeled them "parasites," which attached themselves to the body in the form of unwanted fat and "obstructed its fair, comfortable progress in the path of life."[51] At first, Banting was misunderstood; his critics thought that he had used the term literally and were quick to point out that fat cells were not independent organisms. Banting responded, explaining that he used the term "figuratively"—"as a burden to the flesh."[52] To Banting, fat represented a dangerous excess that drained the body of vital energy. And, indeed, if the formation of fat was not one of the ordinary, daily functions by which the body renewed itself and sustained its life, then corpulence could only be seen as an abnormal or even unnatural surplus, a sign or symptom of disease or dysfunction within the corporeal economy. In other words, fat functioned as a form of symbolic pollution; it underscored the body's vulnerability to foreign substances.

Although Banting was a controversial figure, many doctors agreed with his characterization of body fat as something external to the body and, thus, as surplus. Wadd, for example, describing an autopsy, metaphorically constructs fat as an outside substance found within the body: "The whole of the intestinal canal was imbedded in fat, as if melted tallow had been poured into the cavity of the abdomen."[53] Chambers regards fat not simply as an intruder, but as a pollutant, as seen in his description of fat in the blood stream: "As the blood is, like the Thames at London, at once the common sewer and the supplier of nutrition to the tissues, it is impossible to pronounce whether this fat is the product of decomposition or whether it is a retained secretion."[54] In other words, recently ingested dietary fat, on its way to be combusted, was characterized as nutrition; stored body fat, even when broken down for use, was portrayed as sewage.

For Chambers, not only was body fat worthless to the corporeal economy, but fat bodies were non-productive, and thus worthless, within the economic system. In his search for the limits defining the productive body, Chambers attempted to determine how much bodily weight a man could carry and still perform his economic role; his underlying assumption was that fat would inhibit a man's economic productivity. Chambers thus equated corporeal productivity with economic productivity.

The science of nutrition provided health inspectors with the criteria for judging which foods were needed to maintain and renew the life of the body and which could be considered "useless."[55] It also suggested how to measure each type of nutrient needed for the body to perform its vital work efficiently. Throughout the nineteenth century, experiments were conducted on the inmates of institutions such as prisons and workhouses to determine how the body used various nutritional elements. Nitrogenous matter presented a problem. The body's chemical processes could not be observed directly. Only the effects of chemical reactions on the seemingly solid visible surface of the body were observable. But, as excess nitrogen was thought to simply pass untouched through the body, health inspectors like Smith were able to follow the lead of Haughton and others like him, in measuring waste. Smith conducted a series of tests, weighing inmates and the food they were to consume before meals, and afterwards, reweighing the inmates and their bodily waste. He had to factor in the work each accomplished between weighings in order to discover what percentage of nitrogenous material had left the body without affecting its economy.[56]

For carbonaceous matter, however, the matter was simpler. Excess carbon was stored as adipose tissue. Body fat, therefore, served as the visible sign of excesses of carbon in institutional diet. In fact, to the utilitarian mind, fat on a workhouse inmate represented an additional parasite attached to an already "parasitic" member of economic system. But body fat could be reconverted into useful carbon and thus pressed into the service of the corporeal economy, just as an inmate could in theory reenter the workforce. Smith and his colleagues in other districts assumed a one-to-one correspondence between units of food consumed and fat stored and likewise between units of work performed and fat burned. As Guy explains, the "value" of experimenting with the amounts of carbonaceous foods consumed by prisoners "rests upon the assumption that there is a very intimate relationship existing between increase of food and increase of weight and . . . this relation is not apt to be seriously disturbed by other causes patent or obscure, known or unknown."[57] Smith makes the same assumption when he attempts to measure the fat-burning power of different activities, relying on records of paupers and prisoners weighed before and after exercise: "Hence 1lb of the fat of the body, in the absence of food, would be consumed by less than six hours' labour at the treadwheel, by ten hours of walking at three miles per hour, and by fourteen hours and a half of walking at two miles per hour." Anticipating the calorie-counting of the twentieth century, he attempts to come up with "exactly measured degrees of exertion," assigning a numeric value to each activity, such that walking burned "1.9 units," while rowing consumed "3.33."[58] Thus, the nutritional science, created to resolve problems of workhouse diet, devalued body fat and, by extension, the fat body.

Beyond the Workhouse

In the 1860s, Smith began to publish the results of his studies in nutrition as well as his recommendations for workhouse diet. The knowledge was disseminated in a timely manner, for, by this time, middle-class people desired to become efficient consumers as well. The rise in the popularity of manuals of domestic medicine and instructional pamphlets on health matters served to spread a new nutritional knowledge based on experiments conducted on institutional inmates by public health officials. As Michel Foucault has argued, the eighteenth and nineteenth centuries saw the spread of medical authority into the middle-class home.[59] Corporeal standards constructed within utilitarian public health discourses were appropriated and adapted for use in the resulting discussions about the health and management of middle-class bodies.

Insurance companies provided the immediate cause for the adoption of normative standards of weight by private physicians who treated upper and middle-class patients. Nineteenth-century insurance companies were searching for a way to quantify health so that monetary value could be assigned to human life, and they fixed upon body size as an easily measured indicator of physical well-being. If health were equated with efficiency and efficiency with lack of fat, then health became a knowable, quantifiable phenomenon. It was doctors in the employ of insurance companies who first disseminated utilitarian nutritional knowledge among the middle classes and created in middle-class subjects the desire for efficient bodies. When Thomas King Chambers rose to prominence as the leading expert on diet and weight after he delivered a series of lectures to the College of Physicians in 1850, he was an employee of the Hand-in-Hand Insurance Company. Chambers's writings are informed by the same food-to-work equations that underpinned the work of his contemporaries in the public health field, but his goal is the promotion of health among the middle classes, rather than the feeding of the poor. For example, Chambers shared Smith's interest in finding the "smallest amount of nutriment consistent with the health of the individual,"[60] but for Chambers efficiency was a goal in and of itself.

The insurance companies' desire to reduce the body to a series of equations between diet, weight, and life span reflected a more widespread desire to reduce corporeal anxiety by giving the fantasy of knowledge about, and therefore control over, the dynamic body's tendency toward death. To inhabit the dynamic body was daily to confront anxieties about its maintenance, control, vulnerability and boundaries. As Hinton argues, the process of embodiment must occur "within fixed limits, and in a definite form" in order for health to be maintained:[61] "For the power of the body arises simply from the chemical changes which take place within it; its life consists in the presence of the conditions which those chemical changes demand; and its health is in the perfectness with which those conditions are maintained, and those changes carried on and regulated."[62] The interaction between the dynamic body and these static limits requires a proactive, managerial approach to the body. Dietary regimens supplied such an approach. It is not surprising, therefore, that in the 1860s William Banting's diet plan sparked a reducing craze among middle-class people. Banting's 1863 pamphlet on diet, *A Letter on Corpulence*, went through five editions and sold over 63,000 copies in England, Europe and overseas, and, in the six years following its publication, he received over eighteen hundred letters from "corpulent brethren" who had tried the Banting system.[63]

As the nutritional knowledge created to meet the needs of Poor Law Board inspectors became generalized, the efficient body achieved hegemony, leaving little room for positive resignifications of the corpulent body. Body management practices aimed at eliminating fat, like the nineteenth-century Banting diet, gradually became standard ones. The alimentary discourses that constructed the ideal of the efficient corporeal economy stigmatized corpulence as waste, as opposed to work, and it is this stigma that the fat body still bears today.

Notes

1. Edward Smith, *The Present State of the Dietary Question* (London: Walton and Maberly, 1864), 12–13.
2. William Augustus Guy, *On Sufficient and Insufficient Dietaries with Special Reference to the Dietaries of Prisoners* (London: Harrison, 1863), 240.
3. Edward Smith, *Dietaries for the Inmates of Workhouses: A Report to the President of the Poor Law Board* (London: Eyre and Spottiswoode, 1866), 25.
4. For example, Jeremy Bentham, the father of utilitarianism, advocated a "moral arithmetic," or "felix calculus," for determining what would provide the greatest pleasure to the greatest number of people.
5. "The Dietary Question," Review of *The Present State of the Dietary Question* by Edward Smith, *The Lancet* (22 October 1864), 469.
6. Smith, *Dietaries*, 24.
7. William Wadd, *Comments on Corpulency and Lineaments of Leanness* (London: Ebers, 1829), 13.
8. James Hinton, "Food—What It Is," *Cornhill Magazine* (April 1861), 460.
9. "The Dietary Question," 469.
10. "Practical Dietaries," Review of *Practical Dietary for Families, Schools and the Labouring Classes* by Edward Smith, *The Lancet* (24 December 1864), 722.
11. Smith, *Dietaries*, 3.
12. Ibid., 50.
13. Ibid., 5, 25.
14. James Hinton, "Health," *Cornhill Magazine* (March 1861), 337.

15. Francis T. Bond, "Bodily Work and Waste," *The Popular Science Review*, 3 (1863), 151.

16. Thomas King Chambers, "On Corpulence [part 2]," *The Lancet* (11 May 1850), 559.

17. Bond, "Bodily Work," 151.

18. Edwin Lankester, *Guide to the Food Collection in the South Kensington Museum* (London: Eyre and Spottiswoode, 1859), 5.

19. Judith Butler, *Bodies That Matter* (New York: Routledge, 1993).

20. Bond, "Bodily Work," 152.

21. Ibid., 149.

22. Ibid., 151–154.

23. Smith, *Dietaries*, 6.

24. Bond, "Bodily Work," 154.

25. Smith, *Dietaries*, 29.

26. Bond, "Bodily Work," 153.

27. Hinton, "Food," 471.

28. Hinton, "Health," 338.

29. Ibid., 339.

30. Ibid., 334, 339.

31. Hinton, "Food," 464.

32. Ibid., 463.

33. Ibid., 472.

34. Ibid., 460.

35. Quoted in Ibid., 460–461.

36. Ibid., 463.

37. Wadd, *Comments*, 141.

38. Hinton, "Food," 472.

39. Hinton, "Health," 333.

40. Mary Douglas, *Purity and Danger* (London: Ark, 1984), 36.

41. Wadd, *Comments*, 141–142.

42. Hinton, "Food," 462.

43. Quoted in Hinton, "Food," 462.

44. Quoted in Ibid., 464.

45. Smith, *Dietaries*, 34.

46. Thomas King Chambers, "On Corpulence [part 1]," *The Lancet* (4 May 1850), 524.

47. Ibid., [part 2], 559.

48. Ibid., [part 1], 524.

49. Ibid., [part 2], 558.

50. Hinton, "Food," 462.

51. William Banting, *A Letter on Corpulence*, third American edition (New York: Harper, 1864), 9. See also my "A 'Horror of Corpulence': Bantingism and Nineteenth-Century Fat-phobia," in *Bodies Out of Bounds: Fatness and*

Transgression, Jana Evans Braziel and Kathleen LeBesco, eds. (Berkeley: University of California Press, 2001).

52. William Banting, *A Letter on Corpulence*, fourth American edition (New York: Mohun and Ebbs, 1865), 28.

53. Wadd, *Comments*, 65.

54. Chambers, "On Corpulence [part 1]," 525.

55. Smith, *Dietaries*, 35.

56. Edward Smith, *Practical Dietary for Families, Schools and the Labouring Classes* (London: Walton and Maberly, 1864), 577.

57. Guy, *On Sufficient*, 262.

58. Smith, *Practical Dietary*, 577.

59. Michel Foucault, "The Politics of Health in the Eighteenth Century," in *Power/Knowledge*, trans. Colin Gordon (New York: Pantheon, 1977).

60. Thomas King Chambers, "On Corpulence [part 6]," *The Lancet* (22 June 1850), 748.

61. Hinton, "Health," 337.

62. Ibid., 335.

63. William Banting, *A Letter on Corpulence*, fourth edition (London: Harrison, 1869), xi.

Chapter 3 ∾

KAKAO AND KAKA

CHOCOLATE AND THE EXCRETORY IMAGINATION OF NINETEENTH-CENTURY EUROPE

Alison Moore

O f all the food products that entered the European consumer market as a result of colonial trade, chocolate underwent the most dramatic differentiation from its original form. In Aztec society chocolate was drunk cold, spicy and bitter.[1] So why in the mid-nineteenth century did Europeans turn it into something sweet, sticky, creamy, and solid? The answer to this question lies in an analysis of the physical and symbolic resemblance of chocolate to excrement: that other brown substance that was of such great concern and fascination for European society of the nineteenth century. The contemporaneous emergence of solid eating chocolate as a coveted consumer object alongside the development of sewerage and toilet technology in nineteenth-century Europe was not incidental. Both relate to the development of a new identity amongst middle-class Europeans who were keen to enjoy the exotic delights of colonial produce as much as they were to deny and sanitize the excretory process in response to the crisis of malodorous bodily products produced by industrial urbanization. Both the deodorized sewers of mid century urbanization policies (particularly in Paris and London), and the availability of fragrant, sweet and pungent consumables from colonial trade, were pivotal in establishing a European bourgeois identity that counterposed itself to the excrement-eating primitives from whom chocolate and its compound ingredients had been stolen. This article will show that throughout the late modern era chocolate has been repeatedly associated, both explicitly and symbolically, with excrement. While excretory and anal repression were seen as central to the construction of European identity in a range of late-nineteenth-century texts concerned with differentiating primitive from civilized Man, chocolate was viewed as a consumer symbol of the gold, wealth, luxury, and new class hierarchies purchased through slavery and colonial exploitation in Africa and the Americas. Chocolate then was the symbolic byproduct of the process by which the European consumer classes domesticated the appropriation of wealth from colonial endeavors and controlled excretory processes in construction of the urban sanitary order. This article will discuss how chocolate was mythologized and marketed initially as an exotic aphrodisiac, then infantalized during the nineteenth century, then—from the *fin de siècle* to the present—constructed as the ultimate and most appropriate gift between lovers. Through this analysis I argue that chocolate has consistently appeared as a symbol of the primitive within the civilized, as the child-like, the sexual, the fetishized, the excremental, which European societies have harnessed, channeled, and transmuted throughout the process of urban sanitization.

Oral contact with excrement represents one of the most charged taboos in modern societies.[2] Coprophagia (the eating of excrement) was most famously eroticized by the Marquis de Sade,[3] and has been documented as a practiced sexual variation by sexologists and psychiatrists consistently from the late nineteenth century to the present.[4] In these examples the consumption of excrement is represented as a distinctly obscure, frequently aberrant and most certainly a marginal desire. However, this article will argue that solid eating chocolate has throughout its history been fashioned and marketed in forms visually, sensually and symbolically alike to excrement and that it hence represents a *simulacrum* of the waste matter that Europeans of the nineteenth century saw as so essential to cast out in the name of a clean, odorless and ordered civilization.[5] In combining the cacao once unique to Aztec culture with the sugar harvested by Europeans in the slave plantations of South America, chocolate is a product of colonial domination par excellence.[6] As I will show, just as nineteenth-century urban planners were formulating the notion that the technologized sewers flushing excrement out of sight and out of smell were a true mark of progress and civilization, middle-class Europeans simultaneously developed a compulsive taste for a new brown, fragrant substance, and shaped it, of all things, into eggs, bars and logs, or alternatively into kisses, hearts, and coins. Hence chocolate functioned as symbol of the erotic, the infantile and the feminine aspects attributed to primitivity and which were cast out as waste matter in the masculine, adult work of civilized society and capitalist economic order. Chocolate marketing still today emphasizes class difference with its demarcation as a luxury product even in the face of mass consumer democratization. Packaged in gold and silver foil, in bejeweled boxes, as coins and gold bars, it represents the essential commodity fetishism of high capitalism as identified by Marx.[7] Its kitsch aesthetic reverses the logic of value, turning excrement into gold, making that which is most valueless into the most valuable; that which is most disgusting (because waste matter) into the most covetable of delicious consumables.[8]

Chocolate and Coprophagia

Today the physical resemblance of chocolate to excrement is obvious to schoolchildren of many cultures, who often refer to it euphemistically as "chocolate." In 2001 the chocolate manufacturer Cadbury's capitalized on this resemblance in its Australian marketing of the "picnic" bar, using a barren photograph of the unpackaged brown, lumpy log printed on giant underground-transport posters with the caption "deliciously ugly," with the implication that the chocolate bar resembled a giant turd. A similar variety of humor has been employed continuously since the early modern era in a folk custom of the Auvergne and several other regions of rural France: the marital ritual of the "rôtie," as documented by the anthropological sociologist Deborah Reed-Danahay.[9] According to this practice, a newly-married couple are pursued into the marital bed chamber (and ideally surprised in the act of consummation) by reveling youths who present them with a chamber pot in which chocolate and champagne are placed and which the young couple are forced to consume. The *rôtie* is a mockery of bourgeois notions of taste in its representation of objects of culinary luxury as excremental symbols in a ritual of eroticism and rite of passage.[10] Here again, as Reed-Danahay remarks, the verbal narrative accompanying the metaphor is that although the *rôtie* looks disgusting (*dégoûtante*; *dégueulasse*), it actually tastes very good (*délicieuse*).[11]

The Marquis de Sade fetishized the consumption both of chocolate and excrement.[12] It was widely believed at the time to have been chocolates that Sade used to conceal the aphrodisiac with which two young women were made ill in the scandal that saw the Marquis flee across the Italian border in 1772.[13] Sade was something of a "chocoholic" (by the standards of today's jargon)—we find it included in the meals described in *The 120 Days of Sodom*[14] and in letters he sent from prison to his wife he demanded alarming quantities of it, including ground chocolate for drinking, cacao-butter suppositories to soothe his hemorrhoids, *crème au chocolat,* chocolate pastilles, chocolate biscuits, chocolate-coated sweets, and solid bars.[15] He complained bitterly of his biscuits not tasting chocolatey enough: "The biscuits must smell of it, as if one were biting into a tablet of chocolate," he wrote to his wife on 16 May 1779.[16] As Roland Barthes noted, the consumption of luxury foods is a conspicuous feature of the Sadean sexual universe since they reiterate the eroticized relations of social inequality upon which Sade's libertine fantasy of sexual domination is predicated—the masters are always aristocratic, wealthy and/or genuinely powerful figures in society. The Sadean libertine, as well as being a drunkard, sexually promiscuous and unwashed, is also a "gourmand" (a lover of fine food, or the less flattering translation: a glutton).[17] And yet it is not only the masters who feast in Sade's novels, since the slaves too must be stuffed full of the finest foods (including chocolate) in order to make their excrement both abundant and palatable for the libertine coprophage.[18] The symbolic notion of chocolate as excrement was not lost on Sade either: in a letter of 9 May 1779 he wrote to his wife that he wanted a chocolate cake for his birthday, "black inside with chocolate as the devil's arse is black from smoke."[19]

In these examples, then, it was through its physical resemblance to excrement that chocolate became invested with aphrodisiacal properties, became seen as the most appropriate gift of love and courtship for a man to offer a women, often depicted as indulgent, sinful, guilt-producing, and corrupting; often associated, moreover, with luxury, gold, and wealth. All these symbolic layers are explicable if we consider chocolate specifically as a consumer product that was specifically derived from colonial trade, and hence a product that reveals a range of European projections and prejudices about the nature of the primitive world from which it was taken. But in order to understand chocolate as a colonial consumer product, we must first understand not only the coprophagia that it symbolizes, but also the notion of sexual excess and primitivity associated with those cultures from which the ingredients of chocolate were derived. Coprophagia is an obvious point to consider in relation to the symbolism of chocolate, not only because chocolate resembles excrement and is eaten, but indeed also because erotic arousal was (and still is today) frequently implied in its consumption. From the moment that Europeans observed and identified chocolate within Aztec society they projected upon it aphrodisiacal and primitive properties.[20] Post-Conquest myth from the time of Bernal Diaz del Castillo to the present, has it that Motecuhzoma drank 50 goblets of chocolate a day and always before entering his harem of 100 women.[21] For the Aztecs chocolate was clearly regarded as an intensely nourishing drink, was also a beverage of the upper classes and indeed was widely used throughout the Central and Southern Americas as a form of currency.[22] However the Aztec and Mayan myths of the origins of chocolate suggest that it held an altogether different symbolism to the aphrodisiacal property ascribed to it by Europeans.[23] It is significant that in the transference from Meso-American to European societies chocolate immediately came to be imbued with sexual and primitive power. As the Antillais anti-colonial writer Franz Fanon and more recently the historian Anne McClintock have shown, European colonial domination can itself be read as a sexualized and gendered process in which the colonial Other stands for the sexualized aspect of the European Self that it projects upon this Other.[24] Of all those products that Europeans derived from colonial expansion and which became a feature of the metropolitan consumer market from the end of the eighteenth century, chocolate was both the most excremental in appearance and the most commonly eroticized.

As the ethnographers and anthropologists I will discuss later demonstrate, coprophagy held a special place in the European imagination concerning how sexual perversion intersected with the civilizing process. The "savage" coprophage manifested the quintessential "autoplastic" personality in which, like a child, one revels in the universe of one's own body, whereas civilized Man acted "alloplastically" on the external environment, symbolized by the abjection and rejection of excrement, which was then marked as taboo.[25] Indeed the role of excrement in the construction of civilized identity in nineteenth-century Europe is apparent on a number of levels. As a number of French historians have demonstrated, the mid century technologization of the Paris sewerage system, along with concerns about urbanization and disease, formed a distinct discourse that related cleanliness, odorlessness, and conquest of the filth of city life to the path of civilizing progress.[26] The notion of criminals, the poor in general, and prostitutes in particular as representing the "refuse of society" was a widespread notion at the time that requires no great effort to identify.[27] In the 1830s, the French town-planner Parent-Duchâtelet had explicitly related prostitutes to excrement, noting that an abundance of both was inevitable in an urban district, and hence, "... the authorities should take the same approach to each."[28] Henry Mayhew's sociological study of the London poor in the 1850s placed particular emphasis on the "filth" entailed in urban poverty, hence his detailed focus on "nightmen" and other cesspool workers. Mayhew noted of the Parisian system of draining faecal matter into the *voiries* of Montfaucon that "the evils of this system are not a few"; however the evil of London's system of drainage into the Thames was "far greater, beyond all in degree," since with the tides washing these "evacuations" back into the river:

> ...the water in which we boil our vegetables and our meat, the water for our coffee and our tea...comes to us, and is imbibed by us, impregnated over and over again with own animal offal. We...drink a solution of our own faeces.[29]

In 1848 Great Britain passed the Public Health Act mandating either a flush toilet, privy or ash pit in every habitation. In the same year the government released five million pounds toward research and engineering of new sanitary technology.[30] As Stephen Inwood notes, with at least 140 sewers emptying into the Thames, and the majority of Londoners deriving most of their fresh water supply from that river, London urban life in the mid century had indeed become a "coprophagic" society. Ironically the use of flush toilets compounded the problem of London's water supply by causing the discharge of even larger quantities of unclean water into the sewer system.[31] Hence, although by the mid nineteenth century the era of hot drinking chocolate may have been losing ground to the new fetishization of solid *kakao*, Londoners nonetheless continued to guzzle a range of brown beverages, not always by consent.

In Paris during the same period, although there was not anything like Mayhew's anxiety about the consumption of excrement implied by the poor sanitation of the Thames, there was nonetheless a marked preoccupation with the notion of sewerage technologization reflecting the status of society as "civilized."[32] Donald Reid notes the mentality that emerged under the regime of Napoléon III, during which time the *Préfet de la Seine,* Baron Georges Haussmann, led a major reconstruction of Paris, both above and below ground. The word "cloaque" (cloaca = the singular excretory, urinary, and generative orifice of birds) with its biological connotation was increasingly replaced by the term "égout" (sewer), connoting a technological construction: "...less a natural organ than a natural form subordinated to man's use...."[33] When the Paris sewers were opened for guided tour in 1867, it was the odorlessness of the experience that was trumpeted by its organizers and was seen as the sign of a truly great advancement in European civilization.[34] Alfred Mayer in the *Guide Paris* of 1867 depicted the Paris sewers as having reached the pinnacle of 600-year evolution, and were hence a sign that French civilization at that moment had surpassed the grandeur of ancient Rome.[35] Pictorial representations of *la visite à l'égout* suggest that it was overwhelmingly patronized by men and women of the middle and upper classes dressed in top hats and feminine frilled finery.[36] Georges Vigarello has shown how the microbial vision of disease that emerged in the late nineteenth century created a new emphasis on cleanliness as a sign of social order and reinforced pre-existing perceptions of dirtiness as inherent to the lower classes. "There are fifty times the number of microbes in the housing of a poor person as there are in the air of a sewer," remarked one *fin-de-siècle* urban planner.[37] To the observer of the *visite à l'égout* images today, there is something profoundly kitsch about the finely dressed ladies and gentlemen being trollied off to observe the odorless and civilized manner in which their ordure is being transported through the bowels of the city. One is reminded of Anne McClintock's observation of "imperial kitsch as consumer spectacle."[38] Indeed, McClintock has shown how, in colonial consumer advertising of the nineteenth century, racial whiteness was conceived as cleanliness through the representation of soap as having the power to clean away racial blackness.[39] The cleanliness of the late-nineteenth-century urban bourgeoisie stands in opposition then to the lower classes of European society, to the degenerate, perverse, and criminal aspects within that society, and to the primitive cultures of the colonial world. The sewer visiting scheme was introduced in Paris at the opening of the 1867 *Exposition Universelle,* an exhibition that celebrated the technological developments and expansionist bounties of France as a colonial power. Similarly, at the Great Exhibition of 1851, Londoners had been treated to the world's first display of public flushing toilets, abundantly lit by the massive spectacle of electrical lighting for which the exhibition later became known.[40]

Trade fairs and exhibitions were to be the stage on which both the captured consumable delights and the deodorized subjugated filth of the bourgeois imperial order were displayed. Indeed it was at the Birmingham trade fair of 1849 that the Fry family exhibited the world's first *chocolat délicieux à manger*: the smooth paste set into defined shapes that was made possible by the mechanism (discovered in 1828 and patented by the Dutch chocolatier Coenraad Johannes van Houten) by which the cacao fat could be separated from the solids, remixed into smooth paste with cocoa and other flavorings and then set into logs, bars and other forms.[41] As the anthropologist Sydney Mintz has remarked, chocolate historians have on the whole had very little to say about the one addition to chocolate that was clearly most instrumental for its status as a desirable European consumer good: sugar.[42] The historian James Walvin has noted, however, that Europeans only took any interest in consuming the Aztec chocolate once someone got the idea of adding sugar to it (Joseph Acosta in 1604 had described the drink as "loathsome" and "unpleasant to taste").[43] Chocolate was thus embraced by Europeans "thanks to the efforts of African slaves," since the European sugar market during the seventeenth and eighteenth centuries was overwhelming supplied by slave plantations in South America.[44] As Timothy Morton notes, it was precisely this sense of one's indulgent sweet beverages being morally tainted with the blood of African slaves that caused outrage and abstention amongst a certain class of British writers at the end of the eighteenth century.[45] Sugar made chocolate into a product not only of the original cultural theft from Meso-American civilization, but indeed of an ongoing exploitation of this other major cash crop of the worst manifestation of colonialism in the Americas. The sweetening of chocolate can moreover be seen as a factor further contributing to its excremental resemblance, resulting in a stickier consistency. In John G. Bourke's amateur ethnographic compendium of excrement-eaters (which I discuss later), contemporary (deviant) European coprophages of the *fin de siècle* were depicted in conversation with a Professor Obersteiner who asked them how they found the taste of excrement, and to which one replied "stinking and somewhat sweet," and another stinking and waterishly sweet."[46] According to Lawrence Wright, one sanitary engineer in Britain during 1870s, when describing the subtle range of smells to be found in a household plumbing system, held that of least concern were the dank, ammoniacal or putrid odors, "as there is a close, sweet smell which is even worse."[47] The interesting thing to consider is whether Europeans were so inclined to interpret the aroma and flavor of excrement as "sweet" before chocolate appeared on the consumer market. In other words, it may indeed be possible that coprophagic sexual desire emerged specifically in the post-Conquest European metropolis; that it was the sweetened and eroticized form of excrement represented by *kakao* that showed some Europeans how to find something sexy and tasty in *kaka*. Is there not a curious phonetic similarity, as Freud remarked, of the words *kaka* and *kakao* (*ca-ca* in Romance languages, κακα in Greek, "cacky" in English)?[48]

Within thirty years of the word "cloaca" disappearing from sewer-technology discourse, solid eating chocolate began to appear on the European consumer market in the shape of precisely that which (apart from excrement) is actually expelled from a chicken's cloaca: the egg. Italian chocolate manufacturers first began producing chocolate eggs in 1884 after word spread of the Tsar Alexander III's gift to his bride Maria Feodorovna of the lavishly jeweled Fabergé egg.[49] From this time on chocolate eggs have tended to replace painted real eggs as fertility symbols in cultures that celebrate Easter. There are several layers to the symbolism of this development that require individual treatment. The egg, as the product of a cloaca, is first of all clearly excremental in reference, but the mimicking of the Fabergé egg is also significant as a gift of sexual love, a gift from a man to woman (as chocolate is generally), and as symbol of wealth and luxury. As the cultural historians Wolfgang Schivelbusch and Barbara Lekatsas have noted, drinking chocolate during the eighteenth century was clearly both a beverage of the aristocracy and of the boudoir.[50] As Schivelbusch observes, illustrations of the period show bourgeois families drinking coffee at breakfast, sitting upright, seeking stimulation for the workday ahead, while aristocratic chocolate drinkers contrastingly lie semi-prostrate, dressed still in bed-clothes, often actually in bed. Chocolate, unlike coffee or even tea, thus became associated less with work or rest from work, and more with sheer idleness.[51] Although the analysis of Schivelbusch ignores the gender implications of this division, Woodruff Smith has recently remarked upon it, noting that association of chocolate as a breakfast food as far back as the seventeenth century established it clearly within the realm of the domestic (and hence feminine) sphere.[52] During the nineteenth century, as chocolate became cheaper and more accessible to the middle classes, its marketing symbolism was geared toward a new appeal as a beverage associated with domesticity, with women and especially with children. As David Courtwright remarks, "Cocoa became the breakfast drink of children, chocolate candies tokens of middle-class affection."[53] The technological innovations of solid eating chocolate—of "conching" (the process by which cacao solids could be blended to produce a completely smooth and creamy paste), followed by Daniel Peters's 1879 addition of Nestlé's powdered milk to solid eating chocolate—resulted in a more excrementally-appearing product than ever before.[54] Increasingly, from the end of the 1880s and into the early twentieth century, solid chocolate was molded into eggs, logs, and other indefinable *lumpf*-like forms; packaged in gold and silver foil, shaped into hearts or "kisses" (for example Hershey's "Kisses," or Perugina's "Baci"), marketed as a lover's gift and as a source of luxury, sensual pleasure, and indulgence. While drinking chocolate was increasingly feminized and infantilized during the nineteenth century, solid eating chocolate was increasingly eroticized and excrementalized.[55]

Money, Chocolate, and Sexuality

Given the discursive associations between primitivity and sexual excess in nineteenth-century Europe, it is logical that a colonial product like chocolate should come to be considered an aphrodisiac, a lover's gift, and symbol of sexuality. Indeed it was the metaphor of colonialism that Sigmund Freud used to describe the relationship of the civilized man to his own sexual desire.[56] Equating "the process of civilization" with "the libidinal development of the individual,"[57] Freud claimed that it was only through a collective sublimation of sexual desire that civilization could be achieved, but moreover that the accumulated energy of this sublimated sexuality was necessary to fuel the immense creative work of civilization. "In this respect," Freud remarked, "civilization behaves towards sexuality as a people or stratum of its population does which has subjugated another one to its exploitation."[58] According to the Freudian schema, then, sexuality is itself collectively colonized through the development of civilized society.

There was a fairly widely shared late-nineteenth-century assumption that sexual control had something to do with the establishment of a technologically advanced and morally superior society.[59] If I privilege the Freudian vision in explicating *fin-de-siècle* ideas about civilization and desire it is because Freud, while highly representative of such assumptions, also offered a much more specific consideration of the way in which civilized society itself was constructed out of a process of excretory sublimation in particular. Inspired by anthropologists studying so-called primitive societies, Freud postulated that it was the pleasure of defecating and of anal stimulation that the civilized individual needed to sublimate in order to form both a moral conscience and sense of shame that would ensure social conformity, but also in order to understand the value of money and to want to engage as an adult in relations of finance and commodity exchange. Freud observed that all children have a natural fascination for "the excretory functions, its organs and products."[60] In attempting to treat patients whom he described as "especially orderly, parsimonious and obstinate" (the "anal" character-type as it is known in contemporary popular psychology), Freud claimed that all such individuals confessed to having been highly resistant to toilet-training as children and had been inclined to do "all sorts of unseemly things with the feces" once passed. Such individuals, for whom the pleasure of retention and defecation was particularly strong, required as adults that their anal pleasure be sublimated into an equally neurotic form of behavior, hence the excessive concern with cleanliness and control.[61] However Freud viewed the sublimation of anality as essential even to normative Œdipal development. The boy-child's development of a functional sense of shame and conformity was dependant upon the recognition that his feces, and along with it the sexual desire for his own mother, must be given up as a trade for maintaining the pleasure of the phallus.[62] Hence the feces that he literally "gives up" to the potty, must be also metaphorically rescinded and sublimated into a new form of behavior. Since the child's feces is his first "gift" to his mother,[63] he later transmutes his anal pleasure into a pleasure in gifts, which later becomes an interest in money. Money and excrement then, Freud asserts, are "easily interchangeable" in the Unconscious and in linguistic slang. Someone who hated to spend money was *filzig* (just as we speak of the "filthy-rich" in English), and a wealthy spend-thrift, on the other hand, was a *Dukatescheisser* (shitter of ducats).[64]

In recalling that, according to Freud's schema, childhood sexuality is to the adult what the colony is to the metropolis,[65] it is clear that this notion of the anal origin of money bears a particular implication for European visions of colonial difference and primitivity. Indeed Freud was not alone in seeing the construction of excrement taboos as a sort of universal signifier of capitalist conformity and civilized behavior. The notion that primitive societies all shared a lack of taboo surrounding excrement appears to have been something of a fashionable topic amongst anthropologists and ethnographers of the *fin de siècle*. Peter Beveridge, studying the Australian Aborigines of the Victorian Riverina area in the 1880s, was typical in this regard. Having described his subjects as lacking any sense of "vice or virtue," showing no ability to exercise restraint in the satisfaction of physical desires whether for food or for sex,[66] he then described a "most disgusting remedy" involving the use of communally collected excrement to be ingested as a cure for a sick and dying person.[67] However, the most voluminous study of the excremental tendencies of the "uncivilized" peoples was the 1891 work of U.S. cavalryman John G. Bourke, who surveyed a vast range of ethnographic and anthropological descriptions of coprophagic rituals throughout the world—a clear indication, he implied, of a universal relationship between excrement taboos and the civilizing process.[68] Bourke took particular interest in the claims of seventeenth-century explorers who depicted native American cultures as eating "all manner of vile things," including "the excrement of wild beasts"; or claims such as those of the German Jesuit Jacob Baegert, who described the Indians of lower California as "a race of naked savages who ate their own excrement."[69] Bourke observed also that the Mexican goddess Suchiquecal was an excrement-eating deity, and claimed that this was a sure indicator that the ancient peoples of Mexico had themselves been eaters of excrement.[70] James Frazer in the highly influential 1890 work *The Golden Bough* observed that, in many of the "savage" societies he described, "the conception of holiness and pollution" were "not yet differentiated..."; hence those most highly valued in society (kings, priests, and chiefs) were treated with the same laws of taboo as were those deemed unclean (murderers, pregnant or menstruating women, pubescent girls, hunters).[71] This "inability," then, to distinguish that which is anti-value from that which is of ultimate value was deemed an essential defining feature of non-civilized societies. Coprophagy was thus an innate tendency of primitive culture.

Images of primitivity, racial blackness and sexual excess continue to appear in chocolate marketing today. In 1996 the French chocolate manufacturer Suchard advertised using an image of a seductive black woman naked but for stripes of gold foil painted across her body with the caption "You may well say no but we hear yes."[72] The advertisement was retracted with an apology following feminist complaints that it played on the misogynist myth of women wanting rape. It is clear that the Suchard ad played on an even more specific mythology than this: the notion of chocolate as a symbol of the primitive and excessive sexuality imputed to women generally and to black women in particular.[73]

If the Internet is any kind of reliable gauge, coprophilia appears to be one of the fastest growing fetish fantasies of the twenty-first century, while books about chocolate have been undergoing an extraordinary boom since the mid-1980s.[74] The language used to describe the sensuality of chocolate eating grows ever more sexually vivid: "Soft and smooth, devilishly sweet and, at its best, messy," proclaims Pam Huwig in her review of the 1992 Mexican film directed by Alfonso Arau, *Como Agua Para Chocolate* (based on Laura Esquivel's novel of the same name).[75] "What really pleases both body and mind," writes Tabitha Powledge, "is the chocolate experience itself—its slippery sweetness, its silky sensuality on the tongue," and quoting the experts: "'What a wonderful thing it is in your mouth,' Rozin rhapsodises."[76] In the 2001 Lasse Hallström film *Chocolat* (based on the novel by Joanne Harris), a chocolatier of mysterious ethnicity (played by Juliette Binoche) bewitches a small town in France, wins the love of a "Gypsy" man (Johnny Depp) and awakens the repressed sensuality of the more puritanical, morally uptight, and conformist members of the community, including the character of the Comte de Reynaud (played by Alfred Molina) who consequently is found wallowing lustfully in the chocolate he had so rigidly resisted, in a scene highly reminiscent of scatological sexual play. The suggestion of both these films is that chocolate functions as a symbol of the repressed, and hence of the soulful love of life and all its pleasures (laughter, friendship, passion, music and dancing, sexual desire, freedom, and relaxed values). For Jungian psychoanalysts excrement is deemed to hold a similar significance in the life of dreams and of the unconscious mind. James Hillman notes the recurrence of excrement motifs in dreams and myths and relates these to the psychic Underworld, the realm in which reality is turned upside-down and inside-out, hence excrement is eaten, entering the body instead of exiting it.[77] Another Jungian analyst, Thomas Moore, writes that "anal dreams suggest carnival, a return to the flesh that has been repressed," and interprets the coprophagia of the Marquis de Sade as originating from the drive towards reintegration of the repressed and abjected parts of the self. Psychic excrement in the Jungian model is the alchemical gold of self-transformation.[78] Chocolate, then, like the excrement it resembles, continues to be invested with powerful symbolic meanings relating to identity, sexuality, and the constitution of the self.

The chocolate of Central America, sweetened with the sugar of the African slave-trade, penetrated the mouths of Europeans on a mass scale at precisely the same moment that the management of their excreta began to symbolize a new civilized identity that stood in opposition to the primitive other of colonially subjected peoples. European bourgeois identity was based on a sense of civilized conformity achieved through the sublimation of sexual desire, and on a sense of civilization manifest in the abjection, technologization, and deodorization of excrement. Chocolate coins and truffles, gold-covered treasures that are brown lumps inside, sticky, sickly indulgences invested with addictive and lustful properties—these are truly the fruits of a class culture born out of the domestication of colonialist reality. If chocolate today continues to be imagined in such terms, I venture to suggest that this may reveal something about the persistence of bourgeois identification in Western societies, and about the continued relations of economic inequality and exploitation that divide the world. In so far as this is the case, chocolate will always be a covetable and guilty pleasure; yet even the determined banalization of contemporary books about it will fail to convince the compulsively desirous that there is not some more complex truth hidden deep within the bowels of their lust.

Notes

1. Sophie D. Coe and Michael D. Coe, *The True History of Chocolate* (London: Thames and Hudson, 1996), 88–92.
2. See "Gut Feelings Cry Out for Waste," *Sydney Morning Herald,* 16 November 2000.
3. In particular in *Les Cent-vingt journées de Sodome, ou l'école du libertinage*, D. A. F. Marquis de Sade, *Œvres* 1, Michel Delon, ed. (Paris: Gallimard, 1990). On Sadean coprophagia see Roland Barthes, *Sade, Fourier, Loyola* (Paris: Editions du Seuil, 1971), 25
4. Richard von Krafft-Ebing, *Psychopathia Sexualis, With Especial Reference to the Antipathic Sexual Instinct: A Medico-Forensic Study,* Franklin S. Klaf, trans. (New

York: Arcade, 1998), 123–128. Havelock Ellis, *Studies in the Psychology of Sex*, 5 vols. (New York: Random House, 1936), vol. 3, Part 1, 57; vol.1, Part 1, 52; vol. 4, 120ff; Magnus Hirschfeld, *Sexual Pathology* (New York: Emerson Books, 1940), 157; Dr. Lo Duca (Hrs), "Scatophilie," *Moderne Enzyklopäpie der Erotik M–Z* (Müchen: Verlag Kurt Desch, 1963), 613–614; Brenda Love, "Cophrophagy" and "Coprophilia," in *The Encylopedia of Unusual Sex Practices* (London: Abacus, 1992), 70–74.

5. By the criteria sketched by Baudrillard, chocolate stands in an ideal "simulating" relationship to excrement in that it is simultaneously a "reflection of a profound reality…" that which "masks and denatures …. masks the absence of a profound reality… is unrelated to any other reality and is its own pure simulacra." Jean Baudrillard, *Simulacres et Simulation* (Paris: Editions Galilée, 1981), 17.

6. See Sidney Mintz, *Sweetness and Power: The Place of Sugar in Modern History* (New York: Viking, 1985), 43.

7. Karl Marx, "Economic and Philosophical Manuscripts," *Early Writings,* Rodney Livingston and Gregor Benton, trans. (Harmondsworth: Penguin Books, 1975), 364–365.

8. The notion of chocolate as most ultimately covetable, as a luxury consumer good highlighting sub-bourgeois class aspiration and longing, is nowhere better illustrated than in Roald Dahl's children's novel *Charlie and the Chocolate Factory* (Harmondsworth: Penguin, 1973).

9. Deborah Reed-Danahay, "Champagne and Chocolate: 'Taste' and Inversion in a French Wedding Ritual," *American Anthropologist*, 4 (1998), 750–761. The practice of the *rôtie* was also documented by the folklorist Van Gennep in the 1940s who in turn refers to nineteenth-century commentators on the *rôtie*. Arnold Van Gennep, *Manuel de folklore français contemporain, Tome 1: Du berceau à la tombe* (Paris: Editions A. et J. Picard et Cie, 1946), 560.

10. As Reed-Danahay remarks, "The use of champagne and chocolate to symbolize human waste is an explicit challenge to class-based attitudes toward taste and high culture." Reed-Danahay, "Champagne and Chocolate," 759.

11. Ibid., 750.

12. Scatological scenes appear throughout *Les cent-vingts journées*, e.g. 142, 161–163, 172–173, 182–186, 237, 286, 277.

13. As Barabara Lekatsas and the Coes point out, it was more likely to have been anise-flavored pastilles that were used for this purpose; yet the myth has endured. See Barbara Lekatsas, "Inside the Pastilles of the Marquis de Sade," in *Chocolate: Food of the Gods, Contributions in Intercultural and Comparative Studies* 14, Alex Szogyi, ed. (Westport: Greenwood Press, 1997), 102. Also: Coe and Coe, *True History*, 233.

14. Sade, *Les cent-vingt journées*, 92.

15. Coe and Coe, *True History*, 233–234.

16. Marquis de Sade, *Lettres à sa femme*, ed. Marc Buffat (Babel, 1997), 102.

17. The libertine Julie, e.g., "a de grandes dispositions à la malpropreté, à l'ivrognerie, à la gourmandise et au putanisme." Sade, *Les Cent-vingts journées,* 71.

18. Barthes, *Sade,* 23–25.

19. Marquis de Sade, *Lettres et mélanges littéraires écrits à Vincennes et à la Bastille,* Tome 1, Recueil inédit par Georges Dumas et Gilbert Lély (Paris: Editions Borderie, 1980), (letter of 9 May 1779), 67.

20. Coe and Coe, *True History,* 90.

21. The myth about Motecuhzoma's chocolate consumption appeared in a number of late-sixteenth-century Spanish sources, and is typically recounted in semi-scholarly descriptions of the history of chocolate published today—that curious category of writing about the cultural history and use of foods that is characterized by a purely descriptive chronology, complete lack of referencing and a high level of banalization. See for example Nikita Harwich, *L'Histoire du chocolat* (Paris: Editions Desjonquères, 1992), 23; McFadden and France, *Cook's Encyclopedia,* 60.

22. Coe and Coe, *True History,* 60–61, 98–99.

23. The Coes, e.g., note the importance of the myth of the origins of chocolate in Aztec visions of self-identity, and also its role as a symbol of status and class. Ibid., 79, 90–93.

24. As Fanon remarks of images of black men as rapists and of Orientalist literature: "Le Blanc civilisé garde la nostalgie irrationelle d'époques extraordinaires de licence sexuelle, de scènes orgiaques, de viols non sanctionnés, d'incestes non réprimés." Franz Fanon, *Peaux noires, masques blancs* (Paris: Editions du Seuil 1952), 133. See also Anne McClintock, *Imperial Leather: Race, Gender and Sexuality in the Colonial Conquest* (New York: Routledge, 1995).

25. I am applying here, perhaps somewhat anachronistically, Mary Douglas's terms for describing the dichotomy assumed by early-twentieth-century anthropologists such as Bettelheim, Roheim, and Norman Brown. See Mary Douglas, *Purity and Danger: An Analysis of Concepts of Pollution and Taboo* (London: Routledge & Kegan Paul, 1966), 116–117. Early anthropology, if it did not use these terms, nonetheless already assumed something similar about the relationship of the self to the external world in defining "primitive" man.

26. Alain Corbin, *Le Miasme et la jonquille: l'odorat et l'imaginaire social, xviiie–xixe siècles* (Paris: Editions Aubier Montaigne, 1982), 167–188; François Delaporte, *Le Savoir de la maladie: essai sur le cholera de 1832 à Paris* (Paris: Presses Universitaires de France, 1990), ch. 5; also Dominique Laporte, *L'Histoire de la merde* (Paris: C. Bourgois, 1993); Reid, *Paris Sewers and Sewermen: Realities and Representations* (Cambridge: Harvard University Press, 1991).

27. See Reid, *Paris Sewers and Sewermen,* 20–36. The vision of sewers as the seat of urban crime is of course particularly pronounced in Victor Hugo's *Les Misérables, in Œvres complètes* (Paris: Collection Nelson, 1862).

28. Alexendre Jean-Baptiste Parent-Duchâtelet, *De la prostitution dans la ville de Paris, considérée sous le rapport de l'hygiène publique, de la morale et de l'administration:*

ouvrage appuyé de documents statistiques puisés dans les archives de la Préfecture de police, avec cartes et tableaux (Paris: J.B. Baillière, 1837), Tome 1.

29. Henry Mayhew, *London Labour and the London Poor*, 4 vols. (New York: Dover Publications, 1968), vol. 2, 386.

30. Stephen Inwood, *A History of London* (London: Papermac, 2000), 419–426.

31. Ibid., 421.

32. This is echoed in the overall tone of John G. Bourke's *fin-de-siècle* survey of "primitive" excrement-eating which he interprets as a signifier of the level of civilization of a culture. Bourke, *The Scatologic Rites of All Nations: A Dissertation Upon the Employment of Excrementitious Remedial Agents in Religion, Therapeutiques, Divination, Witchcraft, Love-Philters, etc., in All Parts of the Globe*, Louis Kaplan, ed. (New York: Morrow and Co. Inc., 1994), 3. See also Kelly Anspaugh, "Powers of Ordure: James Joyce and the Excremental Vision(s)," *Mosaic* 27:1 (1994), 2.

33. Reid, *Paris Sewers,* 36.

34. "...l'eau pûre et fraîche...les secretions s'y exécuteraient mystérieusement et maintiendraient la santé publique sans troubler la bonne ordonnance de la ville et sans gâter sa beauté extérieure." Haussman quoted in Alfred Mayer, "La canalisation souterraine de Paris," in *Paris-Guide, par les principaux écrivains et artistes de la France*, ed. Corinne Verdet (Paris: La Découverte/Maspero, 1983), 184.

35. Mayer, "La canalisation souterraine de Paris," 176–184.

36. Reid, *Paris Sewers,* 39–44.

37. Marié-Davy quoted in Georges Vigarello, *Le propre et le sale: l'hygiène du corps depuis le moyen âge* (Paris: Editions du Seuil, 1985), 221.

38. McClintock, *Imperial Leather*, 209.

39. Ibid., 207–231.

40. Lawrence Wright, *Clean and Decent: The History of the Bath and Loo and of Sundry Habits, Fashions and Accessories of the Toilet, Principally in Great Britain, France and America* (London: Routeldge & Kegan Paul, 1960), 138.

41. Christine McFadden and Christine France, *The Cook's Encyclopedia of Chocolate* (London: Lorenz Books, 1999), 16–17; Coe and Coe, *True History*, 241.

42. Sidney Mintz, "Chocs, Coke and Cacao," *The Times Literary Supplement*, 9 August 1996.

43. James Walvin, *Fruits of Empire: Exotic Produce and British Taste, 1660-1800* (Basingstoke: MacMillan, 1997), 90.

44. Ibid., 93. I am obviously indebted to Sidney Mintz's superb analysis of the history of European sugar consumption in *Sweetness and Power*.

45. Timothy Morton, *The Poetics of Spice: Romantic Consumerism and the Exotic* (Cambridge: Cambridge University Press, 2000), 171–206.

46. This particular story does not appear in Bourke's original 1889 manuscript and was probably added by the German folklorist who edited an expanded edition in 1913. Cf. Bourke, *Scatologic Rites*, 31.

47. Wright, *Clean and Decent*, 150.

48. Sigmund Freud, "Character and Anal Erotism," in *The Freud Reader,* Peter Gay, ed. (London:Vintage. 1995), 296–297. As Sophie Coe noted, the word "cacao" was not used by the Aztecs at the time of the Spanish conquest. It is an older Mixe-Zoquean word (from the culture that probably originally domesticated the cacao plant). The Aztecs and Mayans at the time of Cortés used the word "chocotatl." Coe, "Cacao: Gift of the New World," 148. *Theobroma cacao* is the botanical name for the chocolate tree as named by the Swedish naturalist Carl von Linné (Linnaeus) in 1753. Coe and Coe, *True History*, 17–18.

49. McFadden and France, *Cook's Encyclopedia*, 28.

50. Lekatsas, "Inside the Pastilles of the Marquis de Sade"; Wolfgang Schivelbusch, *Tastes of Paradise: A Social History of Spices, Stimulants, and Intoxicants*, trans. David Jacobson (New York: Pantheon Books, 1992), 91.

51. Schivelbusch, *Tastes of Paradise*, 89–92.

52. Woodruff D. Smith, *Consumption and the Making of Respectability 1600–1800* (New York: Routledge, 2002), 183–185.

53. David T. Courtwright, *Forces of Habit: Drugs and the Making of the Modern World* (Cambridge: Harvard University Press, 2001), 25.

54. Of course what Peters could not have known then is that the Nestlé corporation at the end of the twentieth century would come under attack from health advisors and from organizations, such as the International Baby Food Action Network, for violating the World Health Organization code by marketing milk formulas in West Africa (e.g. Togo) that have been shown to offer vastly inferior nutritional value compared to mothers' natural breast-milk. Tony Waterson and James Tumwine, "Monitoring the Marketing of Infant Formula Feeds: Manufacturers of Breast-Milk Substitutes Violate the WHO Code Again," *British Medical Journal*, 326 (18 January 2003), 7381, 113–115.

55. Again see Christopher Herbert, *Culture and Anomie: Ethnographic Imagination in Nineteenth-Century Europe* (Chicago: University of Chicago Press, 1991), 29–73. There is much that could be added here about the gender demarcation involved in chocolate consumption, both in drinking chocolate which contrasts strongly to the public-sphere and masculine association of coffee, and in solid chocolate which, from the late nineteenth century to the present, has been increasingly suggested to be most appropriate as a lover's gift from man to woman. See Terrio, *Crafting*, 253; also: McFadden and France, *Cook's Encyclopedia*, 59; also Diane Bartel, "Modernism and Marketing: The Chocolate Box Revisited," *Theory, Culture and Society*, 6 (1989), 428–438. On women and sugar consumption generally see Mintz, *Sweetness and Power*, 139.

56. Indeed Ranjana Khanna has recently argued that psychoanalysis itself needs to be understood as a form of knowledge arising out of colonial relations, as a "theorization of nationhood and selfhood as they were developed in response to colonial expansion." Ranjana Khanna, *Dark Continents: Psychoanalysis and Colonialism* (Durham: Duke University Press, 2003), 28.

57. Freud, "Civilization and Its Discontents," in *The Freud Reader*, 742.

58. Ibid., 746.

59. This notion is reiterated in *fin-de-siècle* visions of homosexuality as a distinctly barbarous expression of desire as in Sir Richard Burton's theory of "The Sotadic Zone." See, *Sexology Uncensored*, 203–204. An excellent and detailed discussion of attitudes to homosexuality in relation to colonialism has recently been produced by Robert Aldrich, *Colonialism and Homosexuality* (London: Routledge, 2003).

60. Sigmund Freud, "On the Transformation of Instincts with Especial Reference to Anal Erotism," *Freud Collected Papers* 2, Joan Rivière et al., trans., John D. Sutherland, ed. (London: International Psycho-Analytical Library, 1957).

61. Freud, "Character and Anal Erotism," 294–297.

62. Sigmund Freud, "The Dissolution of the Œdipus Complex," in *The Freud Reader*, 661–664.

63. Freud, "On the Transformation," 168.

64. Freud, "Character and Anal Erotism," 295–297.

65. Indeed the notion of colonially subjected peoples as the naïve children of imperial Europe had widespread currency in nineteenth-century thought. French ethnographer Elie Réclus, who considered the destruction of Australian Aboriginal cultures to be a true loss to humanity, nonetheless persisted in seeing them as essentially child-like. Elie Réclus, *Le primitif d'Australie: les Non-non et les Oui-oui, étude d'ethnologie comparée* (Paris: E. Dentu, 1894). Subheadings to Reclus book include "âmes simples," "naïveté du nègre," 131, 339. See Douglas, *Purity and Danger,* 116; Anne McClintock notes that at the *fin de siècle,* " . . . evolutionary progress was represented as a series of anatomically distinct family types, organized into a linear procession, from the 'childhood' of 'primitive' races to the enlightened 'adulthood' of European imperial nationalism." McClintock, *Imperial Leather,* 359

66. Peter Beveridge, *The Aborigines of Victoria and the Riverina as Seen by Peter Beveridge* (Melbourne: M.L. Hutchinson, 1889), 5–9, 12, 23–24.

67. Ibid., 53.

68. John G. Bourke, *Compilation of Notes and Memoranda Bearing Upon the Use of Human Ordure and Human Urine in Rites of a Religious or Semi-Religious Character Among Various Nations* (Washington: U.S. War Department, 1888).

69. Ibid., 13–16.

70. Ibid., 18–19.

71. James G. Frazer, *The Golden Bough: A Study in Magic and Religion,* (New York: MacMillan, 1947), vol. 1, 223.

72. "Pub: non c'est non." *Nouvel Observateur,* 17–23 October 1996, 37.

73. As Susan Terrio notes, for French feminists who objected to the Suchard ad, "the salient issue was rape, not race." Terrio, *Crafting the Culture and History of French Chocolate,* 256.

74. For example, aside from those I have already cited there are (just in English, French, and German) the following scholarly and not-so-scholarly publications: Marcia Morton and Frederic Morton, *Chocolate: An Illustrated History* (New York: Crown, 1986); Robert Linxe et Sylvie Girard, *La maison de chocolat*

(Paris: Robert Laffont, 1992); Nikita Harwich, *Histoire du chocolat* (Paris: Desjonquères, 1992); Marcel Desaulniers, *Death By Chocolate* (New York: Rizzoli, 1992); Allen M. Young, *The Chocolate Tree: A Natural History of Cacao* (Herndon, VA: Smithsonian Institution Press, 1994); Natalie Bayeux et al., *The Book of Chocolate,* Tamara Blonde, trans. (Paris: Flammarion, 1996); Marie-Christine Clément and Didier Clément, *La magie du chocolat* (Paris: Albin Michel, 1998); Serge Guérin, *Le chocolat* (Paris: Milan, 1998); Annie Perrier-Robert, *Le chocolat* (Paris: Editions du Chêne, 1999); John Ashton, *A Chocolate A Day Keeps the Doctor Away* (New York: HarperCollins, 2001); Olivier de Loisy and Katherine Khodorowsky, *Chocolat* (Paris: Solar, 2003); Philibert Schogt, *Der Chocolatier* (Munich: List, 2003).

75. Pam Huwig, "Making Love—and Chocolate," *Curve* September 1999 (9:4), 28.
76. Tabitha M. Powledge, "A Valentine to Chocolate? (Processing of Cacao Beans to Chocolate Candy)," *BioScience*, 48:6 (June 1998), 435.
77. James Hillman, *The Dream and the Underworld* (New York: Harper & Row, 1979), 184–185.
78. Thomas Moore, *Dark Eros: The Imagination of Sadism* (Woodstock, CT: Springwood Publications, 1990), 62–66.

Chapter 4 ↷

AMERICAN GUTS AND MILITARY MANHOOD

Ana Carden-Coyne

In the first third of the twentieth century, campaigns to remedy the digestive system preoccupied physical culturists in Europe and the United States. Concerns about the interior workings of the body had long been the preserve of health and fitness doyens, as well as those disposed to religion, temperance and muscular Christianity. It was in the First World War, however, that the abdomen seemed to face its most perilous test, as its meaningful status confirmed guts as the locus of masculinity. Military manhood encouraged a particular type of masculinity, one that required stronger than usual inner resolve. Inner resolve was seen as a particularly masculine trait that depended upon hardened and healthy stomachs. The state of men's guts authenticated courage and discipline, which had distinct merits for the military machine. At this time, American Professor of Clinical Medicine Dr. John W. Wilce, coined the term "intestinal fortitude." Tellingly, he was a sports coach at Ohio State University.[1] Earlier, the colloquial use of the term "guts" had referred to spirit, energy or force.[2] Physical culture made use of this notion in a number of bodily and mental contexts. During wartime, however, fitness culture and medicine made important social and military alliances that brought into focus the masculinity of guts.

During the war, concerns about gastronomy, its effect upon the male body, and its impact upon masculine standards such as character, strength and courage, entered American military discourse. In the 1920s, American militarists infiltrated the recruiting arena occupied by physical culture, adapting for their own American cultural and military purposes ideas they were exposed to whilst in combat overseas. Alongside veterans and military writers, literary scholars have long understood trans–Atlantic exposure and mutual influence, and historians too have noted that during and after the world war interest in Franco-American relations, culture and history increased.[3] Popular literature, however, has received less attention, and yet was no less significant. War and the expansion of military bureaucracies and ideologies added a new dimension to these networks. In peacetime, American military ideology sought new allies through which to conduct its campaigns.

Militarists and physical culturists alike identified both guts and manhood as acutely troubled areas in need of rehabilitation. War had ensured that masculinity was now entwined in the tissues and shapes of the male abdomen. The militarization of the male body operated not just as a strategy for mobilization, but also reflected a distinct shift in assumptions about the locus of masculinity. Popular phrases pointing out men's "battle with flab" turned from rather benign metaphors into direct militarist messages. Flabby stomachs were a particular focus in attempts to regulate military fitness, both during periods of wartime recruitment and, significantly, in peacetime. After 1918, both soldiers and civilian men were warned "not to fall back into the flabby unpreparedness that was found to be so prevalent before the war."[4] Militarist rhetoric abounds in the literature aimed at making men fit. Weak men were said to be "under attack" from fat and disease. Fat men "cannot fight, and in every sphere of endeavor a fighter is needed. To achieve success as a fighter one must be willing to struggle in order to keep oneself fit."[5] Waging war was a test of masculine ability, and a test of inner resolve as it manifested in the outward shape of the stomach's flesh. Through exertion and ordeal a young man's body "came of age," and stood the tests marking the passage into military manhood. In the United States, the militarist contribution to physical culture was consolidated after the First World War, despite the fact that participation in this overseas war had only lasted eighteen months. Fortifying American masculinity created a new culture of the abdomen, so that the locus of manhood was in the guts.

Today when we think of the "gutsy" American soldier, our minds might cast to films of American war heroes, whether a brawny renegade played by the prototypical John Wayne (*They Were Expendable, The Sands of Iwo Jima*), or a handsome man of courage such as Gary Cooper (*Sergeant York*), or rugged individualists such as Gregory Peck (*12 O'Clock High*), Humphrey Bogart (*Action in the Atlantic*) and George C. Scott (*Patton*).[6] These icons of military manhood were distinctive for their sex appeal and for the way their characters were inculcated in Hollywood's fabrication of the memory of the Second World War, especially under the collaborative influence of the Office of War Information. American soldiers appeared not simply dutiful and heroic, but superior, precisely because they were "rough and ready." Manufactured images were consolidated by real soldiers appearing in films, like the highly-decorated Audie Murphy, the star of *To Hell and Back* (1955). The image of the gutsy American soldier surfaced in cultural representations from the 1940s, when government propaganda had a firm grip upon the cinema industry and cultural representations of military manhood. Through the 1940s, robust and "gutsy" cinematic figures continued to represent the dominant image of manhood, providing a fascinating counter to disabled men like Roosevelt, the wheelchair-bound president, at a time when the American nation was feeling the impact of the Second World War. The body of the screen soldier was of prime value in Hollywood, and yet the scrutiny of men's bodies had a much longer history in military medicine, recruitment tactics and pension assessments. The significance and condition of the internal and external man had an earlier origin in the collaboration between physical culture and the military after the First World War. In this period, America's war experience was seen to expose weakness and military unfitness.

Far from exemplars of rugged manliness and heroic virtue, many American soldiers had come home battered by their first international combat experience. Despite the initial thrill of victory, the war also produced a remarkable disillusionment, one perhaps not even seen following the Civil War. Reformers retreated from prewar optimism, reflecting inwardly that, "the moment the war ceased the bottom fell out of idealism."[7] Strikes, economic collapse, red scares, racial conflict and veteran agitation threatened civil order and faith in American prosperity.[8] Against the rhetoric of reconstruction, many feared the nation was in decline. In addition, public perceptions and media images of veterans shaped the scrutinizing of America's national body. Ongoing discussion of male disability fuelled speculation about the standard of American manhood.

Politics, economics, medicine, and the fitness imperative were closely entwined between the close of the First World War and the beginning of the next one. Throughout the 1920s and 1930s, officials weighed up the ongoing costs of the disabled veteran, especially in the area of the psychiatric. Predicting that treatment for physical injuries would decline over time, John Clark, Professor of Economics at Columbia University, noted an alarming trend that 68 percent of the new cases for recompense were of the "neuro-psychiatric type," a steadily rising figure since 1926.[9] The U.S.

government would be forced to double expenditure on the 15 million dollars already spent on special hospitals and facilities in order to care for such cases.[10] Physical disability appeared to have economic limits, whereas mental disability seemed boundless.

The sense in which numbers were swelling, rather than dissipating, reflected a range of medical and social conditions, and made more urgent the rehabilitation and repatriation of veterans. By the 1920s, medical scrutiny and public awareness of shellshock was widely in place. Shellshock had unhinged the traditional belief in manliness and courage. Increasingly, psychological conditions became entwined in the very notion of possessing "guts." Intestinal fortitude was as much about mental strength as it was physical force, and both these characteristics were imbued with the ideal of manliness.

Treatments of the disabled, discussions about the limits of rehabilitation, and fears concerning the economic burden and social impact of disabled men informed militarist thinking with a much more preventative approach to the strengthening of the male civilian population. As a result, militarists made new alliances with physical culture in order to reconstruct American masculinity. Intertwined with character, the new focus on specific body parts restructured the foundations of American manhood in the wake of war. Americans realized that men's bodies and minds had been shattered in the war, making it impossible to comprehensively resurrect older values of manliness. Military manhood appeared to be at stake now more than ever. The guts would now take center stage in the theatrics of physical culture and military manhood.

Crucially, victory would be squandered if the guts of civilian men were not fortified. Debates about national service centered upon the fitness standards of recruits in the recent conflict. Former and active military personnel flooded popular fitness literature with narratives on recruitment fitness. Surprisingly, much of the discussion began with a denigration of veterans, implying that the low standard of American recruits implicated them in their own injury and illness. War had not turned Doughboys into American heroes. Instead, it had revealed the "rather startling conditions" of the "disconcertingly high percentage of weaklings" making up the drafted recruits. Alarming statistics were reported, such as that 25 percent of recruits were rejected by the Draft Boards, or that another 15 percent were rejected by the army surgeons, and that a total of 55 percent of the recruits were rejected due to "more or less severe" physical defects discovered in the screening process. The "humiliating truth," one commentator wrote, was that only one in five men (or 10 percent) of the draft passed the fitness test.[11]

Rejection statistics were used to imply that solders had to be passed even when their health standards were regarded as low. This was a curious tactic on behalf of the military, given the success of the American campaign on the Western Front.

Victory on the world stage was not necessarily a cause for celebration at home. At a time when the most pressing postwar issue for the military was pensions, the failure of the national body was targeted. Physical culture was set as the remedy for the American male. Militarists, politicians and fitness experts worked together on this. In 1920, the Senate Committee on Military Affairs debated whether to introduce compulsory universal military training as a way of converting the nation's "weaklings into a strong, healthy race of men."[12] Giving evidence at the hearings was Professor Meylan of Columbia University, who had been involved with athletics in the army during the war. Conducting tests on his American students, he pointed not just to defects in the teeth and mouth, but a marked lack of bodily and muscular development. These ailments stemmed from problems with diet, the internal mechanism of digestion, and a lack of exercise. Meylan was convinced that military training could ameliorate these disorders and increase the health of the nation. Instead of confining it to soldiers, the whole nation's men should benefit from its results.

At this time, the issue of compulsory military training reigned as a debate in the mainstream media and popular press. Many physical culture exponents supported the notion of universal military training, despite also being conscious of the effects of mechanized war on the male body. Tales of wrecked and emaciated men returning from war were concluded with happy endings of transformation to virile manhood, replete with the sexual implications of bulging biceps.[13] It was not so much that Americans possessed a lingering sense of the damage caused by the war, but rather that American manhood should be steeled in order to meet the new demands of civilian life and, more significantly, any potential, future wars.[14] War had exposed male weakness and endowed men with new disabilities. America needed to meet this challenge.

Weighing in on the debate, the Surgeon General Rupert Blue argued that military training should be supplemented by *compulsory* physical training for all male and female youths. Not surprisingly, military professionals ignored the latter part of this advice, and turned parents toward training and disciplining their sons. Military officials contributed articles to magazines, providing evidence of American male deficiency, and bolstering the commercial cause of physical culture, at the same time pushing the case for compulsory national military training.[15] Military professionals as high as the rank of general appeared on the covers of Bernarr Macfadden's *Physical Culture* magazine. Provocative headlines addressed parents with the loaded question: "What to do with your boy?"[16] With fitness as the rhetorical answer, the violence and physical damage incurred in war was further obfuscated.

Militarists and physical culturists now made their alliance, which had not been so over in earlier periods. Like war, muscular development was generally regarded as a masculine enterprise. Although in this period women were encouraged to be fit, this was mainly for reproductive purposes which required careful attention not to over-develop muscles for fear of losing the "dainty" feminine figure, and risk being excluded from the marriage market. The gendering of body parts meant that different parts held different stakes for men and women. A strong and muscular abdomen was indeed a specifically gendered body part. Abdominal exercises were a feature of physical culture instruction particularly addressed to men. The efficient functioning of intestines depended upon not just toned abdomens, but especially muscular ones. Today, the "six-pack" on a male body is understood as a sign of beauty, sex appeal, and fitness. This is also true to some extent during the 1920s—muscular men were said to have greater success with women. Many boasted that they were more virile and reproductive in marriage.

Most significant for militarist purposes, muscular stomachs steeled nerves. Since the late nineteenth century, concerns about men's nerves featured in physical culture literature. Unlike the psychiatric and pseudo-medicalized discourses of the same period, women's nerves were not as much of a problem amongst physical culturists. By the end of the First World War, physical culturists attached much meaning to the medical testing of recruits. Anxious reports showed that up to ten percent of men were rejected for "mental deficiency" and a whole range of nervous disorders.[17] Statistical evidence continued to be regurgitated by militarist writings in the popular press during the postwar years. The substance of masculine bravery may have been in men's guts, but this was in turn directly linked to nerves. Alertness to issues of shellshock and war neuroses galvanized the link between strong stomachs and nervous systems.[18] The term "guts," one major wrote, meant being physically and mentally strong, and able to stick to the task at hand. Guts were important whether one was "a soldier, a statesman or the head of a home."[19] Militarists argued that the kind of guts men acquired by completing national service (which entailed physical culture) made one a victor in the battle of civilian life as much as the battlefield.

Since men's guts were the locus of bravery and manliness, it is not surprising that fitness experts appear obsessed with disorders of the digestive system, particularly dyspepsia and constipation. Dyspepsia (or indigestion) was framed as a disorder that drained men of a quality peculiar to the male body: energy. One common therapeutic confessional repeated: "I had dyspepsia and no pep."[20] The American term "pep" was used in the popular vernacular to refer to an energetic and vital spirit—but it also implied an active disposition, which was especially appealing to physical culturists, who translated the "healthy body and healthy mind" notion of the Greeks into a motto about the *active* body and mind. Pep was also regarded as peculiarly male. Men without pep were described as possessing "shrunken, flabby muscles," "lazy circulation," and "shattered nerves."[21] Arthur Gay, who trained George Weber to a world record of 1700 sit ups, suggested that the "vital power" naturally owing to men was based upon good digestion, which could only be achieved by strengthening abdominal muscles.[22] Activity and vitality were indeed two of the main themes of physical culture. Dyspepsia and constipation were both seen as deleterious to the male body, which was supposed to be especially active and vital, for these were the outward signs of masculine virility. Bodybuilder Lionel Strongfort asserted that digestive disorders made young men weak and incapable of marriage.[23] Bernarr Macfadden addressed this problem by producing self-help manuals such as *Manhood and Marriage*, which explained that unhappy marriages were the woes of "weak men" who suffered from "blood-sapping disorders," many of which originated from dysfunctional stomachs causing inefficient elimination of waste products.[24]

Although virility, sexual, and reproductive success were stressed more than ever in the postwar period, the influence of militarist thinking within physical culture allied virility with military strength and preparedness. Virility was now colored by nationalism and militarism combined, and this impacted upon the idealization of men's bodies and the goal of reconstructing American manhood. Why the First World War would make such an impact upon American physical culture and its associated ideals of the national (male) body, when it had only been in the war for such a short time, is not immediately clear. This development was certainly unique in American history. The Civil War did not have the same impact upon notions of virility, masculinity and military manhood. Can we speculate that modern warfare crushed older ideas of manliness? It seems that American culture combined elements of conservative reaction, modern liberal idealism and productive traditionalism.[25] European, particularly French, models influenced some of that extraordinary dynamic. The French had trained the inexperienced American Expeditionary Force, and supplied it with armaments, experiences, and ideologies.[26] Returning Americans brought with them French ideas about the male body, health, and fitness, including digestion and diet. While this requires further investigation, it is clear that French ideas crossed the Atlantic inspiring much of the literature in American physical culture. Contact between American and French military personnel in First World War may have shaped the focus upon men's guts within a military context. Body culture and body consciousness implicated the militarist construction of American manhood.

Alongside specific articles on national service and contributions from army personnel, military discourse and terminology entered physical culture vernacular with regard to men's troubled guts. Sufferers of dyspepsia described their illness as an "internal bombardment" or a "rebellion." Although such metaphors were first used amongst French physicians and writers around the time of the Revolution, it is interesting that physical culturists in the 1920s revived this expression with particular gusto. Military metaphors added urgency to the implication that the male body was under siege from abdominal forces. Mutiny threatened the masculinity of the guts as the "foaming and fomenting and fermenting" stomach produced a "miserable nausea." Against the militarist ideal of austere, regimented, and gutsy American manhood was the rich, indulgent, and flabby civilian. The weakened bodies produced by such civilian gastronomical excess resulted from the modern conditions of sedentary and urban life. Lazy guts reflected the state of civilization itself, choking on its own prosperity and indolence. Pale and flaccid tongues, weak and sluggish bowels anthropomorphized eating, digesting, and fitness—all affirming the image of the constipated, dyspeptic, and obese as men of cultural, social, and dietary excess:

> My bowels remind me of a millionaire—they hold on tenaciously to their accumulations, for the greater time, then with lavishness expend the amounts in great outpourings. My kidneys hold onto their disbursements and what they do allow to escape is weighty and rusty-appearing . . . my brain is befuddled . . . Nerves? I am a bundle of them.[27]

American morale seemed at breaking point from disorders of the stomach and from lack of fitness. Dyspepsia was regarded as a frequent cause of neurasthenia because, as this man put it, of the "constant nagging discomfort . . . which constantly batter the nervous system." Embattled nerves, and their cost to the community, were a peak concern in the aftermath of the First World War. Rehabilitation would prove crucial.

Reeling from the economic and social effects of the war, one of the important consequences of dyspepsia for American men was a greater fear of moral slippage and social dereliction. Governments, the military and medical practitioners were concerned with rehabilitating soldiers and returning them to the status of civilians. President Wilson had dispelled the idea of pensions and welfare, with the rhetoric of capitalist enterprise combined with individual endeavor. Americans, he said, did not want to be "coached and led," but "know their own business, are quick and resourceful . . . and self-reliant."[28] Physical culture literature mirrored this interest in transforming former soldiers into successful businessmen, clerks or self-made men. The importance of social skills for civilian life, however, conflicted with the militarist discourse of turning soft and sickly men into hardy, battle-ready bodies.

Dyspepsia and constipation were both regarded as "social disasters." Advice was offered in order to prevent their related "fatal disorders" from gaining a foothold on the body.[29] Vague disorders such as the "derangement of the nervous system" were said to lead from a general state of nervousness and irritability, to a lack of ambition and "zest for work," and finally to depression.[30] Bernarr Macfadden's book on *Constipation* advocated toning the abdominal muscles through exercises designed to assist waste elimination. Since the turn of the century, the conditions of the modern world, such as sedentary city-living and increased consumption of refined foods, had been seen as the main culprit. Increasingly, lack of physical exercise became the focus for discourses about constipation, especially during and after the First World War. Although French physical culturists had long regarded "the constipation epidemic" a result of the decadence of their national cuisine, the Americans now claimed it as "the greatest American disease."[31] American gastronomy in itself was not necessarily the problem. Indulgence in refined and sweet foods, usually regarded as feminine tastes, reflected a much more endemic lack of strength and fortitude in the American male's guts. Emerging from the trials of war, there could be no place for weakness of will, now so allied to the operation of the guts.

Militarist thinking colored advice given by physicians to physical culture readers. Constipation sufferers were feminized as weaklings, as men effectively lacking strong guts. With a boot-camp tone in his voice, one physician and columnist barked at his imaginary patient:

> The trouble with you is, you are plain lazy. You doubtless have the feeling that you were born to be carried on a bed of roses, that everything good would be handed to you, and that some guardian angel would keep you from all harm. There are a million others like you. You want to do as you please

and expect your body machine to fall into line...You...hamper and interfere with your body's multitudinous duties...you'd make a miserable showing in any position calling for strength and muscular control... Nobody can do for you what you must do for yourself.[32]

Making regular bowel movements was man's duty to his body. Men needed to acquire "roughness" in their diet, which would affect their entire state of being. "Roughness," in the form of foods containing roughage, lent itself to the development of hardened and forceful men.[33]

Although the dietary habits of young American men were occasionally targeted as an underlying problem with guts, after the war these discussions were mostly geared to a critique of social habits associated with diet. Young men were accused of "excessive indulgence in stimulants," not just tea, coffee, and Coca-Cola, but also "the direct action of narcotics." Rather than leading to over-activity, though, these stimulants were regarded as producing fatigue, draining the life force of masculine energy, and breaking down nerves.[34] Indeed, reported draft statistics claimed 46 percent of rejects had alcohol and drug problems.[35] Modern life encouraged men to ingest these poisons, which needed to be expelled from the blood stream and excretory organs. A plethora of articles about constipation and autointoxication filled the literature of physical culture in this period. Toxemia of the blood and lymph was one such complication mentioned as a "destructive by-product of the gases and acids—arising from the retained waste."[36] As well, lack of muscular exercise allowed poisons to accumulate within the "system of end products," instead of being "squeezed out of the muscles" and eliminated through the kidneys and bowels. Appealing to bourgeois sensibilities, constipation advice referred to "educating the bowels" as one would the brain. Physical strength, efficient elimination, and "intelligent attitudes to eating" all provided "brain-power" for the "race of life" where ambition and financial success were all important to be able to compete in the modern world.[37]

Closely related to the inefficient elimination of toxins, obesity was also an obsession of American physical culture. Countless narratives of transformation from fat to muscularity abound. Where some confessed their indulgence in food and lack of exercise, cured men claimed they would rather die than return to "their burdensome blanket of blubber."[38] One doctor argued that men who abused their stomachs should be arrested. Others admonished, "nobody loves a fat man."[39] Fat men were seen as a direct reflection of the degraded state of the nation. The war had made this seem more acute, and the postwar concern to rebuild the image of the national body and to enforce a level of fitness upon young able-bodied men in particular, was a result of recruitment information disseminated from the armed forces through newspapers and popular magazines. It served well the commercial purposes of such physical culture empires as Bernarr Macfadden's, at the same time as acting as propaganda for the military. Gymnasium instructors were nicknamed "solder trainers," helping to work a "heavy battalion" of unfit and overweight men.[40]

Fat boys and men were apparently among the most fearful and anxious of Americans. They were said to "die young" or were simply "afraid of being."[41] Middle-class parents were instructed on adequate physical training for young male children. Rather than through formalized education, commercial strategies would achieve the fitness of the next generation. Identifying the fitness of young boys as a major family, social, and political issue, physical culturists attempted to shift parental focuses to this end. This marked a move away from the usual concerns of wealth accumulation, politeness, and morality that preoccupied middle-class cultures in France and the United States in the early twentieth century.[42] Dying young was reserved for warriors or heroes, identities encoded in the rhetoric of beauty and sacrifice reemerging in European society after the war. Although it seemed that there was no compensation for the fat, ugly, and living, the guts proved a central area for the reconstruction of the male body as the constituent locus of manhood.

Physical culture aimed to reconstruct American manhood in the period following the First World War. The next generation of recruits would be ready for a fight. They would stand as proud exemplars of the fit and prepared national body. The militarist construction of American masculinity during the 1920s entered physical culture discourse, continuing to depend upon the connection between strong guts, reinforced nerves, and manliness. Elsewhere in this volume we see that, around the turn of the century, stomach disorders and flabby bellies were signs of French men's surrender to modern indulgences, and that such a lack of will was perceived as a crisis of masculinity.[43] This powerful discourse made a substantial impact on American physical culture and militarist thinking. To some extent, it has persisted to the present as we continue to regard obesity, simplistically, as a product of lack of self-control and excessive eating. There are gendered implications with this too—fat men are not just flaccid, but are desexualized and almost neutered within current popular imagination. In contrast, fat women, despite being shamefully unattractive, are nevertheless objects of sexual curiosity. Fat women are eroticized for their dangerous and repulsive allure. Their bodies bound to underground perversions, such as

Feederism, the "exotic erotics" of fat women engage historical traditions of gender, sexuality, and power, in a way that (white) men's bodies do not.[44] Constructions of the fat, unfit, asexual man has a history that has been marginal to cultural and historical enquiries into masculinity. Militarism, I would argue, is a significant part of the story and has a specific cross-cultural setting. In the aftermath of the First World War, the connection between manhood and guts was galvanized due to the impact of military service and action. In the United States, militarism infiltrated physical culture discourse transforming the abdomen into the mainspring of courageous and battle-ready masculinity. War, it seemed, would either make or break men, but physical culture assured governments and parents that the essence of American masculinity would be fortified in the guts.

The reformed image of American military manhood stands in direct contrast to concurrent perceptions that masculinity was in crisis. This is an important point to make, for as some historians have recently argued, the rise of masculinity studies often focuses disproportionately on the idea of crisis.[45] Contemporaries, such as the American militarists and physical culturists discussed in this essay, often played this up for their own purposes. In this essay, we have seen that war and disability (both its costs and social impact) raised doubts about military manhood which implicated civilian men. The focus on the poor health standards of draftees, largely recruited from the working classes, enabled the military and government to jettison responsibility for injuries and pensions, on the one hand, and also allowed them to mine new sources of physical talent for the barracks. In this context, masculine crisis was useful rhetoric for the military and the commercial strategies of physical culture. Militarists, however, raised debates about compulsory training in a fitness culture largely servicing the middle classes. Class, then, was a crucial element to the positioning of crisis in American manhood. Militarists used the low standards of draftees to imply that a similar standard existed across the classes, in order to mount a claim for middle-class boys, so that potential recruits would become physically accountable. Militarists had their sights set upon what they already regarded as a better class of recruit, but the poor health standards of the working classes were used as a strategy for shaping new personnel from the mostly untapped reservoir of middle-class youth. The element of class dynamics within the political imperatives of the military therefore provides another dimension to the study of the masculine body in war and its implications in times of peace.

Finally, historians of war and medicine might benefit more from uncovering relationships *between* crisis and recovery. I have suggested here that there is a critical play between the image of the enfeebled recruit, the disabled veteran, the rehabilitated soldier and the fortified civilian. Within the context of military propaganda, the weak state of recruits was continually exaggerated. Military manhood "in crisis" went hand in hand with the vision of the stalwart soldier and war hero. The image of American manhood in transformation, therefore, was a way of demonstrating that military training and physical culture did not just rehabilitate veterans of the recent world war, but rather created a powerful new type of man: the gutsy American.

Notes

1. Hugh Rawson, *A Dictionary of Euphemisms & Other Doubletalk* (New York: Crown Publishers, Inc., 1981), 38–39, 214. I thank Christopher Forth for this reference.
2. John S. Farmer and W. E. Henley, *Slang and Its Analogues* (London: Private Print for John S. Farmer, 1893), vol. 3, 237.
3. Marianne Moore and Kenneth Cornell, *French-American Literary Relationships* (reprint: New York, 1967; New Haven: Yale University Press, 1952); René Taupin, *The Influence of French Symbolism on Modern American Poetry*, William Pratt and Anne Rich Pratt, trans. (New York: AMS Press, 1985); Henry Blumenthal, *American and French Culture, 1800–1900: Interchanges in Art, Science, Literature, and Society* (Baton Rouge: Louisiana State University Press, 1975); Marvin Farber, ed., *Philosophic Thought in France and the United States: Essays Representing Major Trends in Contemporary French and American Philosophy* (New York: University of Buffalo, 1950).
4. W. V. B. Riddell, "Soldierly Fitness in Time of Peace," *Physical Culture* (November 1920), 31.
5. Bernarr Macfadden, "Fat, Disease and Death," *Physical Culture* (January 1920), 44.
6. Similarly, films about World War One made during the 1940s projected this theme of limitless courage, such as embodied in the actor Errol Flynn (*They Died with Their Boots On*). A rare example of showing disability was *The Best Years of Our Lives*. The lead actor's real hands were amputated in the Second World War. His character must reintegrate into civilian life, and face his girlfriend. It presents, however, the disabled hero as a man overcoming adversity. His marriage to his former girlfriend signifies the successful repatriation of his masculinity. For a brilliant analysis of this film, see David Gerber, ed., *Disabled Veterans in History* (Ann Arbor: University of Michigan Press, 2000).
7. John A. Thomson, *Reformers and War: American Progressive Publicists and the First World War* (Cambridge: Cambridge University Press, 1987), 278.
8. Robert H. Zieger, *America's Great War: World War I and the American Experience* (Oxford: Rowman and Littlefield, 2000), 187 ff.

9. John Maurice Clark, *The Costs of the World War to the American People* (New Haven: Yale University Press, 1931), 180.
10. Clark, *The Costs of the World War*, 189.
11. Arthur Capper, "Why We Must Have National Physical Training," *Physical Culture* (May 1922), 20.
12. Richard Winans, "What Do You think About National Military Training?" *Physical Culture* (April 1920), 32.
13. Ana Carden-Coyne, "From Pieces to Whole: The Sexualization of Muscles in Postwar Bodybuilding," in *Body Parts: Critical Explorations in Corporeality*, Christopher E. Forth and Ivan Crozier, eds. (Lanham, MD: Lexington Books, 2005).
14. Winans, "What Do You Think," 32.
15. There were some notable exceptions to this line. Some readers wrote to the editor complaining about its pro-militarist stance. Comparing the American body with the fitness and gymnastic training of German recruits, one reader wrote, "there are ten million dead men in Europe, fifteen million superfluous women in Europe, a few million cripples and venereally diseased men and women, and the best prepared nation got licked." Letters to editor, *Physical Culture* (August 1920), 17.
16. *Physical Culture* (April 1920).
17. Winans, "What Do You Think," 85.
18. W. V. B. Riddell, "Soldierly Fitness," 29.
19. Major John J. Boniface, "Physical Fitness a National Obligation," *Physical Culture* (June 1920), 109.
20. "I Had Dyspepsia and No Pep—Now I Have Pep but No Dyspepsia," *Physical Culture* (April 1924), 58.
21. "I Had Dyspepsia," 59.
22. Arthur F. Gay, "Strengthen Your Stomach," *Physical Culture* (August 1920), 47.
23. "Don't Have a Sour Stomach," Strongfortism advertisement, *Physical Culture* (February 1920), 1.
24. *Manhood and Marriage* advertisement, in *Physical Culture* (July 1920), 134.
25. Hawley, *The Great War*, 147.
26. Robert B. Bruce, *A Fraternity of Arms: America and France in the Great War* (Lawrence, KA: University Press of Kansas, 2003), 142.
27. "I Had Dyspepsia," 59.
28. Cited in Zieger, *America's Great War*, 204.
29. Edith Baker, "Dishes for the Prevention of Constipation,' *Physical Culture* (December 1924), 63; "Constipation: Its Cause, Effect and Treatment," *Physical Culture* (December 1924), 146. See also "Constipated? Here's What You Should Eat," *Physical Culture* (December 1924), 48ff.
30. "Constipation: Its Cause, Effect and Treatment," 146.
31. Edmund Gray, M. D., "These Exercises Will Keep You Cool," *Physical Culture* (July 1924), 59. See also Dr. Frank Crane, "Constipation," *Physical Culture* (April 1920), 16. Interestingly, Australian physical culture literature, which drew

substantially on the Bernarr Macfadden's magazine in style, content, and philosophy, also claimed Australia as "the constipated nation."

32. Edmund Gray, M. D., "Ten Minutes a Day Cured His Constipation," *Physical Culture* (January 1924), 36.
33. Dr. Frank Crane, "Constipation," *Physical Culture* (April 1920), 16.
34. Edwin F. Bowers, M. D., "Avoid Fatigue—Your Greatest Efficiency Problem," *Physical Culture* (June 1920), 22.
35. Winans, "What Do You Think," 85.
36. "These Exercises Will Keep You Cool," 53.
37. Brinkler School of Eating, "Constipation, Brain and Nerves," advertisement, *Physical Culture* (July 1924), 140.
38. Raymond S. Hofses, "I'd Rather Die Than be Fat Again," *Physical Culture* (October 1924), 59.
39. Dr. Frank Crane, "Learn How to Eat," *Physical Culture* (August 1924), 64.
40. *Physical Culture* (September 1920), 34.
41. Travis Hoke, "Why Fat People Die Young," *Physical Culture* (November 1923), 57; Edith Baker, "Mineral Oil Recipes for Fat Folks," *Physical Culture* (July 1924), 63.
42. Michèle Lamont, *Money, Morals, and Manners: The Culture of the French and American Upper-Middle Class* (Chicago: University of Chicago Press, 1992).
43. Christopher E. Forth, "The Belly of Paris: The Decline of the Fat Man in Fin-de-Siecle France," chapter 11 in this volume.
44. Here, I am borrowing from Roy Porter's seminal article on Tahitian women and the Cook voyages, "The Exotic as Erotic: Captain Cook at Tahiti," in *Exoticism in the Enlightenment*, Roy Porter and G.S. Rousseau, eds. (Manchester: Manchester University Press, 1990), 117–144.
45. Bryce Traister, "Academic Viagra: The Rise of Masculinity Studies," *American Quarterly*, 52 (2000), 274–304; Judith Allen, "Men Interminably in Crisis? Masculinity, Sexual Boundaries and Manhood," *Radical History Review*, 82 (Winter 2002), 191–207.

Part II ∾

CULTURE AND THE ABDOMEN

Chapter 5 ∽

THE *PHILOSOPHE'S* STOMACH

HEDONISM, HYPOCHONDRIA, AND THE INTELLECTUAL IN ENLIGHTENMENT FRANCE

Anne C. Vila

"The stomach rules the brain": with that pithy maxim, Voltaire summed up much of the spirit of scholarly endeavor in the French Enlightenment. The stomach did, indeed, seem to rule the life of the mind in eighteenth-century France, a time when social pleasures like fine dining were central to the effort to redefine the modern intellectual as a public-spirited, convivial fellow eager to partake of worldly life.[1] Nowhere, it seems, did the French love of food and the equally French passion for ideas converge more harmoniously than in the mythic "repas philosophique," the imaginary gathering of Voltaire and other famous talking heads that became one of the century's canonical images.[2] However, even in this golden age of intellectual sociability, the connection between the thinker's mental and digestive pursuits was far from simple: although *philosophes* like Voltaire and Diderot were avid gourmands who disavowed the ascetic image of the scholar that had prevailed in the past, they were often ambivalent about the belly-centered excesses of their own era.[3] They seemed, moreover, to regard the Republic of Letters as an institution plagued with indigestion—both the metaphorical indigestion induced by the flood of books issuing forth from writers great and small, and the literal indigestion that tormented those who overindulged in high living, the pursuit of learning, or both at once. The *philosophe*'s stomach was thus the target of two syndromes: hedonism, widely viewed as a driving principle of contemporary culture; and hypochondria, a blanket term for the digestive/nervous ailments held to be rampant among *gens de lettres*—a group that, true to the universalizing tendencies of the Enlightenment movement, was broadly defined to include all manner of authors and thinkers, from belletrists to scientists.

The stomach was not the only means by which the thinker seemed to embody the peculiar effects attributed to thinking in eighteenth-century France: moralists, physicians, and literary authors were just as concerned about the troublesome links they perceived between thinking and the nerves, not to mention thinking and the gonads.[4] However, because it was viewed as a major center of "sympathetic" interaction with all the other organs of the body, the stomach played a privileged role in this period's redefinition of the learned man as both a social and a medical type. Multiple currents in the intellectual climate of this era helped to make a delicate or dyspeptic stomach the defining trait of a genuine intellectual: the star status which doctors granted to *gens de lettres*, first in dietetics and then in the nascent field of psychiatry; growing interest in the abdomen as a seat of illness, especially for disorders associated with over-study; and, last but not least, the intense scrutiny which prominent authors seemed to pay to their abdominal functions and dysfunctions. Broadly speaking, that scrutiny was rooted in motivations that were jointly somatic, philosophical, and social: *philosophes* fretted over their stomachs partly because they were truly suffering, partly because they were fascinated with the body's mechanisms, and partly because having chronic digestive problems facilitated conversation with their high-born benefactors, who tended to complain loudly of their own "flighty" digestion.[5]

Penetrating the tight causal relationship which eighteenth-century French authors posited between stomach disorders and mental application thus entails examining the peculiar physical–moral nature that was then ascribed to *gens de lettres*: their constitution, their passions, their work habits, and their position vis-à-vis the rest of society—most particularly the fashionable upper crust, an epicurean world in which the leading intellectuals of the French Enlightenment moved smoothly, but with varying degrees of wariness or disdain.[6] It also involves exploring the ideas held about the body by *gens de lettres* themselves: that is, both their lived experiences of the stomach–mind relation and their philosophical musings upon it, which ran the gamut from the gastronomic to the scatological.

Because medicine and literature were equally involved in making the stomach crucial to the identity of the scholar or *homme de lettres* in

Enlightenment France, this essay will consider how the mind–stomach problem played out in representative works from both of those fields. Beginning with medicine, I examine hygienic texts from the 1750s to early 1800s that singled out intellectuals as the social group for whom strict, sober dietary regimens were most important. I also delve into the period's specialized discourse on hypochondria and melancholy, which consistently spotlighted studious types while oscillating in its focus between the gastric and cerebral realms. Then, turning briefly to imaginative literature, I analyze the references to the stomach that pervade the writings of Voltaire, arguably the most famous (and famously ailing) *philosophe* of the day. Although Voltaire's approach to his own dyspepsia was idiosyncratic, deviating at times from even his own doctor's recommendations, he nonetheless put the stomach to some inventive social and literary purposes—thereby attesting that physicians were not the only Enlightenment thinkers to regard the abdomen as a topic rich in both practical and theoretical meaning.

Dietetics, Hypochondria, and the Thinking Man

The intellectual life was decidedly double-edged in eighteenth-century France: although *gens de lettres* enjoyed an unprecedented degree of favor in polite company, they also appeared to be an exceptionally frail and sickly lot. At first glance, the shadow of disease that hung over mental labor might seem difficult to reconcile with the period's exuberant reverence for thinkers—a group that, as many historians have emphasized, enjoyed a spectacular rise to prominence in Enlightenment culture.[7] Pathology was, however, an important complicating factor in the so-called "cult" of great men, a movement that turned as much around the intellectual's moral–physical distinctiveness as it did around his integration into fashionable society. Moreover, although the thinker's brain was unquestionably chief among the organs that set him apart from the rest of humankind, his stomach ran a close second in importance.

Scholars were, for example, strongly implicated in the hygienic injunction that capped Anne-Charles Lorry's popular treatise on dietetics, the *Essai sur les alimens* (1754): "one must start early in thinking about one's body, observing exactly the proportion that must exist between the sum of one's excrements and that of one's food."[8] That balance, Lorry insisted, was seriously disrupted when one employed the body for "unnatural" purposes like study: "Philosophy and the lifestyle it entails are the institutions of life most contrary to nature, unless exercise, sobriety, and regularity of conduct repair their defects" (235–236). Lorry was a fashionable Parisian doctor who counted several *gens de lettres* among his friends and patients, yet he nonetheless urged his learned readers to exercise greater caution when engaging in the absorbing, "ecstatic" pleasures of the mind (234). Lorry viewed mental labor as liable to dry out the viscera, make the humors fester, keep the body bent over, and diminish circulation—thus leading to weak stomachs, constipation, and shortened life spans; he also believed that it took a physician far more effort to cure a man of letters "than for a man in any other circumstance" (211–214, 233).

The eighteenth century's pronounced anxiety over the health of scholars was clearly tied to the "expansion of the medicable" into areas like hygiene, a branch of medicine that enjoyed a marked rise in France after 1700.[9] This, as Brockliss and Jones have underscored, was the period when hygiene was first regarded as an important part of the medical curriculum, when self-help manuals on the art of conserving health were published in abundance, and when French physicians began to write on diseases specific to certain professions. To some degree, physicians' focus on the health problems of learned men was an off-shoot of occupational medicine, a field that developed significantly during the final decades of the Ancien Régime.[10] There was, however, something more intense and personal about the medical community's alarm over the bodily dangers of mental application (as compared, say, to the work-related disorders of hatters, spinners, or goldsmiths).[11] That is, even though they themselves belonged to the country's enlightened intelligentsia, French physicians worried greatly over the debilitating effects of social–intellectual refinement.[12] Their approach to the intellectual as a medical type was thus deeply inflected by the period's larger debate over the decadence of civilization, a debate that included but was not limited to the celebrated anti-Parisian diatribes of Jean-Jacques Rousseau.

As with the specialized literature on female vapors (which also proliferated in the second half of the eighteenth century), a broad but not always consistent strand of Rousseauism ran through medical portrayals of the ailing scholar.[13] Some physicians regarded this figure as living proof of Rousseau's dramatic pronouncement that "the man who meditates is a depraved animal."[14] However, in making that pronouncement, Rousseau himself was merely exploiting a centuries-old concern over the violent passions and mental exhaustion brought on by civilized life. Given that medical writers who focused on the diseases of *gens de lettres* were just as apt to cite ancient or Renaissance authors as the famous "Jean-Jacques," it seems safe to say that they were motivated by reasons that went beyond Rousseau's reactionary moral philosophy. Moreover, even when they were overtly Rousseauistic, these physicians often included themselves or their medical colleagues among the ranks of sickly, dyspeptic cerebralists.

Take, for example, Samuel-André-Auguste-David Tissot, whose best-selling book *De la santé des gens de lettres* (1768) probably did more than any other French-language work to popularize the notion of study as perilous to the health of those who engaged in it. As in his almost contemporaneous essay on the diseases of *gens du monde*, Tissot assumed here the stance of a detached, mildly disapproving observer of learned men, whom he depicted as egregious abusers of virtually every category of the "non-naturals"—especially *ingesta*, or food and drink.[15] Tissot's treatise was, indeed, very Rousseauistic in tone: it even included a direct quote of Rousseau's declaration that "library work…wears out the machine, […] destroys the [body's] forces [and] weakens courage."[16] However, four years prior to the publication of *De la santé des gens de lettres*, Tissot himself had been portrayed as prone to severe bouts of work-induced indigestion and depression by his close friend and fellow Swiss physician Johann Georg Zimmermann.[17] Thus, despite his stern rhetorical tone, Tissot's discussion of the health problems of thinkers had a veiled autobiographical quality—one of the many traits of this treatise that would be imitated by specialists of "learned" maladies well into the next century.[18]

Digestion was paramount in Tissot's conception of *gens de lettres*: although he also professed concern over scholars's sedentariness and their tendency toward "literary intemperance" (29), he devoted more than a third of this treatise to dietary matters. Repeating the well-established dictum "a bad stomach follows men of letters like the shadow follows the body," Tissot declared the stomach to be one of the two body parts that suffered the most promptly and gravely from excessive mental application, whose damaging effects went from loss of appetite, to the "absolute cessation" of digestion, to general weakness, and from there to spasms, convulsions, and the destruction of all the sense organs (28–29). To explain this devastating pathological sequence, Tissot underscored, first, that the stomach was endowed with an abundance of nerves that sympathized with the brain when it was irritated, and, second, that thinking diverted the body's humors away from the nutritive functions to supply the scholar's overactive brain (20, 44). He therefore warned his learned readers that their digestion was too slow and their stomachs too sensitive to tolerate either the crude, hearty meals of the robust fieldhand or the rich, spicy, highly varied foods that abounded on the wealthy *mondain*'s table (148,172). Tissot did not, however, go as far as some of his medical contemporaries in limiting the diets of *gens de lettres* to strictly bland foodstuffs.[19] Moreover, he turned the old maxim "the man who thinks the most is the one who digests the most poorly" into something of a compliment for his readers: good digestion, he noted, was usually enjoyed only by "idiots" who hardly think at all (25–26).[20]

Tissot was not original in arguing that there was an inverse relation between high intelligence, on the one hand, and good health and digestion, on the other.[21] However, as the first full-length Francophone treatise devoted to the subject, *De la santé des gens de lettres* crystallized the sense already evident in hygienic discourse that *gens de lettres* needed close medical supervision to counteract the bodily effects of their intense, "intemperate" pursuit of learning. Like most of his contemporaries, Tissot considered those effects to be particularly adverse upon the abdomen, a confederation of organs sometimes called the phrenic or epigastric region. Although he did not explicitly mention the idea of vital regions when describing the interplay of thinking and digestion, Tissot clearly espoused the belief that these two areas of physiological function worked at cross-purposes.

The theory of vital regions owed much of its success in the eighteenth century to the prominence of Montpellier vitalism, one of whose trademark ideas was what Elizabeth Williams has called a "triadic conception" of the body.[22] According to that theory, the organism was dominated by three centers: the brain, the abdomen, and a third organ that was sometimes designated as the chest, and sometimes as the "exterior organ" (roughly speaking, the skin). Although Montpellier doctors often spoke of sympathies when describing intra-organic influences, they tended to use the term "antagonism" to explain the relations of the three vital regions. Louis de Lacaze, for example, argued that the animal economy was driven by contrary currents of oscillation within the ethereal fluid, some of which emanated from the brain, some from the exterior organ, and some from the phrenic region, which he defined as including the stomach, the entrails, and the diaphragm.[23] Because every force in the living body presupposed what Lacaze called a "power of *ressort*" (that is, a quasi-mechanical capacity to react to stimuli), each vital center constantly strove to maintain or renew its own *ressort* while also resisting the actions of the other centers (327, 343). Digestion was thus a key physiological function because "the alimentary mass acts as a sort of ballast or counterpoint that serves to rewind, so to speak, the entire machine by renewing the *ressort* of the stomach" (140).[24] The act of reflection, by contrast, greatly increased the *ressort* of the brain, so much so that the phrenic region might be weakened, thus suspending the ordinary laws of action and reaction necessary for good health (380).

The stomach was also assigned great importance by Lacaze's nephew and occasional coauthor Théophile de Bordeu, one of the most renowned vitalist physicians between the 1750s and 1770s. Bordeu regarded the stomach not just as part of the "triumvirate of life," but also as a dynamic organ that possessed animal intuition, its own distinct tastes and distastes, and, the capacity to play a significant role in most illnesses.[25] Although Bordeu did not focus specifically on the weak stomachs of *gens de lettres*, he did bemoan the "poorly directed" regimens, unhealthy foodstuffs, and perpetual moral agitation of the urban elite—a social category into which intellectuals had become well integrated by the time Bordeu critiqued its bad living habits.[26] The emphasis that Bordeu placed on the stomach in both his physiological and his pathological doctrines had a lasting legacy in French medical thought, inspiring the "gastro-centric" localism of the Restoration medical theorist François-Joseph-Victor Broussais as well as a broader predilection for evoking the phrenic or epigastric region as a site or source of disease.[27]

To some extent, the stomach's role as a determining trait of the intellectual faded in the early nineteenth century, as physicians and philosophers shifted away from purely somatic definitions of psychic disorders toward a more Romantic world view that celebrated the supremacy of the mind even in its diseased state.[28] However, for all of their emphasis on moral versus medicinal therapy, post-Enlightenment physicians did not omit physiology from their accounts of mental labor. To the contrary, they commonly declared that a bodily temperament dominated by the abdominal viscera underpinned the overly "ardent" imagination to which they imputed mental illness in such cerebral types as poets, artists, and musicians.[29] Moreover, pioneering alienists like Philippe Pinel continued to link constipation and over-study within the constellation of causes they cited for hypochondria and melancholy—neuroses that were both gendered masculine in early psychiatric discourse, and differentiated less from each other than from hysteria.[30] The old "bad stomach" complaint therefore persisted in the etiologies which early nineteenth-century physicians proposed for the nervous maladies of intellectuals (now an exclusively male club), even as their emphasis shifted toward the passions and ideas deemed most likely to impair the mind.[31]

The founders of psychiatry were, in short, just as interested as their eighteenth-century precursors in *gens de lettres* as an at-risk medical group: although professional cerebralists had to compete for psychiatric attention with deluded weavers, delirious war veterans, and hysterical women of all stripes, they nonetheless occupied a privileged position in the clinical observations of Pinel and his followers.[32] Like the scholarly health manuals that poured onto the market after 1800, early French psychiatry advanced an image of intellectuals that was at once more spiritualized and more physically deterministic than what had predominated a few decades earlier.[33] According to this new medical image, *gens de lettres* still merited the occasional Tissot-style reprimand for their bad living habits, but they now seemed to float above the common herd by virtue of their "poetic" moral/physical organization. The heightened sensitivity, cerebral intensity, and nervous mobility that had long been associated with intellectuals was now perceived as doing far more than upsetting their stomachs: now it burned up their vital force. As a result, the effort to preserve the health of *gens de lettres* became less a matter of dietetics than of longevity, of modestly rematerializing those whose "heroic souls" had almost stripped them of all carnality.[34]

Belly-Centered Philosophy: The Case of Voltaire

How, then, did the most celebrated *philosophe* of the French Enlightenment live out the experience of his own, digestively troubled carnality? The scope of the question is, of course, enormous, given that Voltaire was famous not only for "doing his body" every morning via vigorous purging, but also for writing volumes of letters about his fragile health, bad stomach, and preference for cassia over rhubarb as a home remedy.[35] Rather than attempting an exhaustive inventory of Voltaire's innumerable evocations of his stomach, I shall undertake simply to sketch the basic patterns they form—and to extrapolate a few insights into how Voltaire conceived of gastric function in relation to the mind, including his own prodigious intellectual labors.

We should, first of all, determine what Voltaire really meant when he coined his maxim on the stomach's power to control the brain. If we go back to the maxim's source, a 1748 epistle which Voltaire dedicated to his niece Madame Denis, it becomes clear that he wasn't referring to *gens de lettres* per se:

> Man the machine, mind that depends on the body
> By eating well rewinds his springs [*ressorts*]:
> With the blood the soul is renewed
> And the stomach governs the brain.[36]

Read in isolation, these four lines might suggest that Voltaire was up to nothing more than setting La Mettrie's man-a-machine thesis to verse.[37]

His epistle was, however, entitled "La vie de Paris et de Versailles," and the machine-like eaters to whom he was referring belonged the "stupid, dangerous, and vain" world of the French upper crust. These eaters, as Voltaire depicted them, were less concerned with savoring their food than with thinking up weak jibes and insipid witticisms that they could utter at the next elegant dinner.[38] Voltaire's remark regarding the mechanical effects of food on the brain was thus originally aimed at idle French aristocrats—a group from which, sociable and ambitious though he was, he strove to keep his distance, especially when he was working on an important literary project (as he almost always was).

Voltaire often used the stomach to pass judgment on the intellectual or moral merits of others: he derided the *anti-philosophe* journalist Desfontaines as a fat, greasy goat who ate and slept happily among his rat-infested books; he consoled Mme du Deffand with the idea that her indigestion proved her superior wit and breeding; he linked the hospitality and affable character of the Président Hénaut to his good stomach; and he commiserated philosophically with Frederick of Prussia over the colic from which they both suffered.[39] Voltaire also interwove his dyspepsia with his celebrity, exploiting both to advance his relations with high-born patrons, to get rid of unwelcome visitors, and to enlist the services of Théodore Tronchin, the renowned Genevan doctor.[40] However, Voltaire truly believed that he had been cursed by nature with a horribly frail stomach that was liable to carry him to the grave at any moment.[41] To prevent such a catastrophe, he employed a regimen that seems inspired more by his own notions of health and the mind–body relation than by any advice he received from Tronchin, a medical and moral conservative who regarded Voltaire's constant worries over his body with a mixture of skepticism, humor, and annoyance.[42]

As a patient, an avid reader of medical books, and a layperson who delighted in playing amateur doctor, Voltaire had a curiously mixed attitude toward his gastric troubles.[43] Although he declared for years that he was dying, Voltaire came to regard his indigestion as the key to both his physical longevity and his prolific literary life. One reason for that shift was the life of retirement which he adopted partly to accommodate his bad stomach, and partly to avoid trouble from the authorities over his writings. It was not until the 1760s that Voltaire explicitly declared that he owed his continued existence to regimen and to retreat; however, even in his early letters, he described his frail health as inseparable from his zealous devotion to intellectual work.[44] In other words, although living in perpetual retreat from the elite social whirl did not always suit Voltaire's temperament, it clearly advanced his mission as a writer and *philosophe*—and his stomach unquestionably played a role in making Voltaire a solitary.[45]

Voltaire's gastric preoccupations also served his intellectual identity in more directly philosophical ways. Although he was half joking when he said "the way we digest almost always determines our way of thinking," he seemed quite convinced that "one must clear out one's entrails to keep the mind clear"—an idea that he set to fiction in his philosophical tale "Les Oreilles du comte de Chesterfield" (1775).[46] This satire, set in England and built around the premise that "fatality implacably rules everything in this world," briefly evokes poor hearing as a determining factor in the lives of its characters.[47] However, the real proof of its premise lies in the realm of digestion—or, more precisely, constipation, a state that the self-purging Voltaire seemed particularly anxious to avoid.

For our purposes, the key moment of "Les Oreilles du comte de Chesterfield" occurs in chapter 7, when, after enjoying a fine meal with two fellow *philosophes*, a surgeon named Sidrac takes over their conversation on the "miseries, stupidities, and horrors that afflict the human race" by reducing all the great dramas in political history to the bowel movements of the leaders involved (680, 685). Constipation, Sidrac argues, has produced some of the bloodiest scenes known to man, including Oliver Cromwell's beheading of Charles I and the Saint Bartholomew's Massacre, authorized by France's Charles IX, whom Sidrac describes as "the most constipated man in his kingdom" (686). To prove his thesis, he employs a decidely bizarre theory of wandering fecal matter:

> What happens to a constipated man? The finest, most delicate elements of his excrement intermingle with the chyle in the veins of Azellius, and go to the portal vein and the reservoir of Paquet. They pass into the sub-clavicular region and enter the heart of the most gallant man, the most coquettish woman. It is like a mist of dried turd coursing through his body. If this mist inundates the parenchyma, the vessels and glands of an atrabilious person, his bad humor turns into ferocity...Don't approach him, and if he is a Minister of State, be careful not to present him with any request [before] discreetly asking his favorite valet if his grace has emptied his bowels that morning. (685)

Digestion, in other words, is the secret engine to the passions on both the grand and the private scale; and history, as Sidrac describes it, would be far better served if historians stopped stuffing their chronicles with platitudes about moral causes and instead paid closer attention to the influence of bodily functions upon the course of human events (687).

Clearly, the digestive fatalism that pervades this Voltairean satire was designed to poke fun at the high and mighty, while also injecting a note of farce into reflection on the human condition.[48] Yet Voltaire's belly-centered philosophy also had a personal edge: his intense purgative regimen—about which he rarely, if ever, joked—may well have been the means by which he strove to resemble what his character Sidrac calls "those persons favored by nature who are sweet, affable, gracious, thoughtful, and compassionate," all because they "defecate as easily as they spit."[49] Purgation may, therefore, have served in Voltaire's mind as a method of redeeming his abject, sickly body by keeping his temper sociable and his intellect sharp—just as he enlisted his stomach ailments to a higher purpose by deflecting the pleasures of the table into literature and conversation.[50]

Although it did not get as much press as Rousseau's melancholy, the image which Voltaire fashioned of his ailing stomach had an interesting legacy in French medical discourse after the Enlightenment.[51] That it not to say that it was merely a fashionable construct: quite the contrary, Voltaire's chronic gastric distress did much to shape his humor, his views on intellectual endeavor, and his emphasis on the hidden, often humble forces at play in human life. Thanks to the obsessive, well-publicized attention which Voltaire paid to his stomach, he became a living embodiment of the idea of "care of the self" that underpinned both the hygiene and the philosophy of eighteenth-century France—fields that converged dynamically in the figure of the frail, suffering *homme de lettres*.[52]

Notes

1. See Steven Shapin's contrast between the traditional, abstemious image of the scholar and the "sociable, merry, and moderately gormandizing philosopher of the eighteenth century," in "The Philosopher and the Chicken: On the Dietetics of Disembodied Knowledge," in *Science Incarnate: Historical Embodiments of Natural Knowledge*, Christopher Lawrence and Steven Shapin, eds. (Chicago: University of Chicago Press, 1998), 43. Many scholars have emphasized the importance of sociability among eighteenth-century French intellectuals—and their aspiration to full membership in "polite" culture: see esp. Emmanuel Bury, *Littérature et politesse: l'invention de l'honnête homme* (Paris: Presses Universitaires de France, 1996); and Gregory S. Brown, *A Field of Honor: Writers, Court Culture and Public Theater in French Literary Life from Racine to the Revolution* (New York: Columbia University Press/EPIC, 2002).

2. Christiane Mervaud discusses this and other engravings by Jean Huber in *Voltaire à table: Plaisir du corps, plaisir de l'esprit* (Paris: Editions Desjonquères, 1998), 9–13.

3. "Diderot Gastronome," in Georges May, *Quatre visages de Denis Diderot* (Paris: Boivin, 1951), 13–33; see Mervaud, *Voltaire à table*, esp. 17–94. On Voltaire, see also Jean Starobinski, "Le philosophe à table," in *Etre riche au siècle de Voltaire*, J. Berchtold and M. Porret, eds. (Geneva: Droz, 1996), 279–293.

4. On the latter subject, see my essay "The Scholar's Body: Health, Sexuality, and the Ambiguous Pleasures of Thinking in Eighteenth-Century France," in *The Eighteenth-Century Body: Art, History, Literature, Medicine*, Angelica Goodden, ed. (New York: Peter Lang, 2002), 115–134.

5. The Montpellier-trained physician Gabriel Venel implied that those who fretted over petty ailments like "digestion fougueuse" suffered mainly from self-absorption: he called them "the people who constantly *observe* or *listen* to themselves." "Digestion," in *Encyclopédie, ou Dictionnaire raisonné des sciences, des arts et des métiers*, Denis Diderot and Jean d'Alembert, eds. (Paris, 1751–1765; reprint, New York: Pergamon Press, 1969), vol. 4, 1002; author's emphasis.

6. Jean d'Alembert, for example, vociferously denounced aristocratic haughtiness toward *gens de lettres* in his *Essai sur la société des gens de lettres et des grands* (1753).

7. Noteworthy studies of this phenomenon include Didier Masseau, *L'Invention de l'intellectuel dans l'Europe du XVIIIe siècle* (Paris: Presses Universitaires de France, 1994); Jean-Claude Bonnet, *Naissance du Panthéon: Essai sur le culte des grands hommes* (Paris: Fayard, 1998); and Darrin M. McMahon, *Enemies of the Enlightenment: The French Counter-Enlightenment and the Making of Modernity* (Oxford: Oxford University Press, 2001).

8. Anne-Charles Lorry, *Essai sur les alimens, pour servir de commentaire aux livres diétiques d'Hippocrates* (1754; second edition, Paris: Vincent, 1757), vol. 2, 210–211. Unless otherwise noted, all translations are my own.

9. Laurence Brockliss and Colin Jones, *The Medical World of Early Modern France* (Oxford: Clarendon Press, 1997), 441–473.

10. Interest in occupational diseases was influenced by Bartholemeo Rammazzini's *Treatise of the Diseases of Tradesmen* (1700; English trans. London: 1705); Ibid., 455. Rammazzini's treatise included a long chapter on "The Diseases of Learned Men" that was commonly cited as a precursor in later medical manuals for scholars.

11. Lindsay Wilson, *Women and Medicine in the French Enlightenment* (Baltimore: Johns Hopkins University Press, 1993), 141–148.

12. Daniel Roche argues that physicians played a fundamental role in the cultivated society of eighteenth-century France—and in the effort to bathe great thinkers in an aura of posthumous heroism via glowing eulogies; see his chapter "Médecins et lumières au XVIIIe siècle," in *Les Républicains des lettres: gens de culture et Lumières au XVIIIe siècle* (Paris: Fayard, 1988), 308–330.

13. On the use of Rousseauean themes by medical vitalists and vapors specialists, see Elizabeth A. Williams, *A Cultural History of Medical Vitalism in Enlightenment Montpellier* (Aldershot: Ashgate Publishing Limited, 2003), 147, 154, 223, 224, 242, 246. See also my study *Enlightenment and Pathology: Sensibility in the*

Literature and Medicine of Eighteenth-Century France (Baltimore: Johns Hopkins University Press, 1998), 236–238.

14. *Discours sur l'origine de l'inégalité parmi les hommes* (1754), in Jean-Jacques Rousseau, *Oeuvres complètes* (Paris: Editions de la Pléiade, 1964), vol. 3, 138.

15. On the manner in which eighteenth-century French physicians used the doctrine of the non-naturals—the six types of things that, according to ancient medicine, determined the body's state of health or illness—see William Coleman, "Health and Hygiene in the *Encyclopédie*: A Medical Doctrine for the Bourgeoisie," in *Journal of the History of Medicine*, 29 (1974), 399–421

16. Rousseau, "Préface à *Narcisse*," cited by Samuel-Auguste-André-David Tissot, *De la santé des gens de lettres* (Geneva: Slatkine, 1981), 33.

17. Johann-Georg Zimmermann, *Traité de l'expérience en général, et en particulier dans l'art de guérir* (original German edition 1763; French trans. by Le Febvre de Villebrune 1797; reed. Paris: A. Delahays, 1855), 480.

18. The practice of self-observation was fairly common among physicians writing on vaporous or nervous disorders: see, for instance, Pierre Pomme, *Essai sur les affections vaporeuses des deux sexes* (1760), cited by Elizabeth A. Williams in "Hysteria and the Court Physician," *Eighteenth-Century Studies*, 32:2 (2002), 249.

19. Light seasoning, Tissot argued, was necessary to provide enough mild stimulation to rouse the "loose fibers" of the scholar's stomach out of their customary sluggishness (164). In the *Encyclopédie*, by contrast, seasoning was denounced as a pernicious worldly fad; see the *Enclopédie* articles "Assaisonnement" (1:765); "Cuisine," by the Chevalier de Jaucourt (4:537–539); and "Non-naturelles, choses" (11:217–224).

20. This saying, a commonplace in early modern medical discussions of the scholarly constitution, was usually attributed to the ancient physician Celsus. See, for example, Ramazzini, *Treatise of the Diseases of Tradesmen*, 148; and Zimmermann, *De l'expérience*, 480. Tissot drew several of his ideas from Zimmermann's chapter "De la trop grande contention d'esprit," 477–488.

21. See, for example, the *Encyclopédie* article "Santé," whose author contended that robust people were rarely *gens d'esprit*—and vice-versa (14:630).

22. Elizabeth A. Williams, *The Physical and the Moral: Anthropology, Physiology and Philosophical Medicine in France, 1750–1850* (Cambridge: Cambridge University Press, 1994), 38–39, 43–44, 51, 59. See also Roselyne Rey, *Naissance et développement du vitalisme en France de la deuxième moitié du dix-huitième siècle à la fin du Premier Empire* (Oxford: Voltaire Foundation, 2000), 164–69.

23. Louis de Lacaze, *Idée de l'homme physique et moral* (Paris: Guérin et Delatour, 1755), 322, 341–343, 353. Lacaze argued that the true source of "philosophical spirit" resided in a "felicitous" disposition of the internal organs (413).

24. Ménuret de Chambaud underscored this aspect of Lacaze's "revolutionary" physiological framework in his article "Oeconomie animale" for the *Encyclopédie*, vol. 11, 366.

25. *Recherches sur les maladies chroniques* (1775) in Théophile de Bordeu, *Oeuvres complètes* (Paris: Caille et Ravier, 1818), vol. 2, 831, 839.

26. Bordeu, *Recherches sur les maladies chroniques*, 2:806.

27. Broussais's *De l'irritation et de la folie* (1828) defined hypochondria and virtually all other mental disorders as arising from gastric irritation. On Broussais's controversial proposition that "knowledge of gastroenteritis is the key to all pathology," see Jean-François Braunstein, *Broussais et le matérialisme. Médecine et philosophie au XIXe siècle* (Paris: Klincksieck, 1986), esp. 38–39.

28. See Roy Porter, "Barely Touching: A Social Perspective on Mind and Body: in *The Languages of Psyche: Mind and Body in Enlightenment Thought*, G. S. Rousseau, ed. (Berkeley: University of California Press, 1990), 45–80.

29. C. A. T. Charpentier, *Essai sur la mélancolie* (Paris: Farge, an XI [1803]), 62–63 and 76.

30. Philippe Pinel, *Nosographie philosophique, ou la méthode de l'analyse appliquée à la médecine* (first ed. 1798; Paris: Maradan, 1813), 85.

31. In his redefinition of hypochondria, Louyer-Villermay emphasized that certain cerebral professions were more likely to induce bad digestion and low spirits than others: namely, those that required an overly uniform, monotonous mental application (like law or administrative work); those that involved serious, severe, and sad ideas (like medicine); and those that required a constantly exalted, "feverish" imagination (like the fine arts); *Traité des maladies nerveuses ou vapeurs*, 290–293.

32. See Juan Rigoli, *Lire le délire: Aliénisme, rhétorique et littérature en France au XIX siècle* (Paris: Fayard, 2001), 434–435 and passim.

33. For example see Etienne Brunaud, *De l'hygiène des gens de lettres* (1819), Joseph-Henri Réveillé-Parise, *Physiologie et Hygiène des hommes livrés aux travaux de l'esprit* (1834; fourth edition [Paris: Dentu, 1843]), and Jean-Marie-François Delabigne-Villeneuve's 1834 medical thesis, *Essai sur l'influence des passions et des travaux intellectuels sur l'économie et la santé de l'homme* (Paris: Didot le Jeune, 1836).

34. "The most poetically organized man is, in truth, almost devoid of material force... As an ancient put it, 'heroic souls have no body.'" Réveillé-Parise, *Physiologie et hygiène*, vol. 1, 104.

35. Ibid., vol 2, 184–185. Voltaire often fretted over whether he could obtain enough cassia to maintain his heavy purgative regimen. See, for example, his letter of 12 October 1757 to Jean Robert Tronchin (Dr. Théodore Tronchin's brother): "The affairs of Saxony can go as they please, but I can't live without cassia... Cassia absorbs all of my ideas." Letter 6720 in *Voltaire's Correspondence*, Theodore Besterman, ed. (Geneva: Institut et Musée Voltaire, 1953–1965), vol. 32, 110.

36. "Épitre 76" (1748), in Voltaire, *Oeuvres completes* (Paris: Garnier, 1877), vol. 10, 344–349, here 346–347.

37. Julien Offray de la Mettrie, *L'Homme-machine* (1747; Paris: Editions Mille et une nuits, 2000).

38. "This, absurd and frivolous troupe, / Is how we spend our all-too-fleeting time. / This is how we waste our days, / Long for idiots, but for those who think, so short." Voltaire, "Épitre 76," 347.

39. On Hénaut and Desfontaines, see Épitre 65 (1744) in Voltaire, *Oeuvres complètes*, vol. 10, 327–328. Voltaire wrote two extensive letters on indigestion and cassia to Mme du Deffand in 1775; see Besterman, *Correspondence*, vol. 90, 34–35 and 174–175. Voltaire's flattering poem on the colic of Frederick of Prussia is reprinted in Starobinski, "Le philosophe à table," 280–281.

40. On Voltaire's relations with the Tronchin family, see Deidre Dawson, *Voltaire's Correspondence: An Epistolary Novel* (New York: Peter Lang, 1994), 101–126. According to André Maurois, Voltaire was well known for using his frailty as a social weapon, exclaiming "Vite, vite, du Tronchin" and feigning indisposition when he didn't wish to receive guests at Ferney. *Dictionnaire des lettres françaises: Le Dix-huitième siècle* (Paris: Librairie Arthème Fayard, 1960), vol. 2, 640, 655.

41. See Besterman, *Correspondence*, letters 214, 642, 1443, 2844, 2962, 3136, 3269, 6731, 8056, 8057, 8058.

42. Brockliss and Jones identify Tronchin as "one of the first advocates of expectant medicine," a physician who prescribed placebos for patients who insisted on being heavily medicated. *The Medical World of Early Modern France*, 572. On Tronchin's attitude toward Voltaire as patient—and his effort to put an end to Voltaire's "frightening" consumption of remedies—see Henri Tronchin, *Théodore Tronchin: Un médecin du XVIIIe siècle* (Paris: Plon-Nourrit, 1906), 149–150 and 160–165.

43. At Ferney, Voltaire took pleasure in "treating" his servants and local peasants when they fell ill, and confessed that he had read "more books on medicine than all the books Don Quixote read on chivalry"; cited in Henri Tronchin, *Théodore Tronchin*, 169.

44. See Besterman, *Correspondence*, letters 144, 146, 642, 1222, 8132, 8133.

45. Voltaire tended to intermingle references to his bad stomach, his intellectual work and his need for solitude; see Besterman, *Correspondence*, letters 3449–3451, vol. 17, 147–151.

46. Mervaud, *Voltaire à table*, 130.

47. Voltaire wrote this tale soon after the death of Philip Stanhope, count of Chesterfield, who suffered from deafness in his final years; see "Note sur 'Les Oreilles du comte de Chesterfield'" in Voltaire, *Romans et contes* (Paris: Garnier Flammarion, 1966), 669. This was not the only text in which Voltaire linked digestion and hearing: Henri Tronchin cites an undated letter to Tronchin in which Voltaire remarked: "when the bowels are clear, the organ of hearing is, too." *Théodore Tronchin*, 368.

48. As Christiane Mervaud notes, Voltaire sounded the same theme in the articles "Déjections" and "Ventre paresseux," which he included in his *Questions sur l'Encyclopédie*; Mervaud, *Voltaire à table*, 131.

49. Voltaire, "Les Oreilles," 686.

50. See Mervaud, *Voltaire à table*, esp. 109–126, and Starobinki, "Le philosophe à table," esp. 283–284. On the redemption of illness through fiction, see Evelyne Ender, " 'Speculating Carnally,' or, Some Reflections on the Modernist Body" in *Yale Journal of Criticism*, 12:1 (1999), 113–130.

51. See, for example, Réveillé-Parise's evocation of Voltaire's ideas on excretion in *Hygiène oculaire* (1816; third edition: Paris: Méquignon-Marvis, 1845), 38; and his detailed analysis of Voltaire's illnesses in *Physiologie et hygiène*, vol. 2, 182–188.

52. See Roselyne Rey's suggestive adaptation of the Foucauldian notion of "souci de soi" to the context of Enlightenment medicine, in "Hygiène et souci de soi dans la pensée médicale des Lumières," in *Communications* 56 (1993), 25–39.

Chapter 6 ∾

COLERIDGE'S DREAMING GUT

DIGESTION, GENIUS, HYPOCHONDRIA

George Rousseau

I am better, than I was. My Spirits are low: and I suffer too often sinkings & misgivings, alienations from the Spirit of Hope, strange withdrawings out of the Life that manifest itself by existence—morbid yearnings condemn'd by me, almost despis'd, and yet perhaps at times almost cherish'd, to concenter my Being into Stoniness, or to be diffused as among the winds, and lose all individual existence. But all this I well know is a symptom of bodily disease, and no part of sentiment or intellect / closely connected with the excessively irritable State of my Stomach and the Viscera, & beyond doubt greatly exasperated by the abruptness & suddenness of my late Transitions from one state to another.

—Samuel Taylor Coleridge, letter to Sir George Beaumont, (1804)[1]

Samuel Taylor Coleridge (1772–1834), the great Romantic poet and symbol maker, would seem to be an odd figure to include in a book about the diverse cultures of the abdomen. Diet, weight, physique, even his own health, are concerns not usually associated with this major figure in Western civilization. Yet, nothing could be further from the truth. Coleridge worried about his health to the point of distraction: it is an understatement to call him hypochondriacal. He situated his gut—specifically the anatomical pathway from stomach to bowels—as the site of all his troubles, to such degree that were he alive today he would be a primary candidate for IBS: irritable bowel syndrome. Rarely overweight, he was nevertheless preoccupied with the look of his *corpora fabrica*, and monitored much that he allowed to pass down his oesophagus. Digestion, above all, consumed him with angst, and he worried about his indigestion in every possible way except along the lines of gender. The idea never crossed his mind, it seems, that he might be in possession of a *female* stomach.[2] He was persuaded that digestion or its opposite—indigestion—was the key to all his troubles in waking and sleeping life; and he eventually developed a theory of dreams that was in large part predicated on the state of the digesting gut at night. The role played by digestion in this context of the body's regimen and its degree of health, forms the heart of my exploration here. And the most curious aspect of Coleridge's dream life is the degree to which he—no committed materialist—paradoxically sought a material cause for his nocturnal afflictions. Hence the place of privilege to Coleridge's dreaming gut in the title of this essay.

I

Some of Coleridge's biographers have, of course, taken an opposite view: the line (correct in my view) that health was of *too much* interest to Coleridge. Earl Leslie Griggs, in the introduction to the first of the invaluable six edited volumes of Coleridge's *Collected Letters*, observed that the correspondence "may at times contain too much of ill health ... too much of remorse and self-justification."[3] Indeed, to work through the letters and notebooks is to discover over and over again Coleridge's boundless fascination with his own soul and body, and in particular the focus of his attention on his stomach and bowels, these as much as his mysticism and system-building. He never overlooked the former (soul) but was far more obsessed with the latter (body). The intestinal tract—stomach, liver, intestines, rectum, the whole of his innards except his penis—proved to be the specific site of endless curiosity and mystery. Here, in the midriff, was the key to his malady, the long disease of his life, and its implied antithesis—health—which he rarely enjoyed. To friends and strangers alike he variously explained the debilitating disturbances in his body—be it constipation, flatulence, vomiting, diarrhea, or simply *pain*—according to a long litany of possible ailments: gout, dysentery, cholera, chronically irritable bowel, or an irritable bladder, influenza, sciatica, rheumatism, cancer, stone, or diabetes.

Other biographers have taken a different tack. Jennifer Ford, for example, focuses on Coleridge's "medical imagination," recognizing how large the lacuna in understanding has been here.[4] But she relies rather too much on Emmanuel Swedenborg (however heavily invested in his mysticism Coleridge was), and on the sense of Coleridge's approbation of Swedenborg's physiology of dreams and nightmares. Coleridge assiduously tried, over many years in prolific annotations that amount to a small book on Swedenborg himself, to concur with the Swedish mystic. But he could not in the end, and hovered all his living days in doubt about a secure theory of dreams. Close textual analysis of the evidence suggests that Coleridge was typically ironic, sardonic, or dismissive, but ultimately unable to agree with Swedenborg's confident theosophical solutions. Coleridge's skepticism about the Swedenborgian interpretation of dreams bears magisterial importance for the evolution of nineteenth-century dream theory from the Romantics to Freud and Jung.

This small caveat notwithstanding, Ford's contribution to the progress of Coleridge scholarship is significant. For the medical imagination has been thoroughly neglected in Coleridge studies, and the lacuna has profound implications for interpretations of his health and, especially, his gut. Considering the role played by the imagination in Romantic (not merely Coleridgean) aesthetics, and, more locally, in Coleridge's landmark *Biographia Literaria*, Coleridge is entitled to be called (Aristotle notwithstanding) the "Father" of all theories about imagination in poetry. But features of this "imagination" have been overlooked. That imagination, as Ford astutely acknowledges, could become deranged and diseased; and such deflections of it could be expected to take a toll on Coleridge's body, as well as his waking and sleeping life. Ford has appealed for a unity of "medical, physiological and poetic imagination."[5] The amalgam enables understanding of the hypochondriacal Coleridge I aim to retrieve here: the Coleridge who was thoroughly *au fait* with the theory of "diseased imagination" as described by late Enlightenment mechanist-materialist philosophers. Building on their theories, Coleridge persuaded himself that his body was in pain, and that the "imagination" was no less crucial in the hierarchical body regime than the visceral organs. This was because it alone constructed the intellectual and symbolic mental order regulating the body. This coupling of medical and philosophical theory paves the way to Coleridge's dream theory, as well as any biographical sense of his health.

Yet what exactly was it that so endlessly troubled Coleridge throughout his life? Sometimes he blamed the effects of bad food or bad weather. Was he diseased, or was he preeminently hypochondriacal, as a number of previous critics have suggested.[6] Or were his discomforts the consequence of his notorious opium habit—opium having a profoundly debilitating effect on the gut, then a convenient shorthand for the vast tubular system extending from the oesophagus to the rectum? Any attempt at a posthumous diagnosis is perilous, particularly one as diagnostically and determinably slippery as hypochondriasis, which has long had a reputation as a non-disease, or at least a condition so problematic in its ambiguity and protean transformations (or at least so heavily conjoined to genius) that it is incapable of definition.

Hypochondriasis was also the complaint of malingerers. As early as 1766, the prolific social commentator and London man-about-town John Hill wrote: "To call the Hypochondriasis a fanciful malady, is ignorant and cruel. It is a real, and a sad disease."[7] Historically, the *morbus hypochondriacus* first spoken of by Galen was a severe disorder seated in the organs of the hypochondria or upper abdomen (the spleen, liver, gall-bladder, etc., the word deriving from *hypo*, under, and *chondros*, cartilage), and was related to melancholia ("black bile") and emotional disorders such as the "spleen" and "vapours."[8] But Hill was the first who wrote in English about the hypochondria diagnosis for lay audiences. Other more ancient commentators than Hill had pronounced on *morbus hypochondriacus* and the difficulties involved in understanding it (e.g., Galen, *On Prognosis*). By the eighteenth century it was principally gendered as a male malady, a counterpart to female "hysteria."[9] Along with other "nervous disorders," hypochondriasis was increasingly being written upon by (male) physicians of eighteenth-century Britain, when it was seen as threatening the well-being of the whole nation.[10] In *The English Malady: Or, A Treatise of Nervous Diseases of all Kinds, As Spleen, Vapours, Lowness of Spirits, Hypochondriacal, and Hysterical Distempers, &c.* (1733), George Cheyne famously recorded that these "nervous Disorders" were "computed to make almost one third of the Complaints of the People of Condition in England."[11] It is unclear from where he derived his statistics, but Cheyne was probably not far off the mark. Two generations later, in 1806, Thomas Trotter in his *A View of the Nervous Temperament* doubled the number: he believed that "nervous diseases" now made up "two-thirds of the whole with which civilized society is infested, and are tending fast to abridge the physical strength and mental capacities of the human race."[12] Hence society—the culture into which Coleridge was born in 1772 and then raised—was growing increasingly nervous. The ill, languorous, hypersensitive body thus quickly became a principal characteristic of the Romantic sensibility. In March 1801 Coleridge—still a young man of 29—apologized to his friend Thomas Poole for having sent him a letter "written in 'a wildly-wailing strain,'" confessing that he had been "horribly hypochondriacal" when he wrote it.[13] Two years later, in October 1803, he even described his friend and poetic collaborator William Wordsworth as "a brooder over his painful hypochondriacal Sensations,"[14] a man becoming "more & more benetted [sic] in hypochondriacal Fancies, living wholly among *Devotees*."[15] The young Coleridge saw the world through hypochondriacal eyes: his culture was by then preoccupied with it so preponderantly that it had filtered down to the household knowledge of educated people.

Roy and Dorothy Porter have identified the "coming-out" (the phrase is mine rather than theirs and is intentionally chosen) of the hypochondriac as a *human* type in late eighteenth-century England as designating an important moment in the cultural history of medicine. It was a dramatic appearance, or "coming out," for the ways in which its stereotypes broke from previous concepts of invalids or *malades imaginaires*. As modern Western society increasingly put a mark on the special, the interesting individual, especially the *genius*, the Porters suggested that the ensuing social tensions "between individual brilliance and polite conformity bred anxieties" which were "somatized into physical complaints, which could be partly owned and partly disowned. Sickliness provides social alibis while suffering purchased the right to be different, to be oneself. Pain commanded a certain social bargaining power."[16] The Romantic *sickly* poet thus became a type, one with legitimate medical credentials. Trotter wrote that "it is to be supposed, that all men who possess genius, and those mental qualifications which prompt them to literary attainments and pursuits, are endued by nature with more than usual sensibility of nervous system." In Trotter's opinion, the power and focus of the mind on higher subjects sapped the "powers of digestion" and reacted upon "the nervous part of the frame." The "literary character" was thus likely to suffer "numerous instances of dyspepsia, hypochondriasis and melancholia."[17] Digestion in its various forms—whether successfully completed or as indigestion and dyspepsia—was crucial to the developing hypochondriac. My point in brief is that if illness was a necessary hallmark of all Romantic writers, hypochondria was the cornerstone of that individual talent because it was, ultimately, an exclusionary strategy.

The idea that the sedentary and studious type hovered in particular danger of illness had been a commonplace in Judaeo-Christian tradition since biblical times.[18] John Hill was only one in a long line of medical commentators, ancient and early modern, who wrote how "The finer spirits are wasted by the labour of the brain: the Philosopher rises from his study more exhausted than the Peasant leaves his drudgery."[19] The sickly writer thus included almost all the prominent British writers in Coleridge's formative mindset: William Cowper, Thomas Gray, James Boswell, Samuel Johnson, Percy Shelley, John Keats. Yet despite Coleridge's own self-fashioning as an incurable hypochondriac (despite his protestations), his incessant ailments, his constant, endless references to his poor health, as well as the further features of the hypochondriacal subject we shall examine below, all combine to suggest an authentic case in its modern sense. Hence Coleridge both suffered the symptoms of which he endlessly complained, as well as sought to ensure that he could be a *malade*: he was both *malade vraiment* as well as *malade imaginaire*. He was the genuine article of the new-style hypochondriac.

II

Coleridge's first physical illness occurred in 1779, when he was only seven and at his first year at school, which was hit by an epidemic of "putrid fever." But more telling than this early encounter with illness was his experience with his immediate family. As the precociously gifted youngest of ten children, with a father of fifty-three and a mother of forty-five, Coleridge was either bullied by or distanced from his eight brothers and spoiled by his parents. He recalled that as a child he "became fretful, & timorous, & a tell-tale—& the School-boys drove me from play, & were always tormenting me." He sought consolation in books, "and I used to lie by the wall, and *mope*—and my spirits used to come upon me suddenly, & in a flood."[20] A significant incident occurred when he was seven, when after an argument with one of his brothers he ran away from home to escape a scolding from his mother. He spent the night out of doors whilst family and friends searched for him. He later recalled that on being found, "I was put to bed—& recovered in a day or so—but I was certainly injured—For I was weakly, & subject to the ague [fever] for many years after."[21] He also recalled "the tears stealing down his [father's] face" when he was brought home, and his mother's "outrageous . . . joy." This event sets a pattern for Coleridge's adult life, of escape and blame, mixed with illness that is not of his own making. As Holmes points out, the importance of this episode is shown by the number of times Coleridge referred to it in later life, and its recurrence in his notebooks.[22] The final traumatic event of early childhood was the sudden death of his beloved father after a heart attack in 1781, a little before Coleridge's ninth birthday. He was soon sent away to school at Christ's Hospital in London, from which date he virtually considered himself an "orphan." The deaths of a brother and sister in 1791 were also particularly emotional blows, provoking the lines:

> Pain after pain, and woe succeeding woe—
> Is my heart destin'd for another blow?
> O my sweet sister! and must thou too die?[23]

My impression is thus of a sensitive, intelligent, highly imaginative youth, but a lonely one too, deeply affected by these early experiences. This is the type of character one might expect to develop into a hypochondriacal adult.

It was in the winter of his final year at Christ's Hospital school, 1790–1791, that Coleridge came down with what he described as "jaundice and rheumatic fever."[24] He spent long periods of time in the school's sick-ward, and was given opium to help him sleep. He recorded his experience in the early poem, "Pain: Composed in Sickness." After this, rheumatism would frequently be referred to as a principal source of pain. An inflammatory disease, rheumatic fever has been described as "an illness of skin, brain, heart, connective tissue, blood and serum, tonsils, and joints."[25] It can make recurrent attacks, and involves such symptoms as joint pains, muscle and abdominal pain, skin nodules, and vomiting. Coleridge's friend and host for the last eighteen years of his life, Dr James Gillman, attributed "all his bodily sufferings" to rheumatism,[26] and this would certainly explain some of the aspects of Coleridge's adult ill health. But it goes no way toward explaining the recurrent problems of the gut, nor the sudden appearance and disappearance of his symptoms, or his obsessive attitude to his condition. The notion of the "English belly" would have resonated in Coleridge's symbol-making mind: it was both larger and smaller than the gut. But the belly, no matter how securely British rather than French or German (the sense of national differences in anatomical organs was rampant by the early nineteenth century), cannot begin to account for Coleridge's difficulties. Indeed, Walter Jackson Bate looks altogether elsewhere, claiming that Coleridge's autopsy "establishes that he had never had anything like 'rheumatic fever' . . . nor in all probability anything else that would *organically* explain protracted physical sufferings as a boy or young man."[27] Yet the biological character of rheumatic fever changed in the very late eighteenth and nineteenth centuries, and heart damage—as well as damage to the brain—is a feature only of this later incarnation of the disease.[28] Nonetheless, whilst rheumatic fever may explain *some* of Coleridge's physical pain, it by no means explains *all* his symptoms.

It was anxiety that Coleridge began to point to as the source of his ailment. In 1794 he informed a friend that he had been "seriously unwell" and "heavy of head & turbulent of Bowels."[29] But at this time Coleridge was also suffering from nervous anxiety associated with his relationship with his future wife, Sara Fricker, a disastrous match encouraged by his friend Robert Southey. When Southey admonished Coleridge for not writing to Sara, Coleridge claimed he had been "taken ill—very ill . . . Languid, sick at heart." and could not write to her then (though he managed to pen an article of "Nonsense" for the booksellers).[30] In 1796 a doctor informed him that his condition was "altogether nervous," originating "either in severe application, or excessive anxiety." Coleridge seized upon this diagnosis: "in excessive anxiety, I believe, it might originate!"[31] He would have known, of course, that the medical practitioners of his time recommended therapeutic techniques aimed at strengthening the constitution of "nervous" patients and hypochondriacs like himself. The correct use of the non-naturals—a regulated diet, sufficient exercise, healthy air—with occasional bleeding, sweatings, purgings, and medication to relieve the buildup of obstructions and facilitate blood flow: these formed the basis of their advice. For Coleridge it became one point of focus following his move to Cumbria in 1800, where the weather and his diet became key ingredients in the higgledy-piggledy recipe of his disease.

In the Lake District Coleridge discovered the potent opium-based medicine known as Kendal black drop, the effects of which were ruinous on his digestion. The effects of his drug-use offer the strongest counter to the argument that he was truly hypochondriacal in the modern sense. Indeed, two of his worst periods of illness, in the early 1800s and the early 1830s, coincide with periods of heavy drug use or attempts to reduce that use. Coleridge appears to have taken opium intermittently during the 1790s, and it appears that his problems with his gut developed at this time. In 1791 he claimed that "Opium never used to have any disagreeable effects on me—but it has upon many."[32] This is a stance he would maintain at least until the later 1800s.[33] When in 1814 Coleridge suggested to Joseph Cottle that it would be best if he were incarcerated in "a private madhouse" for a few months in order to overcome his opium habit,[34] Robert Southey told Cottle that the most "mournful thing" about Coleridge's case "is that while acknowledging the guilt of the habit, he imputes it still to morbid bodily causes, whereas after every possible allowance is made for these, every person who has witnessed his habits, knows that for the greater part . . . inclination and indulgence are the motives."[35] Thus, as opposed to Gillman's claim for rheumatism, Cottle in his *Reminicences* [*sic*] declared that Coleridge's "unhappy use of narcotics" was the "true cause of all his maladies, his languor, his acute and chronic pains, his indigestion, his swellings, the disturbances of his general corporeal system."[36] However, like rheumatism, opium use does not preclude a broader diagnosis of hypochondriasis, as contemporary doctors realized. Trotter, in his account of the nervous temperament, made particular note of the effects the drug had in exacerbating such disorders: "Opium alone gives relief, though it must feed the disease. Such persons seem to compound with their physician for sound nights, and days of ease; and if he does not comply he must be changed. Hard is the task imposed on the medical attendant; he must obey, or starve."[37] In his *Essay on Hypochondriasis*, the physician John Reid similarly noted the danger of the long-term prescription of opium, considering it "a drug which is so likely to become a part of the daily regimen of an hypochondriacal invalid, and which often renders him incurably such." But in Reid's opinion, the malady *antedated* the drug use, "which is often begun to relieve bodily pain," and was a feature of the hypochondriac's intemperate character.[38] Usually it was, and another chapter on the body of melancholics would be needed to disentangle cause and effect here. Suffice it to say that Coleridge was persuaded beyond any doubt that he had drugged himself to relieve these symptoms.

If there were space I could continue to chronicle Coleridge's ailments year by year, observing him among the physicians and as his *own* doctor, identifying his disorders as this or that condition, almost all located somewhere "in the region of the stomach." The point, however, in such a short space is not to compile the evidence but to explain why he is such a prominent candidate for the culture of the abdomen: those conditions located in the gut that he aimed to unify into one totalizing discourse capable of explaining all his maladies and accounting for his talent as well. One without the other would not have suited Coleridge: it had to be both. His defective gut was the proof of his genius and vice-versa. He even permitted his self-diagnosis to guide his momentous life choices. By January 1804, for example, he decided that his delicate constitution could stand the damp climate of England no longer. His illness had not been helped by making his home in the wet countryside of the Lake District, and as rain fell inexorably on the roof of the Wordsworths' Grasmere home, he complained to Robert Southey that his health was "pitiable!... I must go into a hot climate."

Migrate he did, but on reaching Portsmouth en route to the Mediterranean he told the Wordsworths that he believed his ongoing "Hauntings and Self-desertions are, no doubt, connected with the irritable state of my Bowels & the feebleness of my Stomach; but both they & these, their bodily causes, are exasperated by the rapid Changes, I have undergone"—especially in his various travels and escapades since leaving Cumbria.[39] Over and again it is his gut which is the culprit, a body zone still barely understood in the mindset of the Enlightenment and nineteenth century.

Though Coleridge never wrote a book on "distress of the mind," as his letter to the Wordsworths reveals, this period in 1803–1804 was a time of mental as well as physical distress, alongside his increasing enslavement to opium. He was unable to work, was suffering nightmares, was financially embarrassed, and despairing in, and endlessly fretting about, his failed love for Sara Hutchinson. At odds with his "cold" wife, he was clearly depressed. A year's residence in a hot climate, such as Madeira or Sicily, was the answer not just to his problems of health, but to most of his other problems as well. After quitting the Lakes early in 1804, he would not see his wife or children again until late 1806, informing the Wordsworths in November of that year that they had "*determined* to part absolutely and finally."[40] I am thus establishing the picture of a man with obsessive awareness of the state of his gut, seeking in external events and diagnoses potential explanations for his supersensitive abdominal maladies.

III

If Coleridge's ailment was not wholly linked to his opium taking, the suggestion of his most recent biographer, Richard Holmes, that he suffered perhaps from irritable bowel syndrome (IBS) is a promising one, and one that links Coleridge's own focus on anxiety. IBS is a chronic, relapsing functional disorder focused on the small and large intestine, whose "cause and mechanism are unknown."[41] In *Gut Reactions: Understanding Symptoms of the Digestive Tract*, W. Grant Thompson explains that though the "effects of *chronic* emotion or stress on gastric motility and secretion are not precisely known . . . there can be little doubt that they are important in the genesis of symptoms." Certain emotions may be capable of precipitating gastric dysfunctions such as nonulcerated dyspepsia, and it is possible that "a certain personality type with certain previous experiences and associations may undergo changes in gastric function or in awareness of gastric function in response to emotion."[42] As Coleridge declared, it was "Damp without & anxiety, or Agitation, within that cause my Disease." Furthermore, the relationship between the gut and the brain is two-way traffic: one influences the other. The gut can thus "learn" responses from the brain, and a Pavlovian reaction to certain stimuli particular to the individual is possible, though this is as yet unproved. Certain drugs, including opiates and alcohol, "may also cause dyspepsia through unknown mechanisms," and Thompson adds that although hard scientific data is rare, "it is generally accepted that emotion is important in the genesis of dyspepsia."[43] Thompson also explains that nocturnal pain "or spring and fall exacerbations of the pain all tilt the diagnosis toward peptic ulcer,"[44] which would have the potential to explain some of Coleridge's symptoms. Medical research appears to show that IBS sufferers "are more prone to chronic illness behavior and that this behavior is learned.... Such illness behavior may be engendered not only by early life experiences but also by... psychological and personality abnormalities."[45] Again, this appears to fit the pattern of Coleridge's complaint. Many of his attacks coincided with periods of personal emotional anxiety or stressful situations, and would undoubtedly have been exacerbated by his laudanum use, a dangerous mix of opium *and* alcohol. Dyspepsia or IBS would also explain Coleridge's recurrent claim that his bowel problems *preceded* his drug habit.

However, like rheumatic fever, IBS does not provide a full explanation for all the features of Coleridge's case. Hypochondriasis, though, offers an alternative, if quite possibly linked, diagnosis. Unfortunately, like IBS hypochondriasis is an especially problematical condition to pin down, and medical opinion on the exact nature of the disorder remains divided, and it is agreed "that the diagnosis of hypochondriasis is not easy."[46] In the eighteenth century, hypochondriasis was thought to be intimately connected with all operations of the gut, a tradition of belief developing for centuries. The difference is that the tie was sealed by the mid-Enlightenment period: defective guts and sedentary hypochondriacs never again be disjoined. Doctors and especially medical theorists were plummeting to the inner cavities to discover exactly where in the location the seat of the ailing malady— the hyp, as they called it—was located. Robert James in his *Medicinal Dictionary* (1743–1745) defined "Hypochondriacus Morbus" as "a spasmodic-flatulent Disorder of the *Primae Viae*, that is, of the Stomach and Intestines, arising from an Inversion or Perversion of their peristaltic Motion, and, by the mutual consent of the Parts, throwing the whole nervous System into irregular Motions, and disturbing the whole Oeconomy of the Functions."[47] The former naval physician James Johnson in 1827 would also focus his discussion of these nervous distempers on the gut, entitling his rapidly-selling study *An Essay on Morbid Sensibility of the Stomach and Bowels, As the Proximate Cause, or Characteristic Condition of Indigestion, Nervous Irritability, Mental Despondency, Hypochondriasis, &c. &c.* Johnson wrote that "a *morbid sensibility* of the nerves of the stomach and the bowels, with or without the usual symptoms of disordered digestion, was the leading feature of the disease, and the cause of the varied and endless train of symptoms which develop themselves in the mind and in distant parts of the body."[48]

This focus on the guts is clearly useful for a contemporary explication of Coleridge's case. In his seminal work *A View of the Nervous Temperament*, Thomas Trotter, cited above, also observed that these increasingly prevalent disorders included those diseases "commonly called Nervous, Bilious,

Stomach, and Liver Complaints; Indigestion; Low Spirits; Gout, &c." All of these Trotter bracketed together collectively as "nervous disorders," and they were "to be referred in general, to debility, increased sensibility, or torpor of the alimentary canal."[49] As Trotter rightly saw things, the "human stomach is an organ endued by nature, with the most complex properties of any in the body; and forming a *centre* of sympathy between our corporeal and mental parts, of more exquisite qualifications than even the brain itself . . . . In all those disorders whose seat is the nervous system, it particularly suffers."[50] All forms of gout, for example, were "preceded by stomach affection" and attended by dyspeptic symptoms.[51] Hypochondriasis was thus firmly linked by Trotter and other contemporary doctors with the operation of the digestive organs, and was often grouped alongside dyspepsia and indigestion. Individually, these "nervous disorders" were, perhaps, more akin to what would now be identified as IBS, chronic fatigue syndrome, and anxiety disorders rather than hypochondriasis, though they all also feature as frequent diagnoses of the modern hypochondriacal patient.[52]

What exactly is to be understood as hypochondriasis today, this would seem a necessary question, in a discussion about the framing of disease. In the recent study, *Hypochondriasis: Modern Perspectives on an Ancient Malady*, Vladan Starcevic writes that it "can be succinctly defined as excessive and persistent preoccupation with health, disease, and body, which is associated with a fear and suspicion that one is a victim of serious disease."[53] Another characteristic feature, Starcevic claims, is its persistence over many months and years, though with fluctuating intensity. So temporal chronicity is fundamental to the condition. Even when subjects (are they all patients?) possess an organic medical condition, "the symptoms are experienced as far more intense than what could be expected on the basis of the objectively existing, organic pathology."[54] Starcevic observes that whilst there are no symptoms *typical* of hypochondriasis, some symptoms—such as gastrointestinal, dermatological, or those of the central nervous system—are "found more frequently among patients with hypochondriasis."[55]

It may be true, but how (again within the context of weight, diet, and bodily physique, even the more academic framing of disease) shall we understand the victim? And how are the fear and suspicion to be culturally contextualized? Trotter, already sensitive to the pejorative role of alcohol in modern civilization, noted the sensitivity of the hypochondriacal patient in a work on naval medicine, writing how sailors suffering from scurvy recounted to each other their dreams of "green fields, and streams of pure water." These conversations were, he claimed, "as earnestly conducted, as we sometimes observe hypochondriacs in relating their feelings, from any ruffle of temper occasioned by changeable weather, or other slight causes."[56] Other defining features of hypochondriasis include the obsessive bodily preoccupation found in Coleridge, and a constant recourse to medical practitioners. Neither ever let up. Coleridge dismissed many of the physicians he consulted as failures, and wrote significantly in 1796, "I know a *great many* Physicians. They are *shallow* Animals: having always employed their minds about Body and Gut, they imagine that in the whole system of things there is nothing but Gut and Body."[57] Though Coleridge would come to praise some physicians, such as Thomas Beddoes and James Gillman, highly, when he decided that a warm climate was the best solution to his condition it is notable that he had been advised by no less than "*four* medical men" that his only hope for a cure were a "regulated Diet, Tranquillity [*sic*], and an even & dry climate."[58] Perhaps it is no surprise that in 1823 he wrote that he considered it "the chance of my life, that I have counted an unusually large number of medical men (several of them Men of great celebrity & eminence) among my friends."[59]

A fascination with medical texts in an attempt to identify their disorder is another feature of the hypochondriacal personality shared by Coleridge.[60] On a number of occasions he minutely described his ailment according to the symptoms in recently, read books. In 1803 the *Encyclopedia Britannica* provided him with a definition of "atonic gout," a chronic affliction of the whole body rather than merely the gut, which he at first accepted before then rejecting it in favor of an undefined "disease of the skin." Significantly, he blamed his first taking of opium on "a medical Journal [where] I unhappily met with an account of a cure performed in a similar case (or what to me appeared so) by rubbing in of Laudanum, at the same time taking a given dose internally—It acted like a charm, like a miracle!"[61] Miraculous it may have been; yet he continued to compile the symptoms, ordering them into categories and disease constellations, choosing among them, over the years.

These disjointed fragments indicate the range of his concerns for illness, digestion and sleep. His nostalgia after leaving his wife in England must also be included (nostalgia was then at the peak of its trajectory as a diagnosed, if incurable, malady). But his affliction was concomitantly a *hypochondriacal* nostalgia framed by nocturnal visions and encounters with spirits, which had spurred him to consider dreams philosophically in the first place. A nostalgically loaded hypochondriasis rather than a self-feigning excuse not to return to familial responsibilities: the excuse for the failings of a man who has told himself that his nostalgia has made him "ill." In brief I suggest that if hypochondriasis was a vital word and category around 1800, permeated with layers of meaning (however contradictory) for Coleridge and his contemporaries, it was also a concept which permitted him to explain to himself contradictory strands of his life experience that were otherwise impossible to comprehend or reconcile. These certainly extended to his creative, imaginative life, the imagination—as he had been persuaded in Germany—so heavily depended on neuroanatomical processes. Coleridge's hypochondriacal characteristics of impairment thus extended to his many unrealized ambitions and projects, a failure he ascribed to his ill health, exacerbated by opium use taken, he claimed, in his attempts to overcome bad health. This debilitation accounts in part for his contradictory behavior whilst in Germany, especially since the hypochondriac's preoccupation with illness (to put the matter in modern DMS terminology that strengthens the larger point about the modernity of Coleridge's hypochondria) "causes clinically significant distress or impairment in social, occupational, or other important areas of functioning."[62] But even this amalgamation of his hypochondria and nostalgia is only part of the story he was telling himself about his near-Jobean decline.

IV

As time marched, Coleridge increasingly lashed himself for his imminent tragedy as the dupe of opium. Because he labored in such agonies, he had been driven to medicate himself. He heard in 1814 God's accusation: "'I gave thee so many Talents. What hast thou done with them'?"[63] Coleridge would continue to hear the indictment in his profuse nocturnal dream life, whether as death—in life or its reverse. The mariner in his famous poem who cries out, paradoxically, that water is everywhere but he has none to drink, parallels the nocturnal Coleridge driven by spirits who inhibit his sleep. These were the demons of the night who crept into his stomach to pilfer his undigested food. As we shall see, hypochondria and troubled sleep (demons, nightmares, the incubus, and succubus) often went hand in hand in one so addicted to his substance as Coleridge (see figure 6.1).

The foregoing evidence suggests that a diagnosis of hypochondriasis comfortably fits the pattern of Coleridge's ailments. As Arthur J. Barsky writes, "The prominent disease fears, beliefs, and preoccupations of hypochondriacal patients are thought to stem from a misattribution of benign bodily symptoms and normal sensations to serious disease."[64] Hypochondriasis has thus been conceptualized

as a disorder of bodily amplification, in which a wide range of somatic and visceral sensations are experienced as unusually intense, noxious and disturbing. Thus, hypochondriacal individuals may be thought of as especially sensitive to,

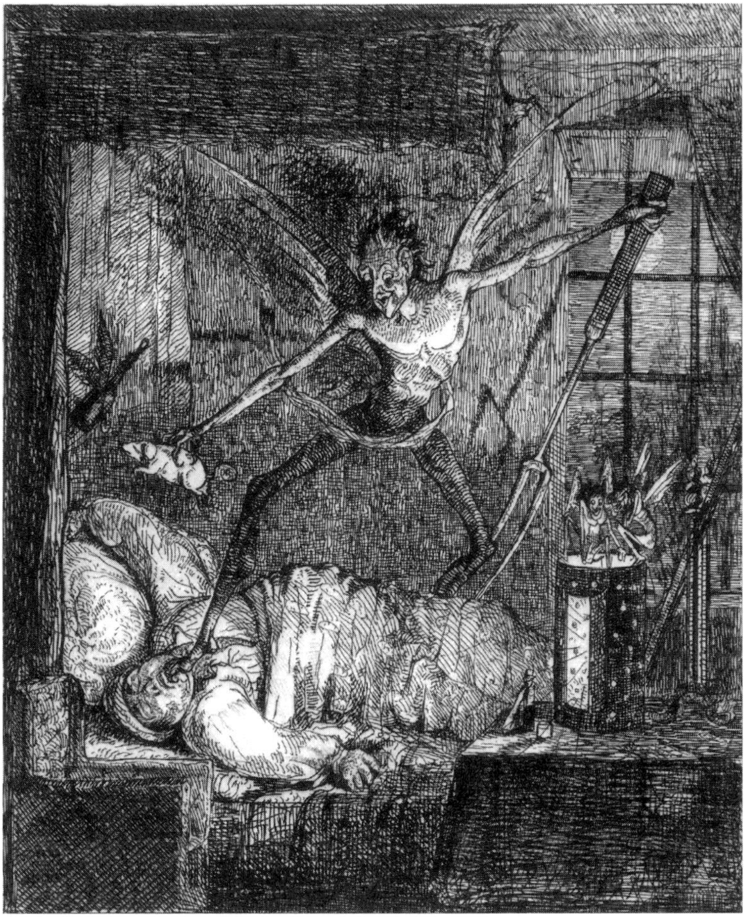

Figure 6.1 A monster, representing indigestion, torturing a man trying to sleep. Etching by H. J. Townsend (Courtesy of Wellcome Library, London).

and intolerant of, bodily sensation in general.... Hypochondriacal people, because their symptoms are so intense and uncomfortable, conclude that these sensations must be abnormal and pathological, rather than normalizing them by attributing them to a benign cause such as overwork, insufficient rest, inadequate exercise, or dietary indiscretion.[65]

Unfortunately, whilst all four of these latter possible attributions apply amply to Coleridge, modern empirical investigation of this thesis has been "relatively sparse." The four also omit the nocturnal dreams that specifically disturbed Coleridge so acutely. As early as 1797, he described his restless self this way: "Frequently have I, half-awake & half-asleep, my body diseased & fevered by my imagination, seen armies of ugly Things bursting in upon me."[66] The symbolism of these ugly objects can be interrupted according to the corpus of pre-1800 dream symbolism, but it is equally significant that Coleridge pauses to comment on his diseased body first. Then there were the observations about his hypersensitivity by those who knew Coleridge, especially the strange way his body had predisposed him. Humphry Davy was only one of many to remark on his friend's "excessive sensibility."[67] Barsky, using modern categories but aiming to account for the same phenomena, notes that anxiety, depression, and dysphoric mood (i.e., chronic discomfort, restlessness, and being ill at ease) all help to amplify bodily distress.

Coleridge himself ascribed his curious condition to chronic anxiety, especially of the type intensified by the demons of the night, and Barsky explains that anxiety "increases self-consciousness, and this apprehensive self-scrutiny amplifies pre-existing symptoms and brings previously unnoticed sensations to conscious awareness."[68] Coleridge's anxiety includes another characteristic of the hypochondriac personality: a vivid fear of death. As Porter and Porter have written, "Coleridge feared sleep, since his nightmares were intolerable. Above all, a paralysing dread of death seized him."[69] Earlier, Erasmus Darwin believed that "the cause of what is term'd hypochondriasis in men" derived from a "general debility" in the stomach and bowels, "which is always attended with so much fear, *or expectation*, of dying, as to induce them to think of nothing but their own health."[70] Darwin thus firmly yoked chronic worry about one's health with the gut. In *Zoonomia* he classified hypochondriasis as a disease of the mind, if not a form of actual madness, though not without forfeiting the gut from the equation, and modern studies suggest that "in the majority (62–88 percent) of hypochondriacal patients, there is at least one comorbid mental disorder," with depressive and anxiety disorders being the most common.[71] Coleridge suffered from both depression and anxiety, and considered his inability to control his opium habit to be "a species of madness."[72] But not without laying sufficient self-evidence on the torments caused him in dreams: his nocturnal life was the clue to his waking reality rather than vice-versa.

So canonical a figure as Coleridge, in whom so much is at stake in the development of Romanticism, cannot lightly be classified, or diagnosed, as imbued with *any* malady unless it has been derived independently by different assessors working toward a common goal. Even for Coleridge there were alternative disease conditions; his need not have been hypochondriasis. Yet I have tried to demonstrate what his decades of concern for his ailments amounted to. His obsession was with the gut rather than any other part of the human body—from the almost daily bouts of intestinal trouble to his perceived sense that he had cholera—and the preoccupation fortified him against the possibility that he was a lesser talent after all. It was not overweight that was the proof but compromised digestion, constant bowel irritation, hellish dreams, the sense that alien devils were picking him over in his bed. As Roy Porter has claimed, hypochondria based on genuine symptoms was the chief sign of the "cradle of genius."[73] Elsewhere I have taken an alternative route by framing his main malady through troubled sleep and nocturnal rituals. This approach reconstructed his contexts of night-thoughts and graveyard sensibility: commencing in the kingdom of sleep this avenue derived Coleridge's genius for the gut and self-diagnosis from nether realms in the land of sleep—or, as was more common for Coleridge, nightly wakening. Here, however, the gut itself, in relation to health and pathology, body and soul, has been my main focus.

My alternative route captured the sleepless Coleridge more ably than I have here, and highlighted what it was like to sleep as little and as poorly as he often did—troubled as he always was by one or another concern—but gave the impression of a different type of hypochondriasis than Coleridge's. Many hypochondriacs and male hysterics warred with themselves at night, experienced one hell after another as they tossed "alone, all alone on a wide, wide sea," but who were not preoccupied with their gut as he was. Read the Coleridge of the letters, the Coleridge of the notebooks and marginalia, and you soon realize that this is a man possessed by the devil of his entrails. He has demonized the gut to the point that it must forever let him down; in doing so it also, through contradiction and paradox, proves to be the site of his greatest imagination, genius, and talent. Whatever he was as a man, and whether philosophical dualist or monist—now proponent of one, now the other, always sparring with the two without coming to any conclusion—he was the possessor of a defective gut that was both his virtue and defect. And he had no embarrassment divulging this to anyone, not even his patrons, as in his numerous letters to his friend and sponsor James Gillman.

Yet another route is found through Coleridge the dreamer—the physiological dreamer. This avenue is the one taken by Jennifer Ford in

Coleridge on Dreaming and it paid handsome dividends,[74] not merely in explaining why Milton and Swedenborg were so crucial for Coleridge's understanding of his own dreams, but in heralding the trumpet call that anatomical and physiological processes could not be omitted. In view of Coleridge's chronic illnesses, the announcement pertained to his medicine, especially his variety of maladies, as well as understanding of the complex processes underpinning them.

There is no space to summarize Ford's important work (discussed at the beginning) or to repeat its findings. Suffice it to invite readers to consult her pages on Swedenborg (147–152) as they form the heart of the post-Cartesian matter about mind–body interaction in the gut, and her last chapter entitled "The Dreaming Medical Imagination" (183–202). This chapter is likely omitted by students of Coleridge's dreaming; yet it represents the conclusions of Ford's own intriguing voyage into the subject and points to the future direction of research in this area. If there is any gap in Ford's conclusions, they lie in gauging Coleridge's tone in his ephemeral notes and marginalia, his announcements of certainty, doubt, and puzzlement, especially in relation to the theorists he was reading: the materialists, dualists, and other philosophers on dreaming from Milton and Swedenborg through Andrew Baxter and the German naturalists.

Coleridge's doubt impelled him to be acerbic and contradictory in these speculations and in marginalia to the thought of others. Select many of the Coleridgean passages cited by Ford in her book and they cannot be construed literally. This is especially true of the comments on Swedenborg, which embody a particular hurdle in Coleridgean exegesis about the understanding of dreams because Coleridge annotated the Swede so prolifically. Yet Coleridge was passionate in his quest to discover the truth about the copula of dreams *and* the gut, or dreaming *in* the belly. Select any of the passages Ford cites on pp. 147–152, even the long letter dated November 1824 to James Gillman about "feculent metempsychosis" and the way "certain foul Spirits of the lowest order are attracted by the precious Ex-viands." You will find a narrator with tongue in cheek only half of whose voice reveals what he literally says. The ambivalence indeed poses a problem for all Coleridge's framing of dreams and—furthermore—for his understanding of his own gut. His dreaming and waking gut cannot be discounted.

This small caveat notwithstanding, Ford's contribution to the progress of Coleridge scholarship is significant. At stake is the vast realm of Coleridge's still unexplored medical imagination, which is so crucial to his whole enterprise that it is worthwhile repeating the comments made in my opening paragraph. When Ford writes that it is "the medical imagination" in all its complexity that has been overlooked in Coleridge studies she puts her finger on a lacuna that could fill not one, but several books.[75] When you consider the role the imagination plays in Coleridge's aesthetics, in literary criticism (especially in the *Biographia Literaria*), and reflect that Coleridge was the Father of theories about the role of imagination in poetry—then Ford's claims that we have overlooked essential features of his notion of that same imagination takes added significance. When Ford recounts, for example, how that same imagination could become "diseased" in the parlance of the late eighteenth and early nineteenth centuries, she treads on the hypochondriacal framing I propose here. When she argues for a unity of "medical, physiological and poetic imagination," she comes close to the hypochondriacal Coleridge who required this sort of "diseased imagination" to persuade himself that his pain was real. What she expends energy trying to demonstrate that "the imagination's power as a translational organ of the body… also creates a poetic world," she connects realms medical and literary in just the sense we have been prescribing.[76] It is, finally, impossible to avoid the conclusion that in his dreams and dream processes Coleridge unified all these views. He could not have done so without his all-important gut.

Notes

1. Samuel Taylor Coleridge (hereafter STC) to Sir George Beaumont, 6 April 1804, in *The Collected Letters of Samuel Taylor Coleridge* (hereafter *CL*), Earl Leslie Griggs, ed., 6 vols. (London: Oxford University Press, 1956–1971), 2: 1122.
2. Stomachs had long been differentiated and gendered by 1800. See apothecary-medic John Hill in *Centaury, The Great Stomachic….* (London: R. Baldwin, 1765).
3. Griggs, *CL*, 1: xxxv.
4. Jennifer Ford, *Coleridge on Dreaming: Romanticism, Dreams and the Medical Imagination* (Cambridge: Cambridge University Press, 1998).
5. Ibid., 194.
6. For instance, see Richard Holmes, *Coleridge: Early Visions* (London: Hodder & Stoughton, 1989), 15; and Walter Jackson Bate, *Coleridge* (London: Weidenfeld and Nicolson, 1969), 102.
7. John Hill, *Hypochondriasis. A Practical Treatise on the Nature and Cure of that Disorder; Commonly Called the Hyp or Hypo* (London, 1766), 3.
8. Esther Fischer-Homberger, "Hypochondriasis of the Eighteenth-Century," *Bulletin of the History of Medicine*, 46 (1972), 391–401.
9. G. A. Ladee, *Hypochondriacal Syndromes* (Amsterdam: Elsevier, 1966), 8.
10. See Roy Porter and Dorothy Porter, *In Sickness and in Health: The British Experience, 1650–1850* (London: Fourth Estate, 1988), 203–210.

11. George Cheyne, *The English Malady; or, A Treatise of Nervous Diseases of all Kinds, As Spleen, Vapours, Lowness of Spirits, Hypochondriacal, and Hysterical Distempers, &c.* (London, 1733), i–ii.

12. Thomas Trotter, *A View of the Nervous Temperament; Being a Practical Enquiry into the Increasing Prevalence, Prevention, and Treatment of Those Diseases Commonly Called Nervous, Bilious, Stomach, and Liver Complaints; Indigestion; Low Spirits; Gout, &c.* (second edition, London: 1807), viii.

13. STC to Poole, 24 March 1801, *CL*, 2: 710.

14. STC to Poole, 3 October 1803, *CL*, 2: 1010.

15. STC to Poole, 14 October 1803, *CL*, 2: 1013. See also Holmes, *Coleridge: Early Visions*, 357.

16. Porter and Porter, *In Sickness,* 209.

17. Trotter, *A View*, 39.

18. See Roy Porter, "Reading: A Health Warning," in *Medicine, Mortality and the Book Trade*, Robin Myers and Michael Harris, eds. (Folkstone: St. Paul's Bibliographies, 1998), 131–152.

19. Hill, *Hypochondriasis*, 6.

20. STC to Thomas Poole, 9 October 1797, *CL*, 1: 347.

21. STC to Poole, 16 October 1797, *CL*, 1: 353–354.

22. Holmes, *Coleridge: Early Visions*, 17.

23. Quoted in ibid., 38.

24. James Gillman, *The Life of Samuel Taylor Coleridge* (London: William Pickering, 1838), 33.

25. Peter C. English, *Rheumatic Fever in America and Britain* (New Brunswick: Rutgers University Press, 1999), xvii.

26. Gillman, *Life*, 33.

27. Bate, *Coleridge*, 103–104

28. See English, *Rheumatic Fever*, 17–31.

29. STC to George Dyer, 11 September 1794, *CL*, 1: 101.

30. STC to Southey, 19 September 1794, *CL*, 1: 105.

31. STC to Poole, 5 November 1796, *CL*, 1: 250.

32. STC to George Coleridge, November 1791, *CL*, 1: 18.

33. Porter and Porter, *In Sickness*, 223.

34. STC to Cottle, 26 April 1814, *CL*, 3: 477.

35. Footnote to Letter 921, Southey to Cottle, no date given, *CL*, 3: 479.

36. Joseph Cottle, *Reminiscences of Samuel Taylor Coleridge and Robert Southey* (New York: Wiley and Putnam, 1847), 351.

37. Trotter, *A View*, 137.

38. John Reid, *Essays on Hypochondriasis, and Other Nervous Affections* (third edition, London, 1823), 178–179.

39. STC to the Wordsworths, 4 April 1804, *CL*, 2: 116.

40. STC to the Wordsworths, ca. 19 November 1806, *CL*, 2: 1200.

41. W. Grant Thompson, *Gut Reactions: Understanding Symptoms of the Digestive Tract* (New York and London: Plenum Press, 1989), 210.

42. Ibid., 82.
43. Ibid., 141.
44. Ibid., 144.
45. Ibid., 191.
46. Issy Pilowsky, "Hypochondriasis, Abnormal Illness Behavior, and Social Context," in *Hypochondriasis: Modern Perspectives on an Ancient Malady*, Vladan Starcevic and Don R. Lipsitt, eds. (Oxford: Oxford University Press, 2001), 254.
47. Robert James, *Medicinal Dictionary* (London, 1743–1745), quoted in G. S. Rousseau, introduction to John Hill, *Hypochondriasis: A Practical Treatise* (Los Angeles: William Andrews Clark Memorial Library, 1969).
48. James Johnson, *An Essay on Morbid Sensibility of the Stomach and Bowels, As the Proximate Cause, or Characteristic Condition of Indigestion, Nervous Irritability, Mental Despondency, Hypochondriasis, &c. &c.* (London: Thomas and George Underwood, 1827), 60.
49. Trotter, *A View*, xvi.
50. Ibid. 205–206.
51. Ibid. 173–174.
52. Vladan Starcevic, "Clinical Features and Diagnosis of Hypochondriasis," in *Hypochondriasis*, Starcevic and Lipsitt, eds., 38.
53. Ibid., 21.
54. Ibid., 23.
55. Ibid., 23.
56. Thomas Trotter, *Observations on the Scurvy; with a Review of the Opinions Lately Advanced on that Disease, and a New Theory Defended* (second edition, London, 1792), 44.
57. STC to Charles Lloyd, Senior, 14 November 1796, *CL*, 1: 256.
58. STC to Beaumont, 2 February 1804, *CL*, 2: 1053 (emphasis in original).
59. STC to Mrs Charles Aders, 30 December 1823. *CL*, 5: 319.
60. See Starcevic, "Clinical Features," 30.
61. STC to Cottle, 26 April 1814, *CL*, 3: 476, 489.
62. See *Diagnostic and Statistical Manual of Mental Disorders* (fourth edition, American Psychiatric Association, 1994), Appendix, point D.
63. STC to Cottle, 26 April 1814, *CL*, 3: 476.
64. Arthur J. Barsky, "Somatosensory Amplification and Hypochondriasis," in *Hypchondriasis*, Starcevic and Lipsitt, eds., 223.
65. Ibid., 224.
66. STC to Poole, 9 October 1797, *CL*, 1: 348.
67. Joseph Cottle, *Reminiscences of Samuel Taylor Coleridge and Robert Southey* (New York: Wiley and Putnam), 293.
68. Barsky, "Somatosensory Amplification and Hypochondriasis," 229.
69. Porter and Porter, *In Sickness*, 222.
70. Erasmus Darwin to Elizabeth, Lady Harrowby, 21 May 1796, in *The Letters of Erasmus Darwin*, Desmond King-Hele, ed. (Cambridge: Cambridge University Press, 1981), 295.

71. Starcevic, "Clinical Features," 34.

72. STC to Cottle, 26 April 1814, *CL*, 3: 477.

73. Roy Porter, *Bodies Politic: Disease, Death and Doctors in Britain, 1650–1900* (London: Reaktion, 2001), 162.

74. Ford, *Coleridge on Dreaming*, n. 4.

75. Ibid., 185.

76. Ibid., 194, 200.

Chapter 7 ∽

IT'S "ALIMENTARY"

FEUERBACH AND THE DIETETICS
OF ANTISEMITISM[1]

Jay Geller

Unlike the extensive discussion and analysis devoted to Ludwig Feuerbach's *Essence of Christianity*[2] and his anthropological materialism, Feuerbach's later "Diet-materialism"[3] has been marginalized, if not outright ignored.[4] The Feuerbach who so influenced Marx by bringing the speculative dialectic from its transcendent perch down to earth by locating the working of the dialectic in the mystification, alienation, and objectification (or projection, *Vergegenständlichung*) of human sensibility and sensuousness is well known. Less well known is the thinker who shifted from seeing human interaction with the external world in the facultative terms of reason, will, and heart to physiological terms such as digestion: the world is incorporated—digested—by the human and thereby transformed into human consciousness. In Feuerbach's later work, "eating" (*das Essen*) replaced "love" (*die Liebe*)[5] as the master trope of human species-being, of the relationship between body and mind, between self and other. Drawing upon the insights of the Greeks before him, who defined animals, gods, and humanity (as well as other peoples) by what they ate, respectively raw food, ambrosia, and bread, Feuerbach would define the human by that fundamental physiological process and practice.[6] Emblematic of this change was his punning coinage of the apothegm, "you are what you eat" (Der Mensch *ist*, was er *isst*: lit. man is what he eats; 1850). Indeed, the *Essence of Christianity*'s anthropological critique of religion so commands the reception of Feuerbach, especially among Anglophones, that his pithy phrase is often mistakenly ascribed to the French philosophical gourmand, Brillat-Savarin.[7]

Eating and food, however, had already played a major role in *Essence of Christianity*, particularly in his discussion of *Judentum*.[8] As many historians of antisemitism acknowledge, Feuerbach's characterization of *Judentum* in terms of utilism (*der Utilismus*), egoism (*der Egoismus*), instrumentalism, exclusive self-interest, and worldly materialism had a great impact on Marx's essay "On the Jewish Question."[9] A few, however, have also called attention to Feuerbach's assertion that "The Jews have an alimentary view of theology."[10] Citing this passage, they have drawn conclusions about Feuerbach's intention to demean *Judentum* from what is in fact George Eliot's mistranslation of the German original, "der Israelite erhob sich nicht über das Brotstudium der Theologie." A more accurate translation would have been "the Israelite did not rise above the exploitation of the study of theology in order to earn his bread."[11] Consequently, *Brotstudium* confirms the accusation of craven Jewish utilism. This article argues, however, that while Eliot missed the meat of the matter she captured the aroma of Feuerbach's stew of traditional antisemitic discourses on Jewish eating habits.[12] Jewish dietary practices, imagined and otherwise, have historically generated a number of largely negative reactions and tropes. An analysis of his texts will demonstrate that Feuerbach had fed from this unsavory repast, leaving in its wake his execrable construction of *Judentum*.

Initially, I set out several of the ingredients that went into this noisome recipe for antisemitism. These include: (1) the notion of the Jewish stench, the *foetor Judaicus* that some Roman and later commentators associated with Jewish consumption of garlic and onions, (2) the pagan and Christian ascription of Jewish misanthropy and arrogant self-righteousness suppos-edly illustrated by their dietary laws, especially the prohibition on eating pork, and the apparent lack of commensality that thereby ensued, and (3) accusations of Jewish ritual consumption of blood that were associated with the blood libel. Once this smorgasbord of anti-Jewish representations has been laid out, the article turns to Feuerbach's discussions of *Judentum* within the context of his developing "Diet-materialism."

Onions, Garlic, and Leeks, Oh My!

When I traveled to Passau, West Germany in 1977 to learn German, I rented a room in the house of a rather elderly couple. One day the Hausfrau prepared an onion tart and in the process of offering me a piece, she remarked: "Sie haben Zwiebeln gern, gell?" (you like onions, right). I soon realized that this was her way of confirming that I was Jewish. Americans, she believed, did not like onions; for Jews, however, onions were supposedly a dietary staple. Onion consumption was a key sign of ethnic differentiation.

Since before the turn of the eras, Jews have been associated with delighting in the consumption of onions and other fragrant plants of the genus *Allium*, notably garlic and leeks. For example, in one of his *Satires* (3.292–296),[13] Juvenal stages the following encounter with a Jew:

> "Where are you from?" shouts he; "whose vinegar, whose beans have blown you out? With what cobbler have you been munching cut leeks and boiled wether's chaps?—What sirrah, no answer?...Say where is your stand? In what prayer-house shall I find you?"

The noted nineteenth-century German ethnographer, Richard Andree, comments in *On the Ethnography of the Jews* (1881) that the ancient Greeks and Romans—unlike contemporary Italians—hated garlic, hence this odious ascription may have become attached to garlic eaters.[14] This custom, he suggests, may well explain the *locus classicus* of the alleged Jewish stench (*foetor Judaicus*), Marcus Aurelius's (in)famous comment on the "malodorous Jews" (*foetentium Judaeorum*) as reported by Ammianus Marcellinus, *Res Gestae* (XXII.5.5). "For Marcus [Aurelius], as he was passing through Palestine on his way to Egypt, being often disgusted with the malodorous and rebellious Jews, is reported to have cried with sorrow: O Marcomanni, O Quadi, O Sarmatians, at last I have found a people more unruly than you."[15] In explicit contrast to such antisemitic polemicists as his contemporary Gustav Jaeger, who claimed that there were particular racial smells,[16] Andree writes that the probable origin of the fabled Jewish stench lies in the Jews' "well-known preference for leeks and the like" (*die bekannte Vorliebe nach Lauchspeisen*).[17] As evidence he cites Numbers 11:5 in which the wandering Israelites bemoan their diet of manna: "Remember how in Egypt we had...leeks and onions and garlic." He continues with reference to Talmudic and East European praises of garlic; the Mishnah, for example advises the eating of garlic on *Erev Shabbat* (Friday evening).

Extensive use of garlic among medieval Jews is evident from Ashkenazic depictions of medieval Jewish couples with garlic and recipes, such as a traditional French one for Passover chicken with forty cloves of garlic to represent the number of years the Jews spent in the desert. Moreover, the image of garlic represented the Jewish medieval communities of Speyer, Worms and Mainz.[18] The early-eighteenth-century compiler of mostly less than flattering Jewish oddities (*Merkwürdigkeiten*), Johann Jakob Schudt, noted how the strong smell of garlic emanated from the homes of wealthy German Jews.[19] Heinrich Heine provides an ironic romantic picture of such medieval Jewish dietary predilections in his prose fragment, *The Rabbi of Bacharach*, when the apostate Don Isaac Abarbanel comments, "my nose is not a renegade. When once, by chance I came at dinner time into this street, and the well known savory odor of the Jewish kitchen rose to my nose, I was seized by the same yearning which our fathers felt when they remembered the fleshpots of Egypt.... I saw once more [in my mind] the steamed mutton with garlic and horseradish, fit to raise the dead." Garlic gravy also graced the meal of Leviathan that the thirteenth-century rabbis of Toledo promised the Franciscan friars in Heine's poem "The Disputation."[20]

Supporters of Jewish Emancipation, such as the French liberal Abbé Grégoire in his *Essay on the Physical, Moral and Political Reformation of the Jews* (1789), also sought to explain the contention that Jews exhale bad smells as an effect of diet. "Others ascribe these effects to the frequent use of herbs, such as onions and garlic, the smell of which is penetrating; and some to their eating the flesh of he-goats; while others pretend, that the flesh of geese, which they are remarkably fond of, renders them melancholy and livid, as this food abounds with viscous and gross juices."[21] Even antisemites in the late-nineteenth century tie the Jewish stench to garlic in the widely disseminated mocking "Song in Praise of Garlic" (*Ehren- unn Lobleid oufn Knoblich*): "Garlic, garlic, bold herb / [you] strengthen your Jew's heart and mind / and profits him with / the genuine, kosher Jewish stench."[22]

Pigs Wallowing in the Mud of Anti-Jewish Representation

In addition to commentary on Jewish customary, if not prescribed, garlic consumption, speculations, implications, and accusations, have also been drawn about the Jewish prohibition on eating pork since before the Common Era. This, for them, strange and unusual taboo fascinated ancient writers. They comment that transgressing the prohibition was what Jews found most abhorrent; Juvenal (*Satires* 14.98–99) depicts a God-fearer for whom eating pork is comparable to cannibalism.[23] A God-fearer was a gentile sympathizer with Judaism who was but a circumcision away from conversion, hence one who follows Jewish customs. Others, like the historian Tacitus, tie Jewish abstinence to the "recollection of a plague, for the scab to which this animal [i.e., the pig] is subject, once afflicted them."[24] Here

Tacitus repeats the Hellenistic-Egyptian historian Manetho's charge that the Jews were not liberated from Egypt but instead were expelled because they were disease-bearers. The Jewish historian Josephus claims that the first century C.E. Greek grammarian Apion denounces the Jews for not eating pork and therefore not partaking of civic sacrifices, hence failing to be good citizens, if not, in fact, traitors.[25] Thus the refusal to eat pork in part contributed to the millennia-long belief that Jews would not be loyal to any gentile government.

Early-eighteenth-century German writers such as Johann Andreas Eisenmenger, whose massive, widely read compendium of Talmudic mis-quotes and of the history of alleged Jewish perfidy, *Judaism Unmasked*,[26] would become the source book of anti-Jewish discourse for the next two centuries and a primary source for Feuerbach,[27] also found the pork pro-scription fascinating. Eisenmenger reports that one of the many derogatory names by which Jews label gentiles is "Pork Devourer" (*Schweinenfleischfresser*). As Feuerbach notes in his major work of appetitive anthropology, "The Mystery of Sacrifice or Man Is What He Eats," Johann David Michaelis, the leading eighteenth-century scholar of ancient Israelite religion, cites in his major work *Mosaic Law* this particular label from Eisenmenger as illustra-tive of the contempt with which Jews hold Christians.[28] An assumption shared by some was that the proscription was so significant to Jewish sep-aration from its neighbors that once the Jews begin to eat pork they would become like any other nation and thus no longer hate humanity.

A widely disseminated Christian legend arose to explain why the Jews abstain from pork. According to the story the Jews once tested Jesus' omni-science by hiding a Jewish mother and her children in a pigsty (one of sev-eral variants on the hiding place). They asked him what lay hidden. When Jesus responded "A woman with children," his examiners mockingly retorted with the lie that only a sow and her piglets were wallowing there. Jesus then proclaimed, "If so let them be sow and pigs," and they were transformed. The conclusion drawn is that Jews abstain from pork for fear of engaging in cannibalism by eating a descendant of those fellow trans-formed Jews. Claudine Fabre-Vassas suggests another set of associations of Jews and pigs surrounding the important role not only played in the rural diet of pork but of the action necessarily performed on pigs to ensure their growth and profitability: castration. Castration is as determinative of the pig as circumcision is of the (male) Jew.[29]

The anti-Jewish iconography of the *Judensau*, the Jewish pig (and its insulting verbal counterpart *Saujude*—Jew pig or dirty Jew) that was dis-played throughout German lands, may have reflected this preoccupation with the Kosher proscription on eating pork. By the dream-logic that informs so much stereotype, the Jews were hence inextricably associated with pigs. Isaiah Shachar in his monograph devoted to the *Judensau* places great emphasis upon another site as the most likely source for this motif: Magnentius Hrabanus Maurus's ninth-century popular encyclopedia, *De rerum naturis*, usually known as *De universo*, that formed the basis of many of the medieval bestiaries. Hrabanus's discussion of the pig draws upon an errant translation of Psalm 17:14 that appeared in the Psalm commentaries of Saint Augustine and Cassiodorus Senator:

> The pig similarly signifies the unclean and the sinners of whom it is written in the Psalm: "Their belly is full with your hid (things). They are sated with swine's flesh [reading '*Saturati sunt porcini*' rather than '*saturati sunt filiis*'—sated with sons—that the Hebrew would dictate and that the Vulgate as well reads] and they leave what is superfluous to them for their children." He [i.e., The Psalmist] says the Jews [are full] of unclean [things] which are hidden by the Lord, that is things which are known to be prohibited. By swine's flesh he means polluted things which are named unclean among other precepts of the Old Testament. They [the Jews] transmitted however the remnant of their sins to their sons when they exclaimed: "His blood be on us and on our children." (MT 27:25)

Here syllogism-like Hrabanus draws the conclusion that since swine symbolize the unclean and sinners, and since the Jews are also unclean and sinners, therefore swine can also symbolize Jews. The *Judensau* traveled from cathedral carving to anti-Jewish broadsheet to nineteenth-century caricatures of the signs of Jewish emancipation that had Jews feasting on pigs.[30]

A noteworthy image appears in one of the famed German physicist and satirist Georg Christoph Lichtenberg's best-known prose pieces, the 1783-published parody of Lavater and the physiognomists, "Fragment von Schwänzen" (On Tails).[31] This brief work begins with an analysis of a pig-tail, more specifically a sow's tail of explicitly Jewish nature. The Jewish character of the tail is so obvious that he admonishes his readers: if they do not recognize in this *Schwanz*(tail)—Lichtenberg says if [you] do not "smell, with your eyes, as if you had a nose in them, the lowly slime in which it grew up at *d* . . ."—they should stop reading right there. Lichtenberg goes on to describe the history of this demonic sow to which this tail was once attached. This pig poisons the streets with her unspeakable stench of manure, desecrates a synagogue, and cannibalistically consumes alive her three piglets. Then when attacking a poor young child she is slaughtered and consumed half-cooked by a gang of young beggars.

In sum, from fast to feast to the object of feasting, Jews and their abstinence from pork sparked the gentile imagination.

The Lack of Commensality

The accusation of Jewish misanthropy (*misanthopia/misoxena nomina*) that was related above to the proscription on the consumption of pork found yet more classical sources in their discussions of the Jews' apparent lack of commensality. Sharing meals were a primary form of sociality in the ancient Mediterranean world. The community formed by strangers breaking bread together exemplified the guest-host relationship that mediated the potentially contentious relationship between self and other. To refuse to eat with another was perceived as an act of disrespect and contempt. Tacitus, for example, comments: "The Jews are extremely loyal toward one another, and always ready to show compassion, but toward every other people they feel only hate and enmity" (*Histories* V.5.1). That the Jews "sit apart at meals" (V.5.2) exemplifies his assertion.[32] Eisenmenger devoted a chapter of his work to this traditional charge.[33]

The ethnographer Andree turns to Jewish dietary customs and how they separated the Jews from other people after concluding that religious differences are an insufficient explanation of the widespread hatred of Jews. He begins his examination of this possible source of antisemitism by citing Heinrich Graetz's classic *History of the Jews*. Graetz wrote that "The withdrawal of the Judaeans [*Juden*] from the repasts enjoyed in common by their fellow-citizens" as well as several other dietary customs, such as:

> their abhorence of the flesh of swine, and their abstinence from warm food on the Sabbath, were considered to be the outcome of a perverse nature, whilst their keeping aloof from intimate intercourse with any but their own coreligionists was deemed a proof of their enmity towards mankind in general.[34]

Andree also calls upon Isaak Markus Jost, whose history of the Jews Graetz superseded; Jost saw a proactive stance in keeping kosher. He comments that Jewish dietary proscriptions were "a powerful means by which the chosen people separated themselves from the surrounding heathens."[35] Andree in his ethnography elaborates further on Jost's and Graetz's particular accounts by noting that "those who are not permitted to eat and drink together can also never befriend one another." With reference as well to the uproar in the Jerusalem Church over Peter's sitting at table with the uncircumcised (Acts 11:3) and to Shylock's rebuff of Bassanio's offer to dine, "I will not eat with you, drink with you" (*Merchant of Venice* 1.3), Andree concludes that such practices can lead to arrogance and to viewing others as unclean. Correspondingly, not partaking of the meals and festivals of the Greeks and Romans led to the perception of the Jews as "a foreign element." Thus, the attitudes generated by Jewish eating practices provide, for Andree, the necessary supplement to any theory of antisemitism's origins.[36]

This lack of commensality also figured prominently in arguments against Jewish emancipation. In response to the Prussian court official, Christian Wilhelm von Dohm's 1781 brief for initiating the process of emancipation for Prussian Jewry, *Concerning the Amelioration of the Civil Status of the Jews*, the biblical scholar Johann David Michaelis wrote:

> The purpose of the Law [i.e., Torah] is to maintain the Jews as a people almost completely separate from other peoples, and this purpose is an integral part of all the laws, down to those concerning kosher and non-kosher food, with the result that the Jews have lived as a separate group during 1700 years of dispersion. As long as the Jews continue to observe the Mosaic Laws, as long as they refuse for example, to eat together with us and to form sincere friendship at the table, they will never become fully integrated in the way that Catholics, Lutherans, Germans, Wends, and French live together in one state. (I am not discussing isolated cases, but rather the Jews as a collective entity.) [37]

Blutwürst and Worse

The alleged Jewish dietary practice that may have most influenced Feuerbach's depiction of *Judentum*, however, was the blood libel. This accusation held that Jews undertook the ritual murder of Christian children in order to secure the human blood necessary for the baking of matzah among other culinary, ritual, and medical purposes. Although Jews had been accused of ritual murder of Christian children in the past, most notably the 1144 murder of William of Norwich (England), the blood libel proper emerged in the German town of Fulda in 1235. Although accusations in German lands peaked in the late fifteenth century, the blood libel continued to be invoked into the nineteenth century, especially in Eastern Europe. Eisenmenger devotes a chapter to the question of whether Jews are allowed to kill Christians in his anti-Jewish encyclopedia and source for Feuerbach, *Judaism Unmasked*. When taking up the issue, Eisenmenger does include arguments from Jewish converts as well as from Jewish texts that the charges are false; these included the Jewish view that blood is unclean and that all blood must be drained from meat when prepared for human consumption. Eisenmenger nonetheless lists a number of instances of the libel and concludes that since some reputable (*wackeren*) authorities claim Jews need such blood—mostly on Easter—that one can suppose some truth to it.[38]

The 1840 Damascus Affair, the arrest and torture of 14 Syrian Jews on the charge of ritually murdering a Catholic priest that resonated throughout European political and cultural life, played a prominent role in at least the second edition of the *Essence of Christianity*. Among the consequences of that particular libel was the instigation of Feuerbach's friend Georg Friedrich Daumer to extend his speculations about an ancient Israelite human sacrificial cult of Moloch/Jehova to the contemporary blood libel accusations. In a January 1842 letter to Feuerbach he describes his forthcoming book, *The Fire and Moloch Cult of the Ancient Hebrews*, with its discussion of Jewish blood consumption. In a postscript to that letter Daumer advised Feuerbach to read the even more vicious antisemitic tractate, *The Human Sacrifices of the Ancient Hebrews*, by Friedrich Wilhelm Ghillany (as well as Eisenmenger's *Judaism Unmasked*).[39] Daumer's letter of January 1843 elaborates on where his studies were taking him. While his first work focused on the Moloch cultus and its alleged identity with the cultus of the Hebrew deity Jehova, he does suggest that, following the accounts of several Jewish converts, the spirit of human sacrifice continues among the Jews. Daumer therefore ties the Damascus and other blood libels to the ancient cult. And in this letter the suggestions of the first text are rendered explicit. Jews of all stripes—among Karaites, rabbinic/talmudic traditions, the Sabbatean sect of Frankists, and the Hasidim—engage in such bloody mysteries. He asserts that "the Jews slaughter their own children and the children of other groups." Then he describes Purim or "the Festival of Hamann" as, at least into the medieval period, a wine pressing festival; that is, the Jews would stick people in winepresses and drink the pressed-out blood as holiday wine.[40]

The next edition of the *Essence of Christianity* testifies to Feuerbach having heeded his friend's advice. Although the original publication of that work and its determination of religion as anthropology, of human species-being as the foundation of religion and therefore of meaning and value had been celebrated by his peers, Feuerbach reissues the work in 1843, having made a substantial number of changes. In particular, his text acquired a significant anti-Jewish tone that is immediately alluded to in the appended preface. Feuerbach concludes this new forward with a delineation of his approach in contradistinction to others. He references the work of Daumer and Ghillany[41] as exemplifying "a merely *historical* analysis of Christianity," whereas he is undertaking "an *historico-philosophical* analysis" (xxi).[42] Feuerbach continues, "The historical critic—such a one, for example, as Daumer or Ghillany—shows that the Lord's supper is a rite lineally descended from the ancient cultus of human sacrifice; that once, instead of bread and wine, real human flesh and blood were partaken. I, on the contrary, take as the object of my analysis and reduction only the Christian significance of the rite, that view of it which is *sanctioned* in Christianity and . . . *that significance* . . . is also the *true origin* of that dogma or institution *in so far* as it is *Christian*" (xxi). He is not disavowing the conclusions of those antisemitic writers who argued that not only had the ancient Israelites practiced human sacrifice but that the practice had not been completely discontinued—quite the opposite. Feuerbach is simply doing something else. His choice of example of a merely historical analysis anticipates the classic site of the historical-philosophic difference between Christianity and Judaism: the role of food. Feuerbach concludes his introduction (and opening two chapters) with a newly added contrast between the Christian and "Israelitish" religion. "In relation to the Israelitish religion the Christian religion is one of criticism and freedom. The Israelite trusted himself to do nothing except what was commanded by God; he was without will even in external things; the authority of religion extended itself even to his food" (32).

They Eat Therefore They Are

In the first edition of the *Essence of Christianity*, Feuerbach had remained true to his second chapter's title: "The Essence of Religion, Considered *Generally*" (emphasis added). The original introduction had concluded with the figure of the perpetual systole and diastole of the human circulation system as a metaphor for the process that constitutes religion. "In the religious systole man propels his own nature from himself, he throws himself outward; in the religious diastole he receives the rejected nature into his heart again" (31). The latter, perceived as the actions of God in, with, through, and upon the individual is the principle of salvation and the source of religion's attraction. In the second edition, Feuerbach adds a specific example: his contrast between Christianity and, following the original, "the Israelites." The use of *Israeliten* instead of the terms *Judentum* and *jüdische Religion* that he had employed (and still employed) in the discussions of the first edition's eleventh and twelfth chapters reflected his recent reading of Eisenmenger, Daumer, and Ghillany's works. While he had already employed *Israeliten* when his primary focus had been on the religious practices of the Hebrews or Israelites of the Bible, the use of *Israeliten* in the revised introduction included his Jewish contemporaries. This is indicated by a section added to the second edition's appendices (§10): "Even the *later* Israelites, scattered throughout the world, persecuted and oppressed, adhered with immovable firmness to the egoistic faith of their forefathers" (298; emphasis added). Feuerbach would omit this passage in his third edition.

The primacy given food and eating in Feuerbach's belittling determination of *Judentum* is anticipated in another, also somewhat incongruous, addition to the second edition's Introduction. When discussing the nature of religious sacrifice, as specifically manifested in the Virgin Mary and the Christian ascetic's renunciation of sensuality, Feuerbach inserts a discussion that shifts the emphasis from the sacrifice to the value of what is sacrificed. "For whatever is made an offering to God has an especial value attached to it. . . . That which is the highest in the estimation of man is naturally the highest in the estimation of his God." He shifts the emphasis from love to food—"The Hebrew did not offer to Jehovah unclean, ill-conditioned animals; on the contrary, those which they most highly prized, which they themselves ate, were also the food of God" (26)—before continuing with his discussion of "the heavenly virgin" (27).

The importance Jews allegedly ascribe to food and eating constitutes a significant part of Feuerbach's only chapter devoted to *Judentum* in *Essence of Christianity*, chapter xi ("The Significance of the Creation in Judaism [*Judentum*]"). It is in this chapter that *Judentum*'s relation to Nature, that is, rendering it "the servant to his will and needs" (112), becomes the index of Jewish egoism. And paradigmatic of the Jewish relation to nature is eating. Feuerbach's extended discussion of Jews and food consists of a string of witticisms and wordplays—one of the rare passages outside the introduction that Feuerbach exercises his sardonic wit—at their expense. In contrast to the Greek audiovisual contemplation of Nature, "the Israelites . . . opened only the gastric sense" (114).

Feuerbach comments then become even more biting: "their taste for nature lay only in the palate; their consciousness of God in eating manna" (114). Following this comment, Feuerbach inserts a passage that had originally been but the beginning—and in the new edition all that remained—of an extended contrast between the humane, philosophic Greeks and the calculating profit-oriented Jews that had followed the discussion of eating. "The Greek addicted himself to polite studies, to the fine arts, to philosophy; the Israelite did not rise above the alimentary view [*Brotstudium*] of theology" (114). This reorganization that grouped together the food-related passages may have led George Eliot to her apparently inaccurate translation, since the retention of the phrasing helped sustain the derisive joke. After two food related biblical citations (Exodus 16:12 and Genesis 28:20), Feuerbach declares "Eating is the most solemn [*feier-lichsten*] act or the initiation of the Jewish religion" (114). Yet in sync with the tone of the passage, Feuerbach ultimately inverts the statement and renders it a profane joke: "Thus with them what the sight of the Supreme Being heightened was the appetite for food" (114).

Feuerbach does employ the dietary trope one other time in the chapter. This passage, obscured by Eliot's translation, may also have a more malevolent significance than the mere repetition of a leitmotif. Feuerbach states that "Men used to suppose that insects, vermin [*Ungeziefer*], sprang from carrion and other rubbish" (115). Where Eliot finds this "so uninviting a source," Feuerbach find a source that is so unappetizing [*unappetitlichen*]. Already reference to Jews as vermin, *Ungeziefer*, had already become part of the menagerie of anti-Jewish representations.[43] Hence, two babbling brooks of anti-Jewish discourse converge on this passage.

Communing with Consumption:
Transformation or Merely Symbolic

Not only would it appear that the belittling and derogatory tone that Feuerbach employs when he discusses the Jewish relationship to food is belied by his later work, but it is also in seeming contradiction with *Essence of Christianity*'s "Concluding Application." The last paragraph of this last chapter commences with "Eating and drinking is the mystery [i.e., its underlying meaning and source] of the Lord's Supper;—eating and drinking is, in fact, in itself a religious act; at least, ought to be so" (277). After a litany of ritual-like proscriptions regarding bread and wine ("Forget not . . . ."), Feuerbach situates his audience in a position that he himself seemed to have assumed when discussing Jewish dietary practices.

> And if thou art inclined to smile that I call eating and drinking religious acts, because they are common everyday acts, and are therefore performed by multitudes without thought, without emotion; reflect, that the Lord's Supper is to multitudes a thoughtless, emotionless act, because it takes place often; for the sake of comprehending the religious significance of bread and wine, place thyself in a position where the daily act is unnaturally, violently interrupted. (277)

He culminates his treatise with a (mocking?) paean to the religious import of these common acts of eating and drinking: "Therefore let bread be sacred for us, let wine be sacred, and also let water be sacred. Amen" (278).

What then is one to make of his earlier comments on *Judentum*? Since the "Concluding Application" had already appeared in the first edition, can one argue that he had not fully integrated systematically all of the additions to the second edition? Quite possibly. As noted above, a number of factors had led to the inclusion of the anti-Jewish passages of the second edition; most important were his readings of the work of his friend Daumer and those works suggested by him: Ghillany and Eisenmenger. The residual uproar over the Damascus Blood Libel as well as the reemerging debates over Jewish emancipation in liberal circles, the events which catalyzed Daumer's and Ghillany's writings, may have also affected Feuerbach's initial positive reception of their claims about human sacrifice among the ancient Israelites and its possible continuation to contemporary times. The tradition of dietary antisemitism as discussed above would only have reinforced his conclusions. Between the appearance of the second and third editions, however, Feuerbach continued his research into the history of religious development.

During this research Feuerbach encountered substantive critiques of Daumer and Ghillany's writings in such works as C. v. Lengerke's, *Kanaan. Volks- and Religionsgeschichte Israels* (Königsberg, 1844) and Ernst Meier, *Die ursprüngliche Form des Dekalogs* (Mannheim, 1846); the latter in particular suggested as well that Feuerbach needed to evaluate the Hebrews' relationship to nature more positively.[44] Perhaps most decisive was his change in attitude toward his onetime friend Daumer. In 1844 Daumer published "Contemporary Anthropologism and Criticism" in *Religion und Theologie* (Nürnberg 1844) that included an attack on Feuerbach's anthropologism, calling it "crazy" (*im Zustande der Verrücktheit*). Feuerbach expressed his displeasure with this "infamous" work in a letter to his brother Friedrich (8 December 1844); he described Daumer as a vain, vindictive, and small-minded obscurantist.[45]

As reflected in his 1846 essay "The Essence of Religion" and its expansion in his 1848 *Lectures on the Essence of Religion*, this additional reading material also led to a reevaluation of the significance of sacrifice. Rather than a sign of the alienation, indeed of the negation of human species-being, sacrifice became viewed as an act of appeasement to and reconciliation with nature after the community had appropriated and consumed its fruits. Consequently, his initial afterthoughts on the value of eating and drinking as reflected in his "Concluding Application" became more central. Discussion of Jews and *Judentum* is all but absent, however; unlike in the *Essence of Christianity* no mention of either appears in the discussion of creation.

To Coin a Phrase

Although Feuerbach makes reference to a number of different groups from the indigenous peoples of the Americas and Africa through the Greeks and Romans to the Christians and rationalists in his 1847 essay, "The Question of Immortality from the Standpoint of Anthropology," his examination of why "all people believe in immortality,"[46] there is a similar absence of discussion of Jews and *Judentum*. While the common but erroneous assumption that Jews do not have a belief in life after death may have created complications for his argument and therefore led to this omission, the essay also marks the first appearance in any form of his apothegm. In this call for the direction of human attention to the fulfillment of existence in this life, Feuerbach poses the question: "Is that which man *is* independent from what he *eats*?" (Ist das, was der Mensch *ist*, unabhängig von dem, was er *ißt*).[47]

Feuerbach answers his question affirmatively when he unveils his alimentary materialism in "The Natural Sciences and Revolution," his 1850 review of Jakob Moleschott's *Theory of Nutrition. For the People.*[48] Feuerbach hoped with this new emphasis to continue the project he had begun with the "often castigated"[49] *Essence of Christianity*, namely, undermining the political and religious presuppositions of the nation-state through the replacement of the deity by diet. As Feuerbach facetiously remarks at the beginning of his review, the state, ironically, fails to censor that which is most subversive to arbitrary social divisions: the natural sciences and its universality. "Aristocratic and bourgeois stomachs are not different."[50] Food and its consumption actualize his monistic speculations. "Food (*Nahrung*) alone is substance, the identity of spirit and nature . . . is the Spinozistic *Hen kai pan* (One and All) . . . . Being is one with eating, to be means to eat." With the exception of this allusion to Spinoza, however, reference to *Judentum* is, in light of the earlier characterizations, surprisingly absent. Feuerbach is not only rendering philosophy in material terms, he is also calling for the materialization of this new philosophy. "A humane diet is the foundation of human development and disposition. Want to better the people, then give them better food instead of declaiming against sin." It is at this junction of his own declamations that Feuerbach provides his punning apothegm what would be its most notorious form: "Der Mensch ist, was er ißt / You are what you eat."[51]

Feuerbach would continue his exploration of the political, religious, and epistemological implications of his "Diet-materialism" in "The Secret of Sacrifice, or Man Is What He Eats," which he first published in the 1866 edition of his collected works. While relishing the outrage directed at him because of his association with the anthropological and ontological claims made by his "scurrilous" saying, Feuerbach proceeds to analyze the most fundamental religious act: sacrifice. He defines sacrifice not in the ascetic terms of the *Essence of Christianity* but in culinary terms: sacrifice is about feeding the gods (*Opfern heißt die Götter speisen*). Here the unity of "I" and "You" (*Ich und Du*) that constituted the essence of religion as well as the highest and ultimate principle of Feuerbach's "Philosophy of the Future" (1843) is founded upon eating and drinking. These common practices "not only hold body and soul together, but also God and humanity, and I and You."[52]

Unlike much of the work, whether addressing eating or not, whether venerating egoism or not, during the last twenty-five years of his life, *Judentum* is more than merely mentioned. While he notes that Michaelis argues that Jewish dietary laws had led to bloody conflicts and that Eisenmenger noted that by calling Christians "Pork Devourers" Jews expressed their contempt for them, Feuerbach also seems to go out of his way to separate the Hebrews from blood consumption whether that of humans or of animals. But he also employs the Jews as negative example of the fundamental import of commensality: "were not the Jews ridiculed and hated by the heathen because they (i.e., the Jews) scorned the foods that they, the heathens, loved." He then pairs a line from an early fifth century C.E. poem by Rutilius Namantianus that describes a Jew as "a creature that quarrels with sound human food"[53] with a passage from Synesius, a roughly contemporaneous Christian neo-Platonist, about the holiness of the table, "because upon it God honors love and hospitality."[54] After this juxtaposition Feuerbach undertakes a series of inversions that betray another side to his apothegm. "Is not the opposite [of Synesius's sentiments] the case, that the God of hatred and enmity is worshipped where commensality is annulled?" He follows up this question with another: "Who does not eat what we *eat, is* he also not what we are?"[55]

The virtual absence of discussion of *Judentum* in Feuerbach's later work may reflect how once eating became the master trope and egoism positively reevaluated[56] then his earlier condemnation of Judaism on these grounds would have been harder to assert. When the occasion arises, however, along with Feuerbach's sardonicism and delight in the chiasmatic, *Judentum* as figure returns to provide the antipode of whatever is the object of his analysis. Where *Judentum* is the originary inversion of Christianity in *Essence of Christianity*, so in this late work it allows him to represent the social negation of his anthropological and ontological claim: "you are what you eat." In effect, his "Diet-materialism" with its dialectics of eating ultimately reproduces the unappetizing history of the dietetics of antisemitism that was already served up in *Essence of Christianity*.

Notes

1. I would like to thank Professor Leonard Hummel of Vanderbilt Divinity School and the editors of this volume for their comments on earlier versions of this essay.
2. *Das Wesen des Christentums*, vol. 5 of Ludwig Feuerbach, *Gesammelte Werke*, Werner Schuffenhauer, ed., 20 vols. (Berlin: Akademie Verlag, 1967–); first edition, 1841; second expanded edition, 1843; third reworked and expanded edition, 1849. Eng. trans.: *The Essence of Christianity*, George Eliot, trans. (Buffalo: Prometheus Books, 1989).
3. The term is borrowed from Marx Wartofsky, *Feuerbach* (Cambridge: Cambridge University Press, 1977), 416.
4. Cf. the dismissive Eugene Kamenka, *The Philosophy of Ludwig Feuerbach* (London: Routledge and Kegan Paul, 1970); and the absence of discussion in Van A. Harvey, *Feuerbach and the Interpretation of Religion* (Cambridge: Cambridge University Press, 1995).
5. Cf. *Grundsätze zur Philosophie der Zukunft* (1843) in *Kleinere Schriften II*, vol. 9 of L Feuerbach, *Gesammelte Werke*.
6. Cf. "Das Geheimnis des Opfers oder Der Mensch ist, was er ißt" (1862/1866) in *Kleinere Schriften IV*, vol. 11 of Feuerbach, *Gesammelte Werke*.
7. Anthèlme Brillat-Savarin's 1825 treatise, *The Physiology of Taste*, bears instead the epigraph: "Tell me what you eat, I will tell you who you are." Wartofsky, *Feuerbach*, 451 n.6, cites an interesting earlier play on "ist" (is) and "isst" (eats) from the late eighteenth century: Friedrich Dicke's pamphlet ""Über ißt und ist: Eine Erklärung des Ursprungs des Opfers" (Concerning Eating and Being: An Explanation of the Origin of Sacrifice), a title not unlike Feuerbach's 1862, "Die Geheimniß des Opfers oder der Mensch ist was er ißt" (The Mystery of Sacrifice, or Man Is What He Eats).
8. Usually translated as Judaism, the German term *Judentum* also includes within its purview the people, Jewry, and their character, Jewishness, as well as their religious practices and beliefs. Because Feuerbach's use of *Judentum* also points to the broader definition, I employ that term throughout this essay.
9. "Judaism is worldly Christianity [*weltliche Christentum*], Christianity spiritual Judaism [*geistliche Judentum*]. . . . Christianity has spiritualized [*vergeistigt*] the egoism of Judaism into subjectivity"; Feuerbach, *Essence*, 120–121.

10. Feuerbach, *Essence*, 114.
11. Cf. Julius Carlebach, *Karl Marx and the Radical Critique of Judaism* (London: Routledge & Kegan Paul, 1978), 104–108; Paul Lawrence Rose, *Revolutionary Antisemitism in Germany. From Kant to Wagner* (Princeton: Princeton University press, 1990); and with the correct translation, Jacob Katz, *From Prejudice to Destruction. Anti-Semitism, 1700–1933* (Cambridge: Harvard University Press, 1980), 162–164.
12. Unfortunately, though, Eliot's translation of the second edition is the only version of *Essence of Christianity* available for Anglophones. Since Feuerbach excised some of his most virulent comments in the third edition, Eliot's translation allowed the stench of his anti-Jewish rhetoric to linger with his English-speaking readership.
13. Cit. Menahem Stern, ed., *Greek and Latin Authors on Jews and Judaism*, 3 vols. (Jerusalem: Israel Academy of Sciences and Humanities, 1980), vol. 2: 98–99.
14. Richard Andree, *Zur Volkskunde der Juden* (Bielefeld: Velhagen und Klasing, 1881), 68–69. Though obviously not a source for Feuerbach, his work serves as a reasonable indicator of the availability of these antisemitic representations and discourses to an educated non-Jew of the nineteenth century such as Feuerbach.
15. Cit. Stern, *Greek and Latin*, 2:605–606.
16. Cf. Gustav Jaeger, *Entdeckung der Seele*, vol. 1, third edition (Leipzig: W. Kohlhammer, 1884), 113; vol. 2 appeared some two decades later.
17. Andree, *Zur Volkskunde*, 68.
18. Maria Diemling presented a paper on "Garlic in Jewish-Christian Polemical Discourse in Early Modern Ashkenaz" at the Fifteenth Klutznick-Harris Symposium on "Food and Jews" in 2002; puffin.creighton.edu/klutznick/ks%2015%20abstracts.htm. "Ashkenaz" is the Jewish term for Germany, geographically the lands that surround the Rhine and Rhône rivers.
19. Johann Jakob Schudt, *Jüdische Merkwürdigkeiten* (Frankfurt, 1714), 349.
20. Heinrich Heine, *The Rabbi of Bacharach*, in Elizabeth Petuchowski, *Jewish Stories and Melodies*, ed. (New York: Marcus Wiener, 1987), 76.
21. In Paul Mendes-Flohr and Jehuda Reinharz, eds., *The Jew in the Modern World*, 2d ed. (New York: Oxford University Press, 1995), 52.
22. Knoblich, Knoblich, toffes Gwarz / Stärkst dien Jüden Sinn unn Harz, / Unn giebst ihn die ganze Wuch / Aechten, koschern, Jüdeng'ruch; cit. Eduard Fuchs, *Die Juden in der Karikatur. Ein Beitrag zur Kulturgeschichte* (Munich: Verlag Albert Langen, 1921), 282.
23. Cit. Stern, *Greek and Latin*, 2:102–103.
24. *Histories* 4.2; cit. Cit. Stern, *Greek and Latin*, 2:18, 25.
25. *Contra Apion* II.137; cit. Stern, *Greek and Latin*, 1:415.
26. *Entdecktes Judenthum*, 2 vols. (Koenigsberg, 1711).
27. See especially appendix 10 that Feuerbach added to the second edition of *Essence of Christianity* (most of the most inflammatory material was excised from the third).

28. Feuerbach, "Das Geheimnis," 28.

29. Claudine Fabre-Vassas, *The Singular Beast: Jews, Christians, and the Pig*, Carol Volk, trans. (New york: Columbia University Press, 1997), 92–94.

30. Isaiah Shachar, *The Judensau: A Medieval Anti-Jewish Motif and Its History* (London: The Warburg Institute, 1974) illustrates this trajectory with over one hundred images of Jews with and as pigs. Hrabanus passage translated on p. 70.

31. In Georg Christoph Lichtenberg, *Schriften und Briefe*, F. H. Mautner, ed., 4 vols. (Frankfurt/M: Insel, 1983), vol. 2, 117.

32. *Histories* 5.1, 2; cit. Stern, *Greek and Latin*, 2:19, 26.

33. *Entdecktes Judenthum*, vol. 2, chap. 12.

34. Heinrich Graetz, *History of the Jews*, Bella Löwy, trans., 6 vols. (Philadelphia: Jewish Publication Society, 1891–1898) 2:203.

35. Isaak Markus Jost, *Geschichte des Judenthums und seine Sekten*, 3 vols. (Leipzig: Dörffling und Franke, 1857–1859), 1:129.

36. Andree, *Zur Volkskunde*, 169–172.

37. "Arguments Against Dohm," in Mendes-Flohr and Reinharz, *Jew in the Modern World*, 42–43. Originally appeared in *Orientalische und Exegetische Bibliotek*, 19 (1782).

38. Eisenmenger, *Entdecktes Judentum*, 2: 227.

39. Letter 282, in Feuerbach, *Briefwechsel II*, vol. 18 of *Gesammelte Werke*, 150–152; Daumer, *Der Feuer- und Molochdienst der alten Hebräer als urväterlicher, legaler, orthodoxer Kultus der nation, historisch-kritisch nachgewiesen* (Braunschweig: F. Otto, 1842); Ghillany, *Die Menschenopfer der alten Hebräer* (Nürnberg, 1842).

40. Letter 347, in Feuerbach, *Briefwechsel II (1840–1844)*, vol. 18 of *Gesammelte Werke* 243–247. This accusation of the necessity for the consumption of the blood of non-Jews during Purim was quite recently reiterated in a 10 March 2003 column in the Saudi government-supported newspaper *Al- Riyadh*. Dr. Umayma Ahmad Al-Jalahma of King Faisal University discussed the use of blood in Purim pastries.

41. All mention of Ghillany, whose antisemitism grew in intensity even as Daumer recanted his earlier position, is removed the third edition of *Essence of Christianity*. Feuerbach also omits many of the anti-Jewish claims of Eisenmenger from his appendix.

42. All page references are to the Eliot translation.

43. Cf. Rainer Erb and Werner Bergmann, *Die Nachseite der Judenemanzipation : der Widerstand gegen die Integration der Juden in Deutschland 1780–1860* (Berlin: Metropol, 1989).

44. Cf. Feuerbach's 28 June 1844 letter to his brother Friedrich (in *Briefwechsel* 18: 361); and Francesco Tomasoni, "Heidentum und Judentum: Vom schärfsten Gegensatz zur Annäherung. Eine Entwicklungslinie vom Wesen des Christentums bis zur Theogonie," in *Ludwig Feuerbach und die Geschichte der Philosophie*, Walter Jaeschke and Francesco Tomasoni, ed. (Berlin: Akadamie Verlag, 1998), esp. 157–163.

45. *Briefwechsel,* 18:420–421.

46. "Die Unsterblichkeitsfrage vom Standpunkt der Anthropologie," in *Kleinere Schriften,* 10:192.

47. Ibid., 10:230.

48. "Die Naturwissenschaft und die Revolution," in *Kleinere Schriften,* 10: 347–368.

49. Forward to the second volume of the 1866 edition of his collected works; *Kleinere Schriften,* 10:191.

50. "Die Naturwissenschaft," 10:351.

51. Ibid., 10:358, 367.

52. "Das Geheimnis," 11:27, 41.

53. Ibid., 11:43, 44; cit. Stern, *Greek and Latin,* 2:662, 663.

54. "Das Geheimnis," 11:44.

55. Ibid.

56. Cf. Harvey, *Feuerbach and the Interpretation of Religion,* esp. 175–179.

Chapter 8 ∽

TOLSTOY'S BODY

DIET, DESIRE, AND DENIAL

Ronald L. LeBlanc

Do not let us stupefy ourselves, do not let us kill our reason with strong food that is not natural to man.

I think that the lust for food is closely linked with sexual lust and serves as its basis.

... the tastes of plain food and fruit ... do not arouse lust. Lust is aroused by ... gourmet dishes.

—L. N. Tolstoy

Recent critical thought on the human body has mounted a serious challenge to the mind/body dichotomy, a construct that has long dominated the European philosophical tradition and that became effectively dogmatized in the wake of René Descartes's writings during the early modern period. Contemporary body theorists, especially those who adopt a feminist perspective, boldly reject the dualistic Cartesian model of the body as a machine distinct from, and subordinate to, the workings of the mind and soul.[1] Lev Nikolaevich Tolstoy's late-nineteenth-century vision of the human body—as an unruly and dangerous "desiring" machine that must be somehow directed and controlled by instructions from the mind and/or soul—would seem to fit perfectly what Bryan Turner has characterized as the Cartesian paradigm of ascetic rationalism, whereby corporeal government (regulation of the body) enables the soul to become liberated from its incarceration within the body.[2] However, the enormity of Tolstoy's worldwide reputation as a great writer, as well as a committed social reformer, political activist, moral spokesman, and religious prophet, often overshadows and conceals his deeply problematic relationship with the impulses of his own body. As we know from his diaries, letters, and literary works (fictional and non-fictional alike), Tolstoy's attitude toward sensual pleasure was deeply ambivalent. On the one hand, he himself seems to have possessed acute sensual sensibilities and strong physical appetites for the pleasures of the flesh; but at the same time, he possessed an equally strong desire for moral and spiritual self-perfection that prompted him to attempt to regulate closely his bodily lusts. His early diaries show him to be at once "over-addicted to self-analysis and self-reproach" and "abnormally sensual."[3] Throughout his life, Judith Armstrong argues, Tolstoy "wages a constant but losing battle with his shameful sexual appetites."[4] "From his youth to his old age," observes another critic, "Tolstoy was body-haunted, obsessed equally by sexual desire and the guilt of sexual satisfaction."[5] One of his contemporaries, the writer and critic Dmitry Merezhkovsky, recognized in this Russian writer's works such a keen intuitive awareness of— and appreciation for—the instinctive, animal life of human beings that he called Tolstoy a "seer of the flesh."[6]

After the midlife spiritual crisis that he experienced during the late 1870s and early 1880s, however, Tolstoy's rich pagan appreciation of earthly delights was eclipsed by deep feelings of moral guilt over the enjoyment of bodily pleasures. The Russian author now came to condemn, quite categorically, those pleasures of the flesh that he had once celebrated so memorably in his fiction, and he began to advocate instead a rigorous brand of Christian asceticism. "When Tolstoy, the sensualist, turned moralist," one critic explains,

> the body with its carnal desires ceased to be the subject of ecstasy and became the target of scorn. Tolstoy, who had once glorified the body, now preached that the flesh had to be forcibly broken to bring about the liberation and salvation of the soul. He demanded the mortification of the body, and he was no less insistent in this demand than Saint Anthony or the pillar saints in the Lybian desert.[7]

Unlike Merezhkovsky, Rozanov, and other Russian religious thinkers at the turn of the century, who advanced the modernist project of rehabilitating the philosophical (and even metaphysical) value of the body by seeking to destigmatize its physiological aspects, Tolstoy instead adopted the bipolar view of medieval Christianity, still espoused by the Russian Orthodox Church during his time, which expressed deep contempt for the flesh and sublime exaltation of the spirit.[8] What predominates in the writings of Tolstoy's post-conversion period, accordingly, is the strict moral imperative to subdue the desires of the flesh, to subordinate our physical urges to our spiritual aspirations, and to transcend our base animal natures in order to allow the divine element that lies buried deep within us to emerge. In his later works it becomes especially clear that Tolstoy now condemns sexual passion as an inherently demeaning, degrading, and destructive instinct within human beings, a brutish animal urge that only impedes people in their quest for moral and spiritual self-perfection.

In this essay I wish to explore how the "moral masochism" reflected in Tolstoy's evolving attitude toward the body and human sexuality—his movement from pagan hedonism to Christian asceticism, from vigorous self-enjoyment to rigorous self-denial—is mirrored by his treatment of gastronomic indulgence.[9] As the carnal pleasures of the flesh came increasingly to be seen as sinful temptations that lure people away from the strait and narrow path of moral righteousness and spiritual self-perfection, Tolstoy tended more and more to regard the gastronomic pleasures of the table with a similar feeling of revulsion and disgust—as bodily pleasures that can no longer be considered morally and spiritually palatable.[10] The gluttonous abdomen, in short, had become as much a seductive demon for the ascetic Tolstoy to exorcise as had the lascivious loins. His advocacy of such radical ideals in sexual matters as celibacy, chastity, and conjugal continence is thus matched by his adoption of extreme dietary measures, such as vegetarianism, abstinence, and fasting. Eating meat and other rich food items, he came strongly to believe, actively stimulates carnal appetite; by removing such culinary luxuries from one's diet, therefore, a person would be able to reduce considerably the incidence and the intensity of concupiscence. Not unlike Sylvester Graham, John Harvey Kellogg, and a number of other health reformers with a religious bent in nineteenth-century America, Tolstoy late in his life adopted a series of dietary practices that were designed to reduce significantly, if not to eliminate entirely, sexual desire. He thus proceeded, much like these "Christian physiologists" from the diet-conscious United States, to wage an ascetic holy war against the body, launching what was essentially a male purity campaign that operated on the assumption that diet can help shape sexual morality.[11] However, Tolstoy's dietary asceticism, as we shall see, ultimately put him at odds not only with an important branch within the Russian vegetarian movement, but also with his own body. This latter conflict emerged in part because his hearty appetite for comestibles that were more gastronomically appealing than the bland peasant diet of oatmeal and cabbage soup never completely abated.

But it also arose because his conversion to a vegetarian diet appears to have exacerbated the gastrointestinal ailments that plagued him throughout the second half of his life. If Tolstoy's moral masochism inclined him toward an anhedronic feeling of "dis-gust" (i.e., a physiological revulsion at, or literally a lack of taste for, physical pleasures), then his body may be said to have responded by reminding him, in a corporeal case of the return of the repressed, that desire is not effectively silenced by mere denial.

Curbing Animal Appetites: Tolstoy's Campaign Against Bodily Pleasure

It was soon after completing the writing of *Anna Karenina* (1877) that Tolstoy experienced the spiritual crisis that made it impossible for him to continue living his life and crafting his art in the same manner he had formerly. As he reveals in his *Confession* (1879), the successful, middle-aged author suddenly became thoroughly disenchanted with his conventional mode of life, calling into question the basic values and fundamental beliefs that had guided his conduct up to this point in his life. The conditions of luxury, idleness, and epicurean indulgence under which the "parasites" from the privileged classes live in late imperial Russia, Tolstoy now realized, make it virtually impossible for them ever to understand the true meaning of life. In keeping with his view of gentry epicureanism as a pervasive and infectious pathological condition, Tolstoy not only advocates eating and living like a simple peasant. He also comes to recognize that gastronomic appetite and sexual desire are powerful libidinal drives that cannot be successfully restrained, moderated or controlled through sheer willpower. The physical pleasures of the flesh and the oral delights of the palate must instead be avoided entirely since they are, by their very nature, so debasing, dangerous, and destructive for any human being who wishes to rise at all above the level of gratifying his or her base animal inclinations. Like alcohol, tobacco, and other addictive drugs, food and sex are seen to "stupefy" us, not only because they stimulate our desire for sensual pleasure, but more importantly because they blur the demands of our moral conscience and thus deaden the spiritual or divine part of our human nature. The deeply disillusioned Russian author thus emerges from his spiritual crisis of the late 1870s and early 1880s as a man fully at war with the physical pleasures that tempt the human body.[12] He now comes to regard both food and sex as highly intoxicating and addictive sources of pleasure whose despotic power over man's will, and debilitating effect upon his life, called for more radical measures than mere moderation and restraint.

   This shift to more radical measures for dealing with the allure of physical pleasures appears to have stemmed largely from Tolstoy's evolving view of the self. In his essay, *On Life* (1888), Tolstoy delineated between two very distinct aspects of the inner self within each human being: (1) an "animal personality" that strives instinctively for the gratification of one's egoistic desires (especially the desire for physical pleasure), and (2) a "rational consciousness" that aspires toward the morally good, concerning itself especially with the welfare of others. As Henrietta Mondry points out, there is a long-standing European philosophical tradition, particularly within Christianity, of equating animality with mere physiology. "European thought has separated animals and humans into binary categories, with the animal as the stigmatized Other," she explains.[13] Tolstoy's model of the self perpetuates these Cartesian dualisms of flesh and spirit, body and soul, animal and divine. The aim of human life, Tolstoy explains in this essay, ought to consist in bringing about "the subservience of our animal body to the law of reason" (XXVI, 348)—that is, we should be seeking to transcend the physical pleasure and corporeal well-being sought by our lower animal self and striving to practice a compassionate Christian love that places altruistic concern for others above selfish concern for oneself.[14] In another of his religious essays, *The Kingdom of God is Within You* (1893), Tolstoy acknowledges that divine perfection is an ideal that human beings can strive for but never actually attain (he calls it "the asymptote of human life" [XXVIII, 77]); yet the striving after divine perfection nonetheless "deflects the direction of man's life from its animal condition" (XXVIII, 78). In our lives, as one of the peasants had advised Levin in *Anna Karenina*, we should be aiming to live not for our belly, but for our soul.[15] The male protagonists in many of Tolstoy's later works of fiction are thus portrayed at various stages of the process of discovering this divine aspect within themselves, trying to renounce their base animal personalities and coarse sensual appetites. In each case, the addictive quality of those intoxicating vices that characterize the idleness, comfort, and luxury of upper-class life are shown to have inured these men to what Tolstoy considered to be the debasing animal activities from which they derive sensual pleasure and enjoyment (especially eating and fornicating), activities that are condoned, if not implicitly encouraged, by the customs, mores, and values of their social milieu.

   The social milieu that existed in late nineteenth-century Russia for aristocrats like Tolstoy was marked by a significant broadening of access to the cultural and material privileges that had traditionally been the exclusive domain of the nobility under earlier tsarist regimes. The Age of Reform, inaugurated with the emancipation of the serfs in 1861, witnessed the launching of a state-sponsored process of rapid industrialization and modernization of the country, where an enlarged public sphere and increased social mobility hastened the growth of a burgeoning middle class (consisting largely of merchants, professional people, and industrialists), eager to share in the bounty of a newly found affluence. New restaurants and department stores appeared in a growing number of Russian cities, along with other forms of retail sales and popular mass entertainment.[16] With the beginnings of a consumer society finally taking root in Russia, however, there also arose a moral backlash generated by anxieties about the public's increasing desire for—and widespread consumption of—these new commodities. Fears about the negative effects that commercialization might have upon Russian society, especially in the sphere of traditional high culture where "boulevardization" (or vulgarization) of art was purportedly taking place, were expressed mainly by members of the intelligentsia, whose ascetic commitment to public service was seriously offended and even threatened by the philistine pursuit of personal comfort, luxury, leisure, and sensual indulgence that they were now observing all around them. Medical and pedagogical literature in Russia from the 1890s and early 1900s, as Laura Engelstein observes, was marked by a preoccupation with male sexual desire, teaching the public the self-restraint and internalized control that were deemed necessary for fulfilling one's civic responsibility.[17]

Tolstoy was among those educated Russians of his generation who feared the disorder and perhaps even destruction that the desire for pleasure—especially sexual and gastronomical pleasure—could engender. In 1881, when he moved with his family to live in Moscow, Tolstoy volunteered to serve as a census-taker in the capital city's very worst slums, undergoing an eye-opening experience that many scholars believe radically changed his view of the existing social order. "Town life was a great trial for Tolstoy," writes one of his biographers,

> the crying contrast between city beggars and the insolent opulence of the rich, at every street corner hungry beggars with hands stretched out for alms, and gluttons gorging themselves in brilliantly lighted restaurants, coachmen shivering on their boxes whilst their masters enjoyed the music of the theatres or churches—all this made his heart ache, imbued as he was with the Christian spirit and seeking for its manifestation around him.[18]

Tolstoy's bitter disillusionment with the existing social order found expression in a scathing essay, *What Then Must We Do?* (1886), in which the author bemoans the fact that tens of thousands of cold, hungry people are forced to suffer while "I and thousands of others like me overeat ourselves with beef steaks and sturgeon" (XXV, 190). The seemingly perpetual holiday enjoyed by the materially wealthy, whom Tolstoy refers to disdainfully as the "ever-feasting" ones, was held to be directly responsible for the abject misery of the poor. Feelings of guilt about enjoying membership in the privileged classes of late imperial Russia prompted Tolstoy to confess that he is a "parasite" and a "louse" (XXV, 246) who feeds upon the labors of others and thus indirectly causes them to die of starvation. In the immediate wake of his census-taking experience in Moscow, Tolstoy endeavored throughout the 1880s to reform radically his own personal life, ultimately renouncing all superfluous pleasures (hunting, smoking, drinking alcohol, eating meat, indulging in sex, etc.) and dedicating himself to productive labor on behalf of the general welfare of others.

Tolstoy's Victorian assault upon the pleasure principle during his post-conversion years finds perhaps its most explicit artistic expression in his highly controversial novella, *The Kreutzer Sonata* (1889). The central character, Pozdnyshev, a jealous, murderous husband who confesses that his swinish animal nature overpowered his more human side, manages to strip carnal love of any emotional or spiritual value it might have, reducing it to a brutish animal lust that dominates, controls, and eventually ruins those who engage in it. The exacerbated concupiscence that results from an unregulated animality, Tolstoy's hero asserts, is not only destructive, but also highly addictive. "I had become what is called a fornicator," Pozdnyshev confesses about his purported sexual addiction,

> To be a fornicator is a physical condition like that of a morphine addict, a drunkard, or a smoker. As a morphine addict, a drunkard, or a smoker is no longer normal, so too a man who has known several women for his pleasure is not normal but is a man perverted forever, a fornicator . . . . A fornicator may restrain himself, may struggle, but he will never have those pure, simple, clear, brotherly relations with a woman. . . . And I had become and I remained a fornicator, and it was this that brought me to ruin. (XXVII, 19)

Wishing to leave no doubt in the reader's mind that the extreme opinions on sexuality, love, and marriage expressed by his deranged protagonist accurately reflect the author's own views, Tolstoy wrote an "Afterword to *The Kreutzer Sonata*" (1890), in which he categorically condemns carnal love and asserts that total sexual continence, "which constitutes an indispensable condition of human dignity in the unmarried state, is still more essential in the married one" (XXVII, 81). Husbands and wives are thus encouraged to live together chastely, like brother and sister, within their conjugal unions.

By questioning the validity of marriage as a Christian institution, by appealing for a non-carnal, compassionate form of love in the relationship between the sexes, and by championing chastity and sexual continence as an ideal for young couples (whether single or married), *The Kreutzer Sonata* launched a very heated debate in Russia during the 1890s over the question of sexual morality.[19] For our purposes, what is particularly illuminating about the highly negative and pessimistic views on carnal love and marriage expressed by Pozdnyshev in *The Kreutzer Sonata*, and later by Tolstoy in his "Afterword to *The Kreutzer Sonata*," is how, in both instances, excesses of sexual debauchery are linked directly and causally with gastronomic indulgence. The young males of Pozdnyshev's social class, for instance, are said to be fed the types and quantities of food that inflame their sensuality. "The men of our circle," Pozdnyshev asserts, "are kept and fed like breeding stallions" (XXVII, 303). The same seems to be true of gentry women, whose main (perhaps even sole) function, we are told, is to bewitch men with their sexual allure. Describing his own wife's animal sexuality, Pozdnyshev says that "she was like a fresh, well-fed, harnessed horse, whose bridle has been removed" (XXVII, 47). The libidinal connection between diet and sex, according to Pozdnyshev, is one of direct cause and effect: eating rich and fleshly foods leads directly and ineluctably to the arousal of sexual desire. "You see, our stimulating superfluity of food, together with complete physical idleness, is nothing but the systematic excitation of sexual lust," he explains.

> The usual food of a young peasant lad is bread, kvas, and onions; he keeps alive and is vigorous and healthy; his task is light agricultural work. When he goes to perform railway work, his rations are buckwheat porridge and a pound of meat a day. But he works off that pound of meat during his sixteen hours wheeling around thirty pound barrow-loads, so it is just enough for him. But we, who consume two pounds of meat every day, and game, and fish, and all sorts of hot foods and drinks—where does all that go? Into excesses of sensuality. (XXVII, 23)

Pozdnyshev thus extends into the realm of diet and sexuality the fundamental moral contrast Tolstoy had described in *Confession* between the authentic peasant way of life (based on hard work and simplicity) and the decadent gentry way of life (based on idleness and luxury). The industrious peasant, who subsists on a basic diet of healthy, wholesome foods, works off his sexual energy in exhausting manual labor; the idle rich, meanwhile, who indulge their aristocratic appetite for all sorts of tasty and stimulating foods (served and consumed in immoderate amounts), are plagued by sexual excitation and carnal lust. "What is really needed," Tolstoy once observed in regard to the necessity of incorporating physical toil into one's life, "is to reject the criminal view that I am to eat and sleep merely for my pleasure, and to adopt the simple and correct view, which the peasants grow up with and hold, that man is primarily a machine, which has to be stoked with food in order to be nourished, and that it is, therefore, shameful, oppressive, and impossible to go on eating without doing any work" (XXV, 388).

In the decadent bourgeois society depicted in *The Kreutzer Sonata*, it is, of course, this "criminal" aristocratic view of the body as a site for pleasure (rather than the "simple" and "correct" peasant view of the body as a machine designed for labor) that prevails within Pozdnyshev's social milieu. Rich foods, as a result, only further fuel the flames of that middle-class crowd's insatiable desire for sexual pleasure. When he accounts for the origins of his own fatal infatuation with the woman he would later wed, grow to hate, and subsequently murder, Pozdnyshev asserts that his carnal love for her was the result, in large part, of "the excess of food I consumed while living an idle life" (XXVII, 24). The direct cause-and-effect connection between gastronomic excess and sexual excitation is reiterated when Pozdnyshev claims that, had he lived in circumstances normal to man, "consuming just enough food to suffice for the work I did," he would not have fallen in love and "none of all this would have happened" (XXVII, 24). In a variant version of *The Kreutzer Sonata* that circulated privately in manuscript form, Pozdnyshev states rather bluntly, "All of our love affairs and marriages are, for the most part, conditioned by the food we eat" (XXVII, 303). In his "Afterword to *The Kreutzer Sonata*," Tolstoy would voice a similar sentiment, castigating upperclass parents for raising their children to behave like animals: they are taught to be concerned only with their physical appetites and well-tended bodies. "And in pampered children, as in all sorts of overfed animals," Tolstoy writes, "there is an unnaturally early appearance of an irresistible sensuality, which is the occasion of the terrible sufferings of these children in adolescence" (XXVII, 82). As a consequence, he adds, "the most terrible sexual vices and diseases are the normal condition for children of both sexes, and they often persist even into adulthood" (XXVII, 82).

Tolstoy's Way of No Flesh: Ascetic Vegetarianism

Given Tolstoy's artistic representation of food in *The Kreutzer Sonata* and in some of his other postconversion works of fiction as a dangerous stimulant that can excite sexual lust, it should not surprise us terribly to find that among the extreme measures against physical pleasure the author came to advocate late in his life (such as his renunciation of hunting, drinking, smoking, and fornicating) he would also include vegetarianism. After all, if the moral and spiritual ideal that we should all be striving to attain is absolute sexual continence, then it follows that we should avoid eating meat, since fleshly food, Tolstoy came seriously to believe, arouses in us sexual passion and carnal desire. And indeed, when Tolstoy writes the essay, *The First Step* (1891), in which he explains his reasons for refusing to eat meat, his motivation for vegetarianism turns out to be more ascetic and religious than ethical or humanitarian. Eating fleshly foods is morally wrong, Tolstoy asserts in this essay, not only because it perpetuates cruelty and brutal violence toward animals (which he addresses near the end of his essay when he describes quite graphically his recent visit to a slaughterhouse in Tula). Meat-eating is also to be condemned, he writes, because it "serves only to develop animal feelings, to excite lust, and to promote fornication and drunkenness" (XXIX, 84). Tolstoy contends, in other words, that a carnal diet stimulates a carnal appetite: that eating animal food arouses animal passions. He argues, in fact, that one should abstain from eating not just meat, but any rich and tasty food item from which one might conceivably derive gustatory enjoyment. After all, gastronomic pleasure, in Tolstoy's chain of reasoning, leads directly and ineluctably to sexual pleasure. Accordingly, he inveighs strongly in this essay against the sin of gluttony (overeating) and he encourages his readers to practice strict abstinence and fasting, rather than mere moderation, in matters concerning the consumption of food and drink.

In the opening sections of *The First Step*, where he refers to some of the ancient Greek philosophers as well as to the early Church fathers, Tolstoy asserts that it is impossible for one to lead a good and moral life—whether as a Christian or as a pagan—unless one begins with abstinence and self-abnegation. Well in advance of Michel Foucault's argument in his *History of Sexuality* (1984), Tolstoy thus draws our attention to the direct continuities that exist between the first Christian doctrines on the body and the moral philosophy of classical antiquity. But where Foucault conceptualizes sexuality in ancient Greece as part of a series of dietetic practices—a "technique of the self," as he puts it—that turned desire into a matter of the proper use of pleasure, Tolstoy seeks instead to subordinate desire to a very rigid moral code.[20] The indispensable "first step" up the hierarchical ladder of moral virtues for both Christians and pagans alike, Tolstoy writes, involves the renunciation of our basic physical appetites and our liberation from the animal lusts that plague us. Tolstoy identifies the three principal lusts that torment human beings as "gluttony, idleness, and carnal love" (XXIX, 73–74). Not unlike Pozdnyshev in *The Kreutzer Sonata*, Tolstoy in his essay on vegetarianism posits a direct cause-and-effect link between food and sex. "The gluttonous person is not equipped to struggle against laziness," he writes, "nor will the gluttonous and idle person ever be strong enough to struggle against sexual lust. Therefore, according to all moral teachings, the striving for abstinence commences with the struggle against the lust of gluttony; it commences with fasting" (XXIX, 73–74). In the same way that the first condition for a morally good life is abstinence, Tolstoy explains, "the first condition for a life of abstinence is fasting" (XXIX, 74). Just as gluttony is the first sign of a bad life, so is fasting "the essential condition for a good life" (XXIX, 74). What lends particular urgency to this need to fast, according to Tolstoy, is the fact that the main interest of the vast majority of people today is to satisfy their craving for food. "From the poorest to the wealthiest levels of society," he writes, "gluttony is, I think, the primary aim, the chief pleasure of our life" (XXIX, 74). Even destitute working-class people, Tolstoy sadly notes, seek to follow the example of the decadent upper classes; they too seek to acquire "the tastiest and sweetest foods, and to eat and drink as much as they can" (XXIX, 74).[21] In a letter he wrote during this same time period, Tolstoy explained to a correspondent: "I think that one of the principal sins, the most widespread and perhaps even the fundamental sin, the one out of which a whole series of other sins develop, is gluttony—gourmandism and worship of the belly—the desire to eat well, to eat at length, and to eat as much as possible" (LXV, 292).

"What is wrong and therefore impoverished in the relationship between the sexes," Tolstoy wrote to another correspondent in March 1890, "is due to the view shared by people of our class that the sexual relationship is a source of pleasure" (LXV, 61). The only effective way to change this view and succeed in curbing our voracious sexual appetite, Tolstoy suggests in his "Afterword to *The Kreutzer Sonata*," is to eliminate any pleasure we might possibly derive from the act of sexual intercourse. Only in this way can we succeed in our efforts to make ourselves what he elsewhere calls voluntary "eunuchs" and thus conquer our carnal lust.[22] The same anti-hedonistic, anti-epicurean reasoning seems to inform the masochistic solution that Tolstoy advances in *The First Step* for curbing our basic animal craving for food: that is, one should strive as much as possible to remove all the pleasure out of the act of eating. One can keep the lust for tasty food under control, he notes, only when one does not eat except in obedience to necessity. "The satisfaction of a need has limits," he writes, "but pleasure does not have any limits. For the satisfaction of one's needs, it is necessary and sufficient to eat bread, kasha, and rice. While for the augmentation of pleasure, there is no end to the flavorings and seasonings" (XXIX, 77). In the lengthy passage that ensues, Tolstoy proceeds to illustrate in considerable detail how, if we continue to eat rich and spicy comestibles (rather than these three bland food items—bread, kasha, and rice), our appetite for gustatory pleasure will never be satisfied but will instead keep growing larger and larger: that is, we will be seduced into piling one more delicious entrée on top of another at a meal. Since eating rich and tasty foods stimulates our desire for additional physical pleasures (both gastronomical and sexual), Tolstoy's solution is thus for us to practice gastronomic abstinence by striving as much as possible to make "unpalatable" the pleasures of the palate, to make "dis-gusting" the delights of the stomach. Our main purpose in eating, after all, ought to be to provide basic, healthy nourishment for the body, not to derive pleasure, enjoyment or stimulation for our taste buds and digestive tract. Nourishment, rather than gustation, ought to be the primary physiological aim of the activity of eating; and a sort of gastronomic "chastity" ought to be the spiritual ideal toward which we strive in matters concerning the palate and the belly. Food addiction, like sexual addiction, thus requires that we adopt austere measures of regulation over what we ingest into the body.

Understood within the context of Tolstoy's ongoing battle against the body (and specifically his campaign against the physical pleasures that tempt the body), *The First Step* reads less like the "Bible of vegetarianism" his Tolstoyan followers made it out to be, than as a moral diatribe against epicureanism in general and gluttony in particular. Although Tolstoy was widely acknowledged at the time as the "father" of Russian vegetarianism, the religious and ascetic orientation that characterized his views on diet ended up putting him seriously at odds with some key members of the fledgling vegetarian movement in early twentieth-century Russia, most notably with those "hygienic" vegetarians (such as Aleksandr and Olga Zelenkov) who advocated a much more joyful, life-affirming brand of vegetarianism. Their motto, "mens sana in corpore sano," with its unmistakable implication that the body needs to be rehabilitated rather than mortified, reflected their goal of creating a healthier and happier life for people through diet reform. This contrasted sharply with the more bleakly evangelical tone and renunciatory Christian spirit of Tolstoy's campaign against meat-eating, which was founded instead on denying the impulses of the body and eschewing any form of gastronomic pleasure.[23] The schism within the Russian vegetarian movement at the turn of the century between Tolstoyan "moralist" vegetarians (*vegetariantsy-nravstvenniki*) and epicurean "hygienic" vegetarians (*vegetariantsy-gigienisty*) mirrors the rift within the American vegetarian movement portrayed in T. Coraghessan Boyle's *The Road to Wellville* (1993) between the health ethos championed by those in the U.S. who followed the latest practices prescribed by German medical doctors (nude sunbathing, manual stimulation of the uterus, etc.) and the male purity crusade led by Christian physiologists from the Anglo-American tradition, such as Sylvester Graham and John Harvey Kellogg.[24] Tolstoy's vegetarian beliefs gravitate, of course, toward this latter abstinence camp. It is not surprising, therefore, that in *The First Step* Tolstoy forcefully condemns the gentry's obsession with gastronomic excess—their daily pattern of gluttonous overeating—as sinful as well as unhealthy. "The educated classes imagine that happiness and health (as medical men assure them, stating that the most expensive food, meat, is the healthiest) reside in eating savory, nourishing, easily digested food," Tolstoy asserts. "The one real, living interest for the majority of both men and women is eating food . . . how to eat? what to eat? when? where?" (XXIX, 74–75).

Tolstoy's Ethics of Diet: Desire, Denial, and Digestion

In his own personal life, as we noted earlier, Tolstoy had by now managed to reject the obscene practice of epicureanism—the gluttonous overeating on a daily basis—that he felt characterized typical gentry life in Russia. In *What Then Must We Do?* Tolstoy had roundly condemned the idle aristocratic life of luxury and comfort that he and his family had long enjoyed, identifying it synecdochally with the excessive amounts of rich foods they consumed at their five-course meals. In addition to the poverty and misery this opulent lifestyle caused for others, the rich foods served at their superfluous meals ruined gentry stomachs by whetting an appetite not for truly nutritious fare, but rather for the types of food that only further irritate one's digestive system. In an angry outburst aimed against the new culture of modern conveniences, pleasantries, and artificial cures that was gaining wide currency in Russia at the time, Tolstoy points to a recent advertisement he had seen for stomach powders designed for the rich, a product whose name, *Blessings for the Poor*, merely confirms his view that only the poor people in Russia (i.e., the peasants and workers) have proper digestion, while the rich need help (XXV, 393). Rather than continue to eat like an aristocrat himself, Tolstoy sought instead to follow a bland and modest vegetarian diet of simple, largely unappetizing foods (mainly basic peasant fare such as oatmeal porridge and cabbage soup) that would sufficiently nourish his body while not pleasuring it or arousing its sensual appetites unnecessarily. In his quest to remove all the pleasure out of the consumption of food and the practice of sex, Tolstoy strove to follow what he perceived to be the admirable example of the Russian peasant, adopting and then maintaining throughout the remainder of his life a highly parsimonious approach toward these two most basic of the physical appetites of human beings. Like the traditional Russian peasant, Tolstoy came to view food exclusively as a source of fuel for the body, rather than as a source of pleasure for the senses.[25] One culinary barometer that tracks this shift in conceptualization and perspective during his lifetime is provided by Tolstoy's changing attitude toward Ankovsky pie. Named after the Swedish doctor (Professor Anke) who first provided the Tolstoys with the recipe, this sweet confection was for many years a favorite family dessert in the Tolstoy home, and a culinary treat that Lev Nikolaevich, it appears, was particularly fond of.[26] After his spiritual conversion, however, and by the time he wrote *The First Step*, Ankovsky pie, according to one frequent visitor to Yasnaya Polyana, had become a term Tolstoy now used in a sarcastic tone to express "his disapproval of our undue hankering after comfort and luxury."[27] Tolstoy's resolve to live simply, chastely, and austerely thus found itself in direct conflict with Ankovsky pie and all that it continued to represent for his aristocratic family.[28]

Ironically enough, however, Tolstoy's adherence at table to a bland vegetarian diet of simple peasant foods coincided almost exactly with the exacerbation of the chronic digestive problems with his stomach that had plagued him since 1865.[29] Although Tolstoy boasted about the inexpensive yet nutritious meatless diet that he followed, his wife complained that this "abominable" and "senseless" diet was having quite a ruinous effect upon her husband's once robust health.[30] In Sophia's opinion, Lev's vegetarian diet did not give him nearly enough nourishment; indeed, she believed that it was directly responsible for his rapidly deteriorating physical condition and his constant bouts with digestive ailments (the doctors had earlier diagnosed him as suffering severe catarrh of the stomach). Moreover, Sophia lamented what she termed his "misdemeanors at table": that is, the immoderate portions of food he ate, the incompatible combinations of dishes he selected, and the haste with which he ate those large servings. According to Tolstoy's utilitarian approach to food, the purpose in following a rather bland vegetarian diet, as we have seen, was to obtain the basic nutritional value of food rather than any pleasing taste. Such an austere, unappetizing diet was also designed to help reduce sexual appetite. His wife's testimony, however, asserts that, in strictly alimentary and physiological terms at least, his functional diet had proven after all to be quite dysfunctional: the food he was eating, she maintained, was making him physically ill, rather than keeping him robust and healthy.

In light of what we know today about the nutritional benefits of a vegetarian diet (not to mention Tolstoy's relative longevity), Sophia's concern for her husband's health may seem rather misplaced. Indeed, Lev's vegetarianism was repellent to her mainly because it was paradigmatic of what she considered the many eccentric ideas her husband had begun to entertain after his midlife crisis, when he seemed to have abandoned nearly all of his earlier values, beliefs, and practices.[31] Tolstoy's abandonment of a normal diet, therefore, struck his wife as but another behavioral eccentricity that she could only hope would prove short-lived rather than permanent. "I should be happy to see him healthy again—instead of ruining his stomach with all this (in the doctor's words) harmful food," she noted sadly in 1891. "I should be happy to see him an artist again—instead of writing sermons which masquerade as articles. I should be happy to see him affectionate, attentive, and kind again—instead of this crude sensuality, followed by indifference" (2:50). As this diary entry strongly suggests, Sophia considered her husband's advocacy of vegetarianism, much like his sexual ideal of celibacy and his religious ideal of brotherly love, not merely counterproductive; to her mind, it was also patently hypocritical. Indeed, she seemed to derive special pleasure out of noting those occasions when the "saint" and "prophet" of Yasnaya Polyana failed—with respect to food and sex—to practice what he preached. With regard to sex, Sophia records in her diary how the physical side of love continued to be inordinately important to her elderly husband, who seems to have remained quite concupiscent even though he had already passed the age of 65 and was publicly preaching absolute marital chastity.[32] Sophia likewise questioned the authenticity of his Christian love, since it was being practiced by a man who seemed to show so little compassion for the members of his own family, especially for his long-suffering wife: "Oh, this sham Christianity, founded on hatred for those closest to you!" (4:119).

The purported sexual and religious hypocrisy on her husband's part, Sophia insisted, was matched by his gastronomic insincerity as well. Although in his publicistic writings he preached moderation in food consumption, abstinence from meat, and simplicity as well as blandness in diet, Tolstoy apparently continued in his private life to succumb to the sinful temptations presented by the pleasures of the table. In her diary, where she in effect chronicles the persistent digestive troubles that Tolstoy experienced during the last part of his life, Sophia repeatedly upbraids her husband for eating enormous amounts of food—often at the wrong time of day and usually on a weak stomach. On more than one occasion Sophia claimed that she had to take steps to guard against her husband upsetting his stomach through overeating. "Being healthy evidently bores him," she noted sardonically with regard to his immoderate eating habits (2:10). As was true with so many other aspects of his life, Tolstoy's indulgent gastronomic behavior in the privacy of his own home seemed to her to be greatly at variance with the rigid principles of abstinence that he preached in public. Even during the final year of his life, she would lament the glaring discrepancy she saw between his ethical tenets on the one hand and his actual personal conduct on the other. Her husband's attempt to improve himself morally and spiritually, through a rigorous brand of Christian asceticism, thus seemed to be undermined by what she considered to be the relatively sybaritic lifestyle that he continued to maintain on his gentry estate. In her opinion, his radical "diet" had turned out to be dysfunctional not only for his physical health, but for his moral and spiritual health as well.

Sophia's perspective on Tolstoy's dietary practices—and, indeed, on his radical Christian beliefs generally—is not without some decided bias, of course. Yet Tolstoy himself confessed on a number of occasions during his post-conversion years to being deeply troubled by the knowledge that he did, in fact, continue to succumb at times to the gastronomic indulgence that he condemned so roundly in the Russian gentry. While food and sex may well have become socially, morally, and spiritually unpalatable for Tolstoy after his conversion, Sophia's testimony and the Russian author's own diary entries suggest that these objects of desire had lost few of their sensual charms and little of their physical attraction for the elderly apostle of Yasnaya Polyana, who continued to have trouble controlling his hungry stomach and his unruly loins.

"All life is a struggle between the flesh and the spirit," Tolstoy had written in 1895, "and gradually the spirit triumphs over the flesh" (LII, 26). Such existential optimism is tempered, however, by the more candid remark he reportedly once made to Maxim Gorky: "The flesh should be the obedient dog of the spirit, running to do its bidding; but we—how do we live? The flesh rages and riots, and the spirit follows it helpless and miserable."[33] Although Tolstoy may have sought in his later years to follow a rigid ascetic diet that he hoped would nourish his spiritual self rather than feed his animal nature and although his followers like to mythologize Tolstoy's purportedly strict adherence to (and deep fondness for) bland peasant food, the Russian author never did lose entirely his hearty physical appetite for both food and sex.[34] He never completely ceased to crave those pleasures of the flesh and delights of the palate that gratified his body rather than nurtured his soul. In his *Confession*, Tolstoy had acknowledged the Socratic truth that one must strive "to be free of the body, of all the evils that result from the life of the body" (XXIII, 22–23), and he had begun during the early 1880s, both in his life and in his writings, to wage a full-scale war against the physical pleasures that mercilessly tempt the human body. Tolstoy in his later years thus epitomized the paradigmatic Christian view of the body as an unruly, passionate, animal, and alien Other that requires strict regulation through the iron discipline of diet and self-denial. But even extreme dietary practices, as we have seen, do not seem to have been quite enough to silence appetite in Tolstoy's case, and the full-scale war he waged upon his body apparently continued right up to the time of the author's death, with no clear victor on either side.

Notes

1. See, for instance, Judith Butler, *Bodies That Matter: On the Discursive Limits of "Sex"* (New York: Routledge, 1993), Susan Bordo, *Unbearable Weight: Feminism, Western Culture, and the Body* (Berkeley: University of California Press, 1993), Linda Nochlin, *Representing Women* (New York: Thames and Hudson, 1999), Janet Price and Margrit Shildrick, eds., *Feminist Theory and the Body* (New York: Routledge, 1999), Alison M. Jaggar and Susan R. Bordo, eds., *Gender/Body/Knowledge: Feminist Reconstructions of Being and Knowing* (New Brunswick, NJ: Rutgers University Press, 1989), and Katie Conboy, Nadia Medina, and Sarah Stanbury, eds., *Writing on the Body: Female Embodiment and Feminist Theory* (New York: Columbia University Press, 1997). For a useful collection of essays that illustrate the current feminist challenge to Cartesian dualisms, see Susan Bordo, ed. *Feminist Interpretations of Rene Descartes* (University Park, PA: Pennsylvania State University Press, 1999).

2. Bryan S. Turner, *The Body and Society* (London: Sage Publications, 1996), 9–11, 17–19.

3. See R. F. Christian, ed. and trans., *Tolstoy's Diaries* (New York: Charles Scribner's Sons, 1985), vol. 2, x.

4. Judith M. Armstrong, *The Unsaid Anna Karenina* (New York: St. Martin's Press, 1988), 18.

5. Ruth Crego Benson, *Women in Tolstoy: The Ideal and the Erotic* (Urbana, IL: University of Illinois Press, 1973), 2.

6. Dmitri Merejkowskii, *Tolstoi as Man and Artist* (Westport, CT: Greenwood Press, 1970).

7. See Rene Fueloep Miller, "Tolstoy the Apostolic Crusader," *Russian Review,* 19:2 (1960), 101–102.

8. Eve Levin discusses the Russian Orthodox Church's medieval views on sex and the body in *Sex and Society in the World of the Orthodox Slavs, 900–1700* (Ithaca, NY: Cornell University Press, 1989).

9. For discussions of "moral masochism," see Daniel Rancour-Laferriere, *Tolstoy on the Couch: Misogyny, Masochism and the Absent Mother* (New York: New York University Press, 1998) and *The Slave Soul of Russia: Moral Masochism and the Cult of Suffering* (New York: New York University Press, 1995).

10. See A. P. Sergeenko, *Rasskazy o L. N. Tolstom: Iz vospominanii* (Moscow: Sovetskii pisatel', 1978), 63. For a fuller treatment of Tolstoy's relationship to food and eating, see my essay, "Unpalatable Pleasures: Tolstoy, Food, and Sex," *Tolstoy Studies Journal*, 6 (1993), 1–32.

11. For an examination of this connection between Tolstoy's views on diet and those held by some of the leading nineteenth-century American food reformers, see my essay, "Tolstoy's Way of No Flesh: Abstinence, Vegetarianism, and Christian Physiology," in *Food in Russian History and Culture* Musya Glants and Joyce Toomre, eds. (Bloomington, IN: Indiana University Press, 1997), 81–102.

12. Following his conversion experience, Donna Orwin argues, Tolstoy "rejected the body, and, therefore, nature, as the source of or even a possible participant in higher human goodness." See *Tolstoy's Art and Thought, 1847–1880* (Princeton: Princeton University Press, 1993), 217.

13. Henrietta Mondry, "Beyond the Boundary: Vasilii Rozanov and the Animal Body," *Slavic and East European Journal*, 43:4 (1999), 653.

14. L. N. Tolstoi, *Polnoe sobranie sochinenii*, 90 vols. (Moscow: Khudozhestvennaia literatura, 1928–1958), vol. 26, 348. All quotes from Tolstoy's works, letters, diaries, etc. come from this ninety-volume jubilee edition of his complete works. References are listed parenthetically by volume (Roman numerals) and page (Arabic numbers). All translations from the Russian, unless otherwise indicated, are my own.

15. "If a man will consciously strive to live not for the stomach, but for the spirit," Tolstoy writes to his friend Vladimir Chertkov on 9 October 1888, "then his relationship to food will be what it ought to be" (LXXXVI, 177–178).

16. For a wide-ranging discussion of the socio-economic and cultural changes taking place in late imperial Russia, see Catriona Kelly and David Shepherd, eds., *Constructing Russian Culture in the Age of Revolution: 1881–1940* (New York: Oxford University Press, 1998).

17. Laura Engelstein, *The Keys to Happiness: Sex and the Search for Modernity in Fin-de-Siecle Russia* (Ithaca, NY: Cornell University Press, 1992). See especially chapter six, "Eros and Revolution: The Problem of Male Desire," 215–253.

18. Paul Birukoff, *The Life of Tolstoy* (London and New York: Cassell and Co., 1911), 97.

19. For a discussion of this debate on sexual morality in late nineteenth-century Russia, see Peter Ulf Møller, *Postlude to the Kreutzer Sonata: Tolstoj and the Debate over Sexual Morality in Russian Literature in the 1890s*, John Kendal trans. (New York: E. J. Brill, 1988).

20. This aspect of Foucault's argument is developed most successfully in the second volume of his three-volume *History of Sexuality*. See Foucault, *The Use of Pleasure*, Robert Hurley, trans (New York: Vintage Books, 1985).

21. Tolstoy was especially distressed by the gluttony he saw in his own pampered children. "They eat to excess and amuse themselves by spending money on the labors of other people for their own pleasure," he wrote angrily to Chertkov in 1885 (LXXXV, 294). "You look for the cause; look for the remedy," he lectured his wife a few days later. "The children can stop overeating (vegetarianism)" (LXXXIII, 547).

22. See Leo Tolstoy, *The Relations of the Sexes,* Vladimir Chertkov, trans (Christchurch, UK: The Free Age Press, 1901), 37–38.

23. See my essay, "Vegetarianism in Russia: The Tolstoy(an) Legacy," *The Carl Beck Papers in Russian and East European Studies*, 1507 (2001), 1–39.

24. T. Coraghessan Boyle, *The Road to Wellville* (New York: Penguin, 1993). For critical studies of the nineteenth-century American health reform movement, see Stephen Nissenbaum, *Sex, Diet, and Debility in Jacksonian America: Sylvester Graham and Health Reform* (Westport, CT: Greenwood Press, 1980), Jayme A. Sokolow, *Eros and Modernization: Sylvester Graham, Health Reform, and the Origins of Victorian Sexuality in America* (Rutherford, NJ: Fairleigh Dickinson University Press, 1983), and James C. Whorton, *Crusaders for Fitness: The History of American Health Reformers* (Princeton: Princeton University Press, 1982).

25. For an excellent study of the Russian peasant diet, see Cathy A. Frierson, "Forced Hunger and Rational Restraint in the Russian Peasant Diet: One Populist's Vision," in *Food in Russian History*, 49–66.

26. Ankovsky pie, in the words of one critic, served as "an indispensable attribute of the festive table in the Tolstoy household" and became for Tolstoy himself "a symbol of a life put right and sanctified once and for all." See Vladimir I. Porudominskii, "L. N. Tolstoi i etika pitaniia," *Chelovek*, 2 (1992), 115.

27. S. A. Behrs, *Recollections* (London: Heinemann, 1893). I am quoting here from Aylmer Maude, *The Life of Tolstoy* (London: Constable & Co., 1910), vol. 2, 336.

28. Porudominskii explains the demise of Ankovsky pie in the following way: "Whereas earlier it signified for Lev Nikolaevich the joyful stability of the family hearth, it became for him an image of an earlier stagnant, idle, and unjust way of life, one that was incompatible with the goals and ideals which he would like to serve." See Porudominskii, "L. N. Tolstoi i etika pitaniia," 115.

29. A. P. Sergeenko maintains that Tolstoy had liver and stomach ailments as early as 1865. See *Rasskazy o Tolstom*, 68.

30. "Lev Nikolaevich is unwell," Sophia records in her diary on 14 March 1887. "He has bad indigestion and stomach aches, and yet he eats the most senseless diet: first it is rich food, then it is vegetarian food, then rum and water, and so on." See Sof'ia Tolstaia, *Dnevniki Sof'i Andreevny Tolstoi* (Moscow: Sovetskii pisatel', 1928–1936), vol. 1, 139. All further references to Sophia's diaries will come from this four-volume edition and will be noted parenthetically in the text (by volume and page number).

31. "Sofia Andreevna's quarrels with her husband over food issues possess a culinary character only in outward appearance," explains Porudominskii. "These were actually quarrels about [competing] worldviews." See "L. N. Tolstoi i etika pitaniia," *Chelovek*, 3(1992), 132–133.

32. "I often suffer because his love for me is physical, more than emotional," she would write as late as 1897, when Lev Nikolaevich was almost 70 years old (2:132).

33. Maxim Gorky, *Reminiscences of Tolstoy, Chekhov, and Andreyev*, S. S. Koteliansky and Leonard Woolf, trans. (New York: Viking Press, 1949), 53.

34. A. P. Sergeenko, describing the modest meal he saw Tolstoy eat in his guest room at the Optina Pustyn monastery just ten days before his death in 1910, writes that Tolstoy's "typical peasant nature was underscored now by the fact that he ate the usual national meal of the Russian peasant—cabbage soup and kasha." See *Rasskazy o Tolstom*, 79.

Part III ی

FAT AND SOCIETY

Chapter 9 ༄

WEIGHT LOSS IN THE AGE OF REASON[1]

Ken Albala

It is typically assumed that the modern anxiety over obesity is a relatively recent phenomenon, stretching back at best no more than a century. In fact, this concern has a much longer history and the first medical discourses addressing the topic date from the seventeenth century, a time when fat was fashionable. By calling attention to the dangers of excess weight, medical professionals were to a great extent responsible for generating a nascent fear of fat. Their recommendations for weight loss are ultimately to blame for the gradual shift in meaning of the word *diet* from a general program of health maintenance to a regimen specifically designed to cure excess weight, which was increasingly defined as a pathological state. The various disagreements among different schools of medical thought only intensified the urgency with which they addressed the topic and losing weight eventually became fashionable, as it remains to this day.

Although Hippocrates and Galen in ancient times did address topic of obesity, among their heirs, the dietary writers of the Middle Ages and Renaissance, there was almost no interest in the topic. Excess fat was merely considered the result of the phlegmatic constitution, something with which a person was born. Naturally, the effects of this imbalance could be mitigated by alterations in diet and the other so-called non-naturals, but excessive fat was not considered a sickness. Only in the case of extreme obesity was there a definite perceived danger, and this focused primarily on the way the condition compromises movement, breathing, the circulation of fluids through the body, and reproduction. This seems to have been rare enough that most medical writers either never spent time discussing it, or mentioned it only as a passing curiosity, or marvel of nature.

There was, of course, a long tradition of inveighing against gluttony, both as a moral concern among theologians as well as a health issue among dietary writers. Eating and drinking too much, consuming too great a diversity of food and without any order or at the proper time, was considered the source of innumerable diseases. But revealingly, obesity was not among them. Oddly enough, most nutrition writers believed that gluttons were poorly nourished, their systems being tossed into such a state of disarray that little food would be properly processed. The surfeit of food was thought to overload and extinguish the heat that facilitates digestion.

Even among theologians, the sin of gluttony was more closely related to greed and lust than any kind of personal defilement, because it involved eating too much while others went hungry. Most exegesis focused on the glutton in Luke (16.19–31) whose real sin was not stuffing himself silly, but neglecting to perform acts of charity, which then made his sin mortal. For refusing to share his feast, he was later consigned to fast in hell. Fat itself was not conceptually linked to gluttony, even though in the popular consciousness, and especially in contemporary depictions gluttons were pictured as fat. Hieronymus Bosch's depiction of Gula (Gluttony) in the rondel of Seven Deadly Sins is one good example. Eating too much might make you fat, but fat itself was no sin.

Why then the topic should have become of major concern after the mid seventeenth century and the subject of several dissertations, inaugural addresses and public disputations, is not entirely clear. It is tempting to suppose that this may have been the first time that there were a significant number of obese people to warrant medical attention. Perhaps it was the first time that enough people in one area had enough expendable income to seek a cure, making obesity a lucrative medical specialty and the object of medical controversy. In the physicians' estimation, it was precisely the sheer number of fat people, particularly in Germany where most of them were writing, that demanded they address the topic. Although it is doubtful that many lay people read these disputations, their proliferation suggests that physicians were increasingly making treatment of obesity a regular part of their medical practice.

An equally plausible cause for the sudden interest is that the flurry of competing physiological theories in the wake of chemical and mechanical discoveries threw the whole question of how and why fat accumulates up in the air, not to mention how to cure it. In other words, the evolution of medical theory itself brought obesity into the limelight as a hot topic. Although there is no precise way of telling when and how these ideas affected popular attitudes toward fat, it is clear that more individuals were seeking innovative means of girth control, and physicians were happy to supply them with solutions. Then as now it was the quick and easy remedies that seem to have captured popular interest rather than the difficult long-term solutions and permanent changes in lifestyle.

Although there are anecdotal references to obesity scattered through sixteenth-century medical texts, mostly gawking at what they referred to as the monstrously obese, the first major work to discuss fat in the early modern period derives from a disputation held in 1580 in Heidelberg between M. Michael Schenkius and the renowned physician (and Protestant theologian) Thomas Erastus. It survives in his collected works, published posthumously in 1595.[2] The disputation is not so much on obesity, but rather why and how fat accumulates on the body. The discussion is still overwhelmingly humoral as at this point new physiological theories had not had much impact on standard Galenism. Erastus, as a good Galenist, had notoriously attacked Paracelsus' chemically-based physiology as well. It is interesting, though, in that it raises a point of contention over whether fat congeals as a result of cold, as Galen would have claimed for the phlegmatic constitution, or from heat. The latter idea is really just a logical deduction of another basic Galenic idea that along with milk and sperm, fat is merely the result of an excess of nutritive matter converted from blood. Since no sound nutrition or sanguification (the conversion of aliment to blood) can process without heat, it follows that only sufficiently hot bodies can accumulate fat.

Erastus counters this notion by drawing extensively from Galen and Aristotle themselves, that of course native (internal) heat is necessary for the process of nutrition, but fat is generated from the most humid part of blood.[3] This humor can only be congealed in a cold atmosphere. It seems his analogy is drawn from the properties of butter and other fats outside the body which are liquid if hot but solid at colder temperatures. Heat can, in fact, make some substances solid, but this results from drying up and concentrating the humors, not what he calls "concretion" but "incrassation" or what might be called thickening or reduction as with a sauce. Again his analogies appear to be drawn from the kitchen.[4] Most importantly, fats cannot be reduced and only become solid with cold. As in the body, fat is generated with heat, but congeals, accidentally, with cold.

In the end, the entire discourse serves only to support the idea that it is only those with phlegmatic constitutions who become fat. It was not yet considered a specific and life-threatening medical condition. The discussion is important, however, because later writers will refer to it as a base point for their departures from Galenic orthodoxy.

In the early seventeenth century, practical dietary writers were still silent on the topic of fat. The only exception is one Gaspard Bachot, among the few physicians in the Galenic tradition to broach the topic, and his advice is both for those who want to become thin as well as those who want to become fat. For the latter he suggested not exercising, eating rich meats and fatty soups, drinking a lot, sleeping long hours, and not studying too much.[5] Obviously the opposite applies to those who want to slim down.

Bachot did consider the ideal body size to be neither too fat nor too thin, or what he called being "en-bon-point." Embonpoint implied a hearty and stout figure though, not an average frame. He also conceded that women are generally fatter than men because of their colder constitutions, and fat tends to congeal around the stomach because it is further from the source of vital heat and gets less exercise than the extremities. Naturally those who "vivent à gogo" and overindulge become fat.[6] Bachot disagreed with Aristotle, though, that fat is always the result of personal habits. He believed there is also a natural fatness to which individuals with certain constitutions are prone, especially the phlegmatic and sanguine, who are more likely to grow fleshy than fat. Some people are naturally fat regardless of how much they eat, and he even relates the story of one man who became sick on a diet, failed to lose weight, and in the end died.[7] Sometimes it is best not to radically alter one's habits, despite the inconveniences of body shape.

On the topic of fat as a sickness, Bachot goes no further than to say that fat people tend to have shorter lives because the constriction of their veins prevents the flow of blood and spirits, which hastens old age. The fat also tends to suffocate the vital heat, pressing on the veins and arteries and causing shortness of breath.[8] This is one of the earliest hints that early modern physicians were beginning to consider excessive fat an actual threat to health, and offer corrective regimens.

Other writers in the early seventeenth century offer little more, apart from the brief anecdote such as Tobias Venner's when he remarks that biscuit is good for phlegmatic people and those "that desire to grow leane" because it dries the body out.[9] For all authors in the Galenic tradition it appears that fat was seen as a natural consequence of a complexion tending to the cold and moist, something which could be corrected, but not considered an illness that demanded serious attention.

One of the most important theoretical shifts that would have an impact on attitudes toward fat stemmed from the work of Santorio Santorio in the early seventeenth century and his efforts to quantify nutrition. Although Santorio does not seem to have been anxious about being overweight himself, he did consistently define health as the maintenance of body weight. With the use of a weighing chair he measured his own weight and calculated the difference between the weight of food ingested and excreted in "sensible" evacuations and decided that "insensible perspiration" accounted for the difference. In fact, he concluded that insensible perspiration through the skin and via the breath makes up the greater proportion of bodily waste. If a healthy man, for example, consumed eight pounds of food in one day, a full five pounds would be excreted through insensible means. Perspiration was a sign that the body had properly refined and assimilated the nutritive matter of food and drink. An excess of perspiration indicated that the body was beginning to waste away, too little was a sign that crude deposits were being left in the body. Maintenance of weight was considered ideal. "Health continues firm as long as the body returns daily to the same weight by insensible perspiration . . . ."[10] Following Santorio, many writers would naturally assume that increased perspiration itself serves to slim the body.

What is perhaps stranger, though, is that Santorio insisted that the accumulation of fat was not a simple matter of eating too much. "He who eats more than he can digest, is nourished less than he ought to be, and [becomes] consequently emaciated."[11] That is, just because food is eaten does not mean it is digested or offers nutrition, a way of thinking totally foreign to our sensibilities, and one that would be abandoned along with Galen in the coming generations.

Drawing on Santorio's ideas Walter Charleton sought to explain the physiological differences between fat and thin bodies. The volume of blood was thought to be a crucial factor, and it was a generally accepted fact that thin people have more blood than fat ones. He used this idea to defend his position that blood is not what nourishes the body, as earlier schools believed. "Men that are fat and plump, have but little blood; and such as are spare and lean, have abundance: which could not be, if blood were matter of nourishment." Paradoxically, he contends that "in a gross body, where are more parts to be nourished, there ought to be more bloud to nourish them: but grosse men, for the most part, eate much lesse, than lean; because they have lesse veins, and being inclined to sedentary and unactive lives, they consume but few spirits."[12] That is, according to his theory that the nerves actually transport highly refined, fermented, and distilled nutrients throughout the body, fatter people need less food because their nerves are large, moist, open, and spongy, which means that nourishment is distributed and assimilated much more easily. Charleton was among the first to work Santorio's mechanical ideas into his theory of obesity, and authors on the topic would continue to be influenced by him for the next century.

In fact, by the next generation Santorio was being hailed as the founder of a whole new understanding of the physiology of the body as a machine. As the first historian of nutritional science, James Mackenzie, writing in the 1750s put it, "He opened a whole new scene in physic, to which physicians and philosophers were in a great measure strangers before this time; and, upon experiments made with amazing diligence and assiduity for thirty years, has established the laws of insensible perspiration."[13] In other words, in discovering a way to quantify metabolic activity, body weight became a medical issue in a way it never had been before. Being overweight was now a sign that something had gone wrong with the body.

Presenting his dissertation at the University of Strasbourg, at almost the same time Charleton was writing, Antonio Udalrico Gosky discussed various forms of weight change. Interestingly the title distinguishes between healthy and unhealthy weight loss and gain (*Solemn disputation on wasting, or decay: that is thinness and slenderness among the healthy people and the sick. Natural fat and corpulence among the healthy and in sickness*).[14] It is not surprising that his arguments are totally Galenic given that his advisor was Melchior Sebizius, the last great dietary writer in a long line of orthodox Galenists.[15] Gosky considered obesity to be especially prevalent in his own region both for men and women, but not necessarily life-threatening.[16] Essentially fat is defined here as the oily and aerial parts of blood separated and congealed accidentally by a cold phlegmatic constitution. The aerial part accounts for the softness of fat compared with more solid terrestrial substances. His remedies are simple and could easily have been empirically validated. They involve eating less quantitatively and eating less nourishing foods, getting more exercise, and perhaps odder to our minds are sleeping less, venesection, and provocation of hemorrhoids, and various medicinal baths designed to extenuate the body.[17]

Despite these cures, he still categorized obesity as a natural state, not necessarily dangerous to health. The section on what he calls "crassness" in sickness describes various swellings that occur on the body as the result of specific diseases, but it does not include plain obesity. In other words, in the mid seventeenth century, it is still not entirely settled whether obesity should be considered a pathological state or not. Traditionally minded theorists like Gosky and his mentor thought not, while the neoterics making use of the new mechanical and chemical theories, as we shall see, believed it was a disease. That is to say, changes in theory played a significant role in recategorizing obesity, and ultimately brought forth new cures based on those theories.

In 1670, Johann Friedrich Held defended his dissertation at Jena on the topic of obesity. He was, as far as I know, the first author to define obesity by belt size, insisting that a waistline over three feet, or thirty-six inches with a full stomach, is technically obese.[18] He was also the first of the doctoral candidates to take account of the latest chemical theories and the implications these have for the topic of fat. Naturally he indicated that an abundance of nutrition as well as the poor quality of food are prime factors, as is faulty insensible perspiration.[19] His insistence that it is only one particular part of the nutrient-rich blood that can be converted to fat, namely the oily and aerial part, puts him squarely in the iatro-chemical camp. How and why fat accumulates on some bodies and not others was a more difficult question, especially without the standard humoral explanation to fall back on. Held mentioned that Boerhaave had claimed that a chemical imbalance is responsible, in particular an excess of the sulphurous part of blood.[20] Others claimed that it was an imbalance of alkali in the stomach, which makes sense. A lack of stomach acid would lead to faulty digestion, or fermentation in this case, and the crude oily parts of the food would accumulate in the body. This happens all the more readily with fatty foods that are difficult to break down, and also with beer, which he identified with the "beer belly."[21]

Held also offered specific remedies based on this chemical understanding of fat. First was to consume less meat, and hence less fat. He rejected venesection, a standard Hippocratic remedy based on the assumption that less blood would equal less nutrition and hence weight loss. He also considered surgery far too dangerous, though he had read about various attempts to excise body fat. Much safer and effective are the chemical remedies, the various purgatives, emetics, and sudorifics that would speed the passage of food through the body and hence prevent the accumulation of fat. He gave recipes for vomits, clysters (or suppositories), laxatives—anything that would void the body from any opening. One would assume that it might be easier to just eat less, and in fact he did eventually suggest this. In general his dietary recommendations are a little stranger, though: "vegetables, biscuits moistened with vinegar, bran, salted foods and whatever descends quickly through the stomach and intestines through peristaltic action." Added to this are "aromatics . . . salted fish, roasts, smoked meats, lamb, acid fruits and anything bitter."[22] The logic of these is anything that will pass quickly through the body, offers little nutritional value, and in the case of salted and smoked foods, it seems those that will dry up the body or "extenuate" it. Capers, he concluded, are the ideal dieting food.

Obviously Held was citing the new chemical theories second-hand. In the case of Michael Ettmuller, his comments on obesity were at the fore-front of chemical research. In his dissertation (here meaning disputation, taking place in Leipzig in 1681) on excess corpulence, he put forward a more explicit theory of faulty fermentation in the stomach. A simple excess of food stifles the internal vessel, exactly as it would in brewing beer, pre-venting food from breaking down and being refined.[23] These crude ele-ments are then deposited throughout the body's vessels, causing not only constriction but a variety of diseases. How fats specifically congeal he explains through an analogy which seems both chemical and culinary. It is certainly easy to imagine. An accumulation of acids perhaps mixed with some nitrous elements breathed in through the air binds with the fluid fats creating coagulation or, as we might say, an emulsion, just as acids react with oils, or as lye does with fats in soap-making. These are then deposited in special vessels throughout the body.[24] Furthermore, the wider and more lax the body's passages and pores are, the more easily fat is deposited. So loose-ness, or lack of tension in the nervous fibers is another reason some people become fat and not others.

Ettmuller also entered into a discussion of the nature of nutrition itself, which had been contested among anatomists and physiologists. Some sug-gested that it was only blood that nourishes, others the lymph flowing through nervous vessels, and others a kind of milky serum or fatty part of the chyle contained in the blood. But fat is not merely generated from fats. Bread, raisins, nuts, as well as milk, butter, and eggs can be fattening.

Ettmuller's remedies include eating less, and preventing the food from remaining too long in the body. As with Held, anything that quickly evac-uates the body can be useful—including salivation provoked by medicinal woods or mercury, or even by chewing tobacco.[25] Substances which accel-erate fermentation, promote circulation and prevent the coagulation of fats can also be useful. Chemicals which make food more homogenous also aid in this process, again mercury. With less violence, change of air can help, not as with humoralists to counteract the cold constitution, but rather to aid internal fermentation and insensible perspiration with heat. Of food, he offers the typical advice to eat and especially drink less, and to season food with acrid and acid flavors: vinegar, citron, salt, and also with spices like pepper, cloves, cinnamon, ginger, and cress, mustard, and radishes.[26] All these were considered incisive condiments that cut through the body, an idea that stretches back to classical antiquity. Vinegar with absinth or rue, both intensely bitter, has a detergent cleansing effect and works even better. Lastly, he offers dozens of pharmaceutical remedies as well—tartarous, nitrous, and vitriolic concoctions meant to scour the inside of the body and flush it out. The perennial recourse to laxatives seems deeply embedded in the popular consciousness to this day.[27]

Shortly after Ettmuller, and in nearby Jena, Karl Christian Leisner submitted his doctoral dissertation on the topic of obesity. What makes his argument unique and particularly interesting for the historian, is how he explains that fat has not had any negative social stigma attached, in fact exactly the opposite in the Western tradition. He seems very sensitive to the fact that among peoples perpetually facing hunger, fat can be a form of life insurance. Even among his own German countrymen, he knows that peasants value fat and even find it beautiful. He relates how in Venice, girls before matrimony are intentionally kept cooped, as it were, and fattened up with unctuous and sweet foods to make them more appealing and Venus-like.[28] The ideal female figure, if judged by Titian's somewhat corpulent Venuses, supports Leisner's contention that fat was anything but embarrassing.

Leisner is also explicitly aware that he is trying to change the reigning opinion by pointing out all the threats to health that obesity poses. "Praise of obesity can be easily disparaged if we weigh the dangers" he claims, which provides fairly good evidence that fear of fat was introduced into peoples' minds by physicians, rather than any new standard of beauty.

Obesity is not, as old physicians claimed, merely a neutral condition, but one that impedes all bodily functions and is itself a morbid state. It prevents proper movement of the body, constricts the veins, clogs the body's passages leading to clogs and putrefaction, breathing ailments such as asthma, sterility, and even fear, and stupidity as the free passage of spirits in the brain is prevented. That is, fat is not merely the concretion of deposits in certain parts of the body but throughout the whole.[29] He also believed that Germans were especially prone to obesity given the northerly latitude as well as their propensity to indulge in excessive food and drink. But at the same time, he recognized that people are anxious to find cures, many of which are themselves dangerous. He offers examples of women who abuse various therapies designed to dry out the body, ultimately causing obstructions of the viscera. Although anecdotal, this provides some evidence that people had begun to diet in the modern sense of that word. Another case mentioned here involves a person who overdosed on chickpeas boiled with salt, one of Held's recommendations. In the end, Leisner is skeptical whether obesity really can be cured. It is always best to proceed with caution.[30] One can only guess if this comes from his awareness of the failure of more drastic therapies.

Venesection, Leisner believed, may have the opposite effect intended, as in trees that fruit better when the sap runs, because the body is emptied, tempered, and more apt to receive nutrition. He did approve of the standard aromatics and diuretics, and evacuants like sarsaparilla, sassafras, and guiac root—as well as chewing tobacco, which he traces back to Borelli, but smoking too can be useful for asthma, often associated with obesity.[31] External remedies that open the pores can also be useful, including hot baths or standing near ovens and freshly baked bread. But the safest remedy is merely to eat less and eat foods that nourish less—especially lettuce and endive in salads, vegetables, and fish. Acidic fruits like cherries, plums, barberries, currants, pomegranate, lemons, and sour apples are ideal, along with capers, olives, and pickles.[32] All of these, once again, scour the body and cut through fat.

Although Leisner included among his remedies some of the stranger new fads, his voice was one of reason among the flurry of new and in his mind dangerous diets. Just as today, late-seventeenth-century Europeans were not only confused by conflicting medical advice, but they also seem to have taken recourse to the quickest, easiest and most drastic weight loss regimens. From this point down to the present the interest in slimming diets would only intensify.

In the eighteenth century the popularity of obesity as a topic for disputation reached its real heyday. George A. Bray has identified no less than 34 doctoral dissertations in the course of the century.[33] I focus on two of the earliest of these, partly because they are indicative of the ways in which coverage of the topic would change.

In 1701 Ernest Fecht presented his inaugural disputation on obesity at Rostock. Like Leisner, he began by insisting that the ancients, Galen in particular, were mistaken in not classifying obesity as a disease. It is not merely a state of body somewhere between the phlegmatic constitution and an unnatural disorder, but is itself a pathological state demanding a physician's intervention. "The obese are not healthy, nor jolly."[34] This is another example of a physician consciously criticizing popular associations of fat by imposing his own medically-based discourse and thereby inciting anxiety, guilt, and ideally a visit to the professional for a remedy.

Fecht's discussion differs from those of the seventeenth century, in making fuller and more explicit use of the latest iatro-mechanical theories to explain fat. First, he quickly dispenses with the errant opinion of one chemist who believed that fat accumulates from an excess of salts in the body, which because of their sharp angles abrade the tissues and cause nutritive matter and ultimately fat to be lodged therein. The more common chemical explanation, he notes, depends on acids to coagulate the fats, apparently also the opinion of Sylvius de la Boë, one of the leading iatro-chemists.[35] In the end, however, he settles on the greater importance of physical laxity of the body's finest passages. If these are wide and loose, the body's fluids pass slowly and nutritive matter accumulates more easily than in those with taut and rigid body fibers and narrow vessels. That is, a particular body type causes obesity rather than personal habits, and the speed of these fluids' passage explains everything. Nonetheless, this body type requires careful medical supervision.

Fecht's remedies are nothing very new: aromatics and spices, diuretic foods like parsley, asparagus, celery, carrots, and fennel. It is his interesting combination of chemical and mechanical explanations that not only keeps this topic controversial, but in the minds of physicians and their patients. The ability to pick and choose among rival systems, or even combine features of several, meant that dieters could find one that suited their own particular tastes. If one diet condemns bacon and meat, there is sure to be another somewhere that recommends it.

The dissertation of Daniel Wilhelm Triller at the University of Halle in 1718 is similar in its eclectic mixture of various theories along with the latest microscopic and anatomical discoveries, but much simpler in its conclusions. To his credit, Triller was among the first to describe fat as a kind of storage system for the body, derived from whatever nutrients are available and unused—not merely fats. It can be drawn on to nourish the body in times of need, and will necessarily accumulate in any body if there is an excess of nutrients.[36] Naturally, therefore, the only reasonable cure is fasting. Unfortunately the author did not feel he had the time to discuss unnatural fat, so there is not much discussion of obesity per se. But his work does point in one of the directions that would be taken up in the course of the eighteenth century: practical and simple advice, and conclusions drawn from careful observation, reason, and self-help. Unfortunately it appears that the demand for quick and simple remedies, then as today, kept the other theories and remedies in circulation. If anything the thriving medical trade in curing obesity encouraged newer and more outlandish remedies.

One need only think of what became of this kind of practice in Great Britain. Thomas Short's full length *Discourse Concerning the Causes and Effects of Corpulency*, for example, while acknowledging that many of his countrymen consider fat fashionable, lashed out (much as the Germans did) in detailing the dangers of obesity.[37] As for the causes, he threw every possibility into the pot: bad air hindering perspiration, the mechanical effect of eating sweet and fatty foods, which easily accumulate in the fat vesicles, or foods that are only broken down with difficulty and thus linger in the body too long, such as eggs, rice-milk, and shellfish. Then there are the standard old non-naturals, without the humors: too little exercise, too much sleep, excessive sexual activity. Above all it is looseness of the body's fibers and excessive dilation of the passages, a mechanical defect. And as a cure he recommends anything that will tighten and tone the body, giving it more solidity and tension: "simple and earthy Aliments . . . as Eggs, Panados, rough Wines" along with austere and acid medicines, exercise, and cold baths.[38] Further along he also suggests detergent grains like oats, rye, or barley baked into bread, less nutritious foods like fish and herbs, and sharp wines and stale ale rather than smooth liquors, which presumably stick to the ribs more easily.[39] He also recommends bitter, aromatics that promote perspiration, vinegar, guiac, and sassafras, as well as smoking tobacco. In other words, he has the full panoply of remedies drawn from various different schools based on completely different theories. Perhaps he does not go overboard like his countryman Cheyne with his milk and seed diet, with which he claimed to have reduced his own "crazy carcass" of 400 lbs.[40] Nor like Jeremiah Wainewright does he suggest good strong black coffee without sugar, milk, or butter.[41] Or to top them all, there is Malcolm Flemyng who will recommend eating soap to clean out the digestive system.[42] But it is clear that the melee of opinions and rival theories, especially in their being jumbled together by medical writers choosing bits of this and that, can only have impossibly confused the poor patient seeking help. And seek help they apparently did if the enormous popularity of the genre from the eighteenth century to the present is any indication, and if peoples' perpetual search for simple solutions and quick remedies was neither effectively disappointed nor completely satisfied.

Notes

1. The dissertations and disputations cited in this essay, housed in The National Library of Medicine, were brought to my attention by an article by George A. Bray entitled "Obesity: Historical Development of Scientific and Cultural Ideas" in *Obesity*, Per Bjorntorp and Bernard N. Brodoff, eds. (Philadelphia: J. B. Lippincott Co., 1992).

2. Thomas Erastus, *Disputationum et epistolarum medicinalium* (Tiguri: Ioannem Wolphium, 1595), 67–78.

3. "Sequitur ex dictis causam pinguedinis effectricem, esse calorem nativum qui concoctionis author est. At non quilibet calor, sed moderatus et humidus sanguinis partes tenuiores in pinguedimem transmutat." Erastus, *Disputationum*, 69.

4. Erastus, *Disputationum*, 70–73.

5. Gaspard Bachot, *Erreurs populaires touchant la medecine at regime de santé* (Lyon: Barthelemy Vincent, 1626), 203, 405.

6. Ibid., 394–419.

7. Ibid., 402.

8. Ibid., 419.

9. Tobias Venner, *Via recta ad vitam longam* (London: Edward Griffen for Richard Moore, 1620), 23.

10. Santorio Santorio, *De medicina statica* (Paris: Natale Pissot, [1611] 1725), cited in James Mackenzie, *The History of Health and the Art of Preserving It* (Edinburgh: William Gordon, 1758), 265.

11. Mackenzie, *History of Health*, 275.

12. Walter Charlton (*sic*), *Natural History of Nutrition, of Life, and Voluntary Motion* (London: Henry Herrington, 1659), 53–55.

13. Mackenzie, *History of Health*, 252.

14. Antonio Udalrico Gosky, *Disputatio solennis de Marasmo, sive marcore. Macilentia item et gracilitate sanorum. Macilentia et gracilitate aegrotantium. Crassitie et corpulentia sanorum naturali. Crassitie et magnitudine corporis morbosa aegrorum* (Strasbourg: Typis Eberhardi Welperi, 1658).

15. Regarding Sebizius' *Alimentorum facultatibus*, see my *Eating Right in the Renaissance* (Berkeley: University of California Press, 2002).

16. "Vasta, crassa, corpulenta, et quadrata, pingua item et obesa corpora visuntur quotidiè, praesertim in regionibus septentrionalibus, utroque in sexu, masculino et feminino." Gosky, *Disputatio*, fol. F3.

17. Ibid., fol. G3v.

18. Joann Fridericus Held, *Disputationem medicam de corpulentia nimia* (Jena: Typis Nisianis, 1670). "Filum ab umbilico per ilia circumdictam, si venter cibis debitè sit distentus, trium pedum mensuram attingat oportet. Hanc igitur, qui admodùm excedunt, ventriosi, corpulenti, et obesi dicuntur," fol. A2.

19. "Corpulentia nimia est molis corpoeae, ex carnis et pinguedinis augmento, nimium incrementum, ab abundante nutrimento inductam...." Held, *Disputationem*, fol. A4v.

20. Ibid., fol. B3v.

21. "Circa thoracem non solum intercostales, sed et alios, vis infimum ventrem praecipuè musculosos abdominis cum pinguedine, inter cutem et panniculum carnosum interjacente..." Ibid., fol. B2. The reference to beer, which he considered high in oily and sulphurous parts, is on fol. A4.

22. Ibid., fol. D4v, Ev.

23. Michael Ettmuller, "Dissertatio VIII: De corpulentia nimia" in *Opera Omnia*, vol. 1, (London: Sam Smith, 1688), 90.

24. Ibid., 93. In the French translation it reads as follows "en un mot ce n'est qu'une huile ou un beurre compacte qui se prend et se coagule fortement. Cecy est illustré par les experiences des huiles que les acides coagulent une substance adipeuse." *Practique speciale de medicine,* second edition (Paris: Jean Guignard, 1698), 640.

25. Ettmuller, *Practique*, second French edition, 663–664.
26. Ettmuller, 98 in Latin edition, 670 in French.
27. I would not, however, agree with James C. Whorton that the concern has always been one of constipation. Among humoralists it was corrupt raw matter in the stomach during concoction that was feared, and needed to be sped along. In the tracts discussed here, it is not so much emptying the waste products from the intestines, as flushing the entire circulatory system which contained both processed nutrients and potential or actual fat deposits. *Inner Hygiene: Constipation and the Pursuit of Health in Modern Society* (New York: Oxford University Press, 2000), ch. 1.
28. "Puellae, ait, apud Venetos cum matrimonio copulandae sint, lautè admodum tractantur, ut habiliores fiant; utuntur triticô nutritô cum lacte; longius in diem dormiunt, valde otiosae extra aërem vivunt, ut tandem caponum instar pinguescant: ideò et unctuosis ac dulcibus vescuntur cibis, ut ita magis delicatulae ac venustae suis sponsis dedicari possint." Carol Christian Leisner, *Dissertatio medica de obesitate exsuperante* (Jena: Typis Gollerianis, 1683), 4–5.
29. Ibid., 26–33.
30. Ibid., 65. "Verùm historiae Medicae non planè impossibilem vel dubiam esse obesitatis curationem nobis persuadent, licet eadem cautam ac prudentem Medici opem requirat."
31. Ibid., 75–76.
32. Ibid., 95–96.
33. Bray, "Obesity: Historical Perspective," 283.
34. Ernestus Henr. Fecht, *Disputatio medica inauguralis de obesitate nimia* (Rostock: Typis Joh. Wepplingii, 1701), 5–6.
35. Ibid., 12–13. The author in question here is one Fr. Bonamicus in *De alimentis*; "Plures Neotericorum materiam nutritam ad partes delatam coagulatione verti in nutrimentum et pinguedinem statuunt, eumque in finem blandum quoddam acidum in partibus excogitarunt, quae etiam mens Sylvius est," 18.
36. "Hoc ut probemus, ad ipsos statim provocamus pingues et obesos, qui inediam facilime ferre solent et possunt, ex nulla alia, opinor, ratione, quam quod natura ex superfluo hoc succo nutritio sive pinguedine, illud retrahere quasi vel resorbere potest, quod ad amissum restaurandum sufficiebat." Daniel Wilhelm Triller, *De pinguedine ceu succo nutritio superfluo* (Halle Magdeburgicae: Typis Christiani Henckelii, 1718), 14.
37. Thomas Short, *A Discourse Concerning the Causes and Effects of Corpulency* (London: J. Roberts, 1727), iv. "The great Desire and Inclination which too many discover, to attain a corpulent Habit of Body. . . there is a Modishness or Pleasure in it, and that it challenges Respect from others; little considering the Danger they run, in procuring such a Habit, or the many Inconveniences that attend it."
38. Ibid., 57.
39. Ibid., 72.

40. Cheyne, *An Essay of Health and Long Life* (New York: Arno Press, 1979), xvi.

41. Jeremiah Wainewright, *A Mecanical Account of the Non-Naturals* (London: Ralph Smith, 1708), 185.

42. Malcolm Flemyng, *A Discourse on the nature, causes, and cure of Corpulency* (London: Printed for L. Davis and C. Reymers, 1760). That this absurdity was actually taken seriously, one may trust William Wadd who in his own book on obesity relates this story: "a near relation of mine, many years ago, was requested by a gentleman in the country to purchase him a quarter of a hundred weight of Castile soap, for the purpose of eating it . . ." William Wadd, *Cursory Remarks on Corpulence* (London: J. Callow, 1816), 25.

Chapter 10 ✑

USELESS AND PERNICIOUS MATTER

CORPULENCE IN EIGHTEENTH-CENTURY ENGLAND[1]

Lucia Dacome

The Age of Corpulence

Thomas Wood, a miller of Billericay, in Essex, was born of intemperate parents on 30 November 1719. As a child, he suffered from various disorders, but after he recovered from smallpox at the age of thirteen, he remained healthy until about the age of forty-four. During this period, he voraciously ingested fatty meats three times a day, consumed large quantities of butter and cheese, and drank strong ale. When about forty years old, Wood began to grow very fat but continued to be healthy and "digested his food without difficulty." In his forty-fourth year, however, "he began to be disturbed in his sleep," complained "of the heart-burn," and was afflicted by "frequent sickness at his stomach, pains in his bowels, headache, and vertigo." He became sometimes costive, but at other times went to "the opposite extreme," was almost constantly thirsty, had a "great lowness of spirits," and suffered from "violent rheumatism, and frequent attacks of the gout." His illnesses also caused him two epileptic fits, and he recurrently experienced a sense of suffocation, especially after his meals.[2]

Dramatic as it might look, Wood's story of corpulence and sickness was by no means uncommon. Corpulence was on the rise in eighteenth-century British consumer society, and warnings were issued about the consequences of "intemperance and excess."[3] In 1727, for instance, Thomas Short, physician in Sheffield, noticed that people had never been so fat. "I believe," he asserted, "no Age did ever afford more Instances of Corpulency than our own."[4] In order to show the "many Advantages which a thin or middling Habit of Body is entitled to," Short then published a treatise in which he warned the increasing number of corpulent people against the dangers of "such an undesirable Load of useless and pernicious Matter." Besides its troublesome nature, propensity to disease, and tendency to shorten life, in Short's view a corpulent body could scarcely be kept from putrefaction, even while the soul still inhabited the "clayie Cottage."[5] Short's account of corpulence is striking. His association between excessive fatness and material corruption is all the more disquieting. Why did Short use such macabre language to describe corpulence? What medical views did he endorse in his rhetoric of decomposition and death? Corpulence made the body grow to an extraordinary size and brought about a host of ills. In eighteenth-century Britain its significance as a phenomenon that brought together uncontrolled physical growth and precocious death extended beyond the medical domain. By the mid century, corpulence was discussed in arenas as different as *The Gentleman's Magazine*, *The Philosophical Transactions*, and dictionaries as well as in the medical literature. And by the time George Baker, Fellow of the College of Physicians and of the Royal Society, published the account of Wood's case in the *Medical Transactions* of 1772, excessive fatness had found a stable place among eighteenth-century concerns.

Among those who wrote on corpulence in this period, the physician George Cheyne was acclaimed as an ex-corpulent man who had dieted his way into the world of the thin and healthy. Similarly to Short, Cheyne maintained that corpulence could be cured through low regimen, and from the 1720s, he made a name for himself as "Dr Diet."[6] In 1724, his *Essay of Health and Long Life* sanctioned his popularity as a guru of alimentary temperance.[7] Some years later, Cheyne famously published in *The English Malady* (1733) his own personal battle against corpulence and the temptations of lavish food, and provided an influential account of his body now growing exceedingly corpulent and now losing weight. In recent years, Cheyne's description of his corpulence and its related illnesses has been the object of considerable research. Attention has been drawn to the relationship between Cheyne's mystical background and his mechanistic philosophy, to the bearing Cheyne's medical and religious tenets had on his views of the body, and to Cheyne's pursuit of medical authority through a skilful blending of medical expertise, personal experience and caring advice.[8] However, still little is known about the role of corpulence in the setting in which Cheyne's own account of the corpulent body and its ills was developed and disseminated.

What follows explores the place of corpulence in eighteenth-century British society. Attention is drawn to views of corpulence as an impairment of the bodily economy and an affection of the balance between ingesta and excreta. The corpulent body is accordingly examined as one of the sites in which standardized views of the body and codes of social and moral integrity were discussed and negotiated.

A "Singular Distemper"

As corpulence gained in visibility, practitioners started to wonder about its causes and looked for remedies. In 1727, Short devoted his work on corpulence to the discussion of the origins and cure of this "troublesome, unhealthy, and generally unactive Habit of Body." He pointed out that as corpulence was caused by disturbances in physical evacuation, its cure largely rested on the regulation of bodily discharges. While the immediate cause of corpulence was an accumulation of blood that was not "sufficiently attenuated and discharged by Perspiration," remote causes included the bad quality of air and excessive food and drink. This meant that factors such as "warm and foggy Air," the "Air of wet, flat, and marshy Countries, as *Holland*, some Parts of *Lincolnshire*, *Essex*, and *Cambridgeshire*," "City Air" and "Plenty of Eatables and Drinkables, of a soft, smooth, balsamick Nature" all contributed to the development of this disturbance.[9] According to Short, in order to cure corpulence, one had to counteract on its causes. This included choosing to live in a clear, serene air, using exercise and labor, following a moderate and spare diet, and dedicating oneself to "all those Things which promote insensible Perspiration" such as "the Use of Flannel Shirts," cold baths, "friction with a Flesh-Brush, Hair or hard Cloth," "Gentle Evacuations," and the "Smoking of Tobacco."[10]

Elaborated within the Galenic tradition linking nutrition with transpiration, in the early modern period the notion of insensible perspiration informed a widely shared image of a porous body whose health depended on the control of secretion and discharges.[11] It also lay behind the tenet that corpulence was the outcome of a stoppage in the bodily economy and the view that its cure required proper management of the "non-naturals," namely, those environmental factors including air, food and drink, exercise, sleep and wake, and the passions of the mind, whose regulation was considered essential for the pursuit of health. Well into the eighteenth century, the non-naturals continued to play a part in the world of healing and in the literature on self-help that was addressed to the lay.[12] Short's own remarks on the endemic perishability of the corpulent body due to the accumulation of unperspired matter were consistent with contemporary views of the correlation between health, the management of the non-naturals, and the regulation of bodily excretion. His advice on how to cure corpulence was accordingly addressed to the lay rather than to the "Gentlemen of that Profession."[13]

Along with Short, other writers on corpulence, including John Fothergill, maintained that a moderate and spare diet constituted the best method to cure this "singular distemper."[14] But in 1760 Malcolm Flemyng praised the beneficial effects of diuretics, and advocated the use of soap.[15] Like Short, Flemyng maintained that excessive fatness was caused by factors like the immoderate ingestion of food, "especially of the rich and oily kind," and defective evacuation through the outlets of the body.[16] In the same way as Short, moreover, Flemyng believed that remedies against corpulence included a moderate diet based on lean and plain food, cold bathing, and proper bodily discharges through urine, feces, sweat, and insensible perspiration.[17] Unlike Short, however, he maintained that corpulence consisted in an accumulation of fat rather than of blood.[18] As such, it could be cured by soap, namely, "a composition consisting of a vegetable, fixt, alcaline salt, made by incineration, and oil or fat, whether animal or vegetable, with the addition of quick-lime." Soap was "entirely dissolvable in soft water." As much as it helped to eliminate oil and fat from clothes, and restored them "to cleanness, sweetness, and whiteness," it could also wash away the unnecessary fat of the body.[19]

In so far as the quality of soap was concerned, Flemyng preferred the Spanish soap from Alicant. But Castille soap could also do. And Flemyng recommended a course of at least three months based on the daily ingestion of no more than four drachms of soap.[20] In 1763, Dr. Wade, physician in Lisbon, declared himself perplexed by Flemyng's remedy, having once met a gentleman who had ingested soap for several months, and who ended up fatter than ever, having in fact been "emaciated when he began that course."[21] Flemyng, for his part, assured that his cure was corroborated by success. He had personally treated an extraordinarily corpulent physician who had grown fat by insensible degrees, but had ended up in grief as he became so corpulent that he was "obliged to ride from house to house to visit his patients in the town where he practised, being quite unable to walk an hundred yards at a stretch; and was in no small degree lethargic." Thanks to Flemyng's cure based on soap, the corpulent physician had recovered. After two or three months during which he "took every night at bed-time, a quarter of an ounce of common home-made castile soap, dissolved in a quarter of a pint of soft water," he "could walk a mile with pleasure."[22]

Fat Doctors

That physicians were among the ranks of those mainly affected by corpulence may have not been reassuring. And nonetheless, in eighteenth-century Britain, fat doctors were common in kind. Some of them gave rise to the image of the physician who was too corpulent to walk and check patients. This was the case, for instance, of George Cheyne, whose bodily growth to overwhelming fatness coincided with a personal and professional crisis.[23] As a distemper that made one lose control over one's actions and movements, and could be cured by means of self-control, corpulence impelled something of a moral call. In this sense, Cheyne's own story of overwhelming fatness ended up being an edifying one. As the Italian physician Antonio Cocchi (1695–1758) recalled in his analysis of excessive fatness, even in a case apparently as hopeless as Cheyne's there had been a happy ending: thanks to his conversion to vegetarian dieting and low regimen, Cheyne finally managed to lose so much weight that he could roll the skin of his belly over to his back, and could climb up the stairs and see his patients.[24]

In 1733, Cheyne dramatized his own experience as a corpulent man for the readers of *The English Malady*, his work on nervous distempers. Advocating the necessity of alimentary temperance and moderate life, the account of his own case became a memorable token of the relationship between excessive fatness, the benefices of dieting and the moral implications of the pursuit of health.[25] In it, Cheyne narrated how his own body had epitomized the whole cycle of corpulence and leanness as a cycle of viciousness and virtuosity.[26] Having been fat and greedy, Cheyne railed against "the robust" and "the high feeders." Having been a gourmand, he pronounced a final curse upon gluttony. Associating the "putrefying and cadaverous" state of his overgrown body with his addiction to excess, he evoked a state of alimentary innocence and purity. In his autobiographical piece, Cheyne confessed that being "naturally of a large Size," his insatiable appetite had caused him to grow "daily in *Bulk*" to the point of getting excessively "*fat, short-breath'd*" and lethargic. Upon the undertaking of a proper regimen, he recovered. After some time, however, he relapsed, became again "*Heavy, Dull* and *Lethargick* to an extreme Degree," and famously swelled to thirty-two stone (448 pounds).[27] Recalling his corpulence in a letter to his patient and correspondent Samuel Richardson, he wrote:

> I had been so exceedingly fat, unwieldy, and overgrown beyond any one I believe in Europe, that I weighted 34 Stone, this had so stretched my Skin and Belly, that when my Fat and Belly was shrunk to a common Size by

many repeated Vomits (at first once or twice a Week), want of Sleep, a perpetual Lowness, Loss of Appetite, and Inability to digest any Thing but Milk and Bread, my Gouts fell out through the Cawl where the Spermatic Vessels perforate it and made a Kind of Wind Rupture which was some Years a Breeding unheeded.[28]

Further evoking the excruciating days of his illness, Cheyne described his body as "a putrefied overgrown Body from Luxury and perpetual Laziness, scorbutical all over, a regular St. Anthony's Fire every Two Months, regularly the Gout all over Six Months of the Year, perpetual Reaching, Anxiety, Giddiness, Fitts, and Startings."[29] In this miserable state, he had resorted to vegetarian dieting. Having converted to low regimen, he dieted his way into his personal accomplishment as a patient and his successes as a physician and an author: he lost more than half his weight and capitalized on his condition as an ex-corpulent who had managed to overcome his sickness. Thanks to his writings, he became a much-cherished protagonist of the dissemination of low regimen and moderate life. Having spent the last part of his life as the prophet of alimentary temperance, at the age of seventy he wrote to Richardson that he felt better than ever.

Corpulent Minds

By linking his suffering as a corpulent man addicted to excess with his mental distress, Cheyne warned the "*polite* and *delicate*" readers of *The English Malady* that corpulence was not just harmful to physical health.[30] His choice to conclude his work on "Nervous Diseases of all kinds" with the account of his own case was in fact telling of the fashioning of corpulence as a particular instance of the correlation between bodily impairment and mental disorder. Corpulence provoked an irresistible sense of lethargy and gave rise to nervous distress. In doing so, it ran the risk of making one lose control over the mind.[31] Not surprisingly, Cheyne's liaison between nervous disorder and over-embodiment became particularly successful at a time in which symptoms traditionally associated with scholarly melancholy were being reconceptualized as typical vexations of affluent and urban life. As Cheyne himself observed, one third of the elite of the increasingly prosperous British society was in mental distress.[32] Now obstructing, now relaxing, and now irritating and consuming the nerves, nervous disorders widely afflicted the wealthy and the leisured, whose sedentary life, comfort, and excessive refinement made inclined to fall prey to nervous distress.[33] As excessive consumption and inactive life were included among the factors that contributed to threaten genteel minds, anti-luxury campaigners appealed to moderation and restraint as an anti-dote to the risks of the overconsuming order.[34] They exemplified these risks by presenting apocalyptic scenarios of overconsumption in which they displayed the effects of excessive ingestion on the body and its econ-omy: while they fashioned the overconsuming body as a body that was bound to perish, they warned that an overconsuming society was a society affected by a terminal disease.[35]

A number of medical treatises and manuals of polite conduct placed controlled consumption at the intersection between medical views on the benefits of low regimen and the fashioning of moderation as a crucial value of the culture of politeness. As early as 13 October 1711, Joseph Addison, prophet of the culture of politeness and editor of *The Spectator*, praised tem-perance as a "great Preservative of Health," and condemned gluttony as a symptom of present-day degeneration.[36] Well into the eighteenth century, dancing masters brought together polite manners and bodily discipline by presenting dancing both as a crucial element of a polite education and an antidote against "the gathering of those gross and foggy humors which in time form a disagreeable and inconvenient corpulence."[37] As dieting became a fashionable model of self-care, reference to Cheyne's views on regimen appeared in Chambers' *Cyclopaedia* (1728) in entries such as "abstinence," "diet," "drink," "evacuation," "exercise," "food," and "pas-sion."[38] As self-restraint, controlled ingestion, moderate exercise, and polite manners were increasingly fashioned as means of class-identification against the "vulgarity" of ungentlemanly behavior, the advocation of alimentary temperance became fashionable among that section of the genteel society that, as Lord Chesterfield put it in a letter to Cheyne of April 1742, approved of Cheyne's "physical" principles while it remained hesitant towards his metaphysics.[39]

As historians have suggested, eighteenth-century calls for low regimen, moderate exercise, and self-control may be regarded as one of the ways through which the urban elite sought to reconfirm its role in society.[40] Warnings about the impairing consequences of corpulence may accordingly be situated in a setting in which the moral dimension of self-control was meant to legitimate the claims of leadership advanced by the elite.[41] It is sig-nificant, in this sense, that the cases of corpulence that were publicized in the mid eighteenth century largely concerned men. This does not mean, of course, that women were not addressed by anti-luxury campaigners, who in fact targeted them as compulsive and uncontrollable consumers. Nor does that necessarily imply that women were not affected by corpulence; for, in fact, eighteenth-century writings on excessive fatness occasionally included cases of corpulent women as well as of corpulent men. Yet, to a large extent, eighteenth-century corpulence gained visibility as a distemper that mostly affected men.

In so far as corpulence was associated with nervous disorder, the presentation of corpulence as a predominantly male affliction may be read in the context of the gendering of nervous distempers such as hysteria and hypochondria; the former being conceptualized in terms of natural constraints inescapably affecting women's physiology, and the latter being fashioned as the consequence of improper conduct, and thus calling for a reform of men's lifestyle on the basis of higher moral grounds.[42] One may add that, alarming as they might have been, images of corpulence had a part to play in the making of the polite gentleman. While politeness constituted a crucial requirement of gentlemanliness, it also raised anxieties about the adoption of models of behavior that were associated both with the feminized culture of sensibility and the effeminate manners of French politeness. As historians have shown, an implicit tension informed eighteenth-century views of the polite gentleman with the question: could men be at the same time polite and manly?[43] This tension ran the risk of challenging the claims of moral superiority (and, therefore, entitlement to leadership) that were advanced within the culture of polite gentlemanliness. If politeness meant adopting the manners that characterized women and the French, could gentlemen legitimately aspire to the guidance of the nation? Questions such as this lay at the center of the conflicts and contradictions that accompanied the rise of polite culture in a society characterized by a dramatic increase in the access to consumption. Not surprisingly, the preparation and intake of food became one of the arenas in which such anxieties were articulated and discussed. As such, it informed the famous polemics on French cuisine, setting defenders of the wholesomeness of English cookery (corresponding to English simple and plain manners) against the lasciviousness of French dishes instantiating, according to critics, French sophisticated manners and effeminate affectation.[44] By the mid eighteenth century, one could read in polite manuals that French dishes were pernicious to the stomach.[45] In works such as in *The Trial of the Lady Allurea Luxury* (1757), French cuisine was furthermore associated with luxury, and the French "Allurea Luxury" was tried for having "most wickedly and maliciously plotted and conspired the Destruction of this Land, by corrupting the Morals of our People." One of its faults was to have covered the "old *English* hospitable Table" of a "true *Englishman*" with "nothing but Frenchified disguised Dishes" so that "high-seasoned Ragouts and masqueraded Poisons" had replaced the "honest roast

Beef and Plumb-Pudding, and the noble Bacon Chine and Turkey."[46] As the outcome of indulgence in the traditional pleasures of the "true Englishman" fond of beef, butter, mutton, and ale, corpulence could then implicitly evoke an ideal of masculinity which, once duly subjected to an appropriate course of moderation, could still comply with the demands of polite behavior without falling into the pitfall of effeminacy. As the target of moral and medical warnings about the benefits of self-control, it also made a powerful case for the social, moral, and physical implications of giving in to luxury and excessive consumption.

As calls for low regimen shaped a model of the body that was meant to guarantee well-being, new patterns of moral integrity were defined against views of the physical impairment of the corpulent body. Looming at the horizon of eighteenth-century polite and commercial society, images of abnormal embodiment came to constitute a threat to the standards of conduct that were supposed to grant the equilibrium of individual and social bodies. They also provided the basis for the formulation of criteria of normality and their correlative notions of physical health and mental balance. The model of embodiment that ensued from these criteria was construed against views of embodiment that did not match these standards. While the allegedly nervous and delicate female body was by default excluded from such standards, at the margins of this operation of normalization, corpulent bodies were fashioned as extraordinary. They were presented in association with images of intemperance, sin, deformity, overwhelming materiality, decomposition, and death. In the literature linking moderate behavior with health and mental stability, the normal body was then created along the series of oppositions that set those who were capable of regulating their bodily discharges against those who were not, and those who successfully pursued self-knowledge against those who were at risk of losing their minds. The corpulent body was accordingly presented as unnatural, pathological, preternatural, and deadly.

Extraordinary Bulks

By the mid eighteenth century, representations of corpulence had reached a new climax. In 1727, Thomas Short presented in his *Discourse* the case of a "young Lady, who died of Corpulency in the 25th Year of her Age," weighed 500 pounds, and "was a Monster in nature for Bulk" alongside that of a corpulent man, who "was to her as a Man of a middle Habit is to one exhausted by an Atrophy."[47] In 1740, moreover, Johann Georg Keysler wrote to have met in Savoy a corpulent *Englishman*, who was "said to have weighed five hundred and fifty pounds," and was then forced to employ twelve chairmen to be taken around. He then paired this case with the story of "the young Englishman of Lincoln," who was thought to eat eighteen pounds of beef every day and "weighed five hundred and thirty pounds."[48] And this was just the beginning.

In May 1751, Dr. Coe, physician at Chelmsford, discussed in the *Philosophical Transactions* the case of Mr. Bright, "the fat Man at Malden, Essex" as an example of a man who was "so extremely fat, and of such uncommon bulk and weight" that there could be "very few, if any, such instances to be found in any country, or upon record in any book."[49] Although Bright's own ancestors had been greatly inclined toward corpulence on both his parents' sides, none of them had quite matched Mr. Bright's bulk. Bright's body had in fact grown so corpulent as to become legendary. In 1751, *The London Magazine* emphasized that Bright's body appeared to be "of an astonishing bulk, and his legs were as big as a middling man's body."[50] In the same year, Coe provided a quantified account of Bright's dimensions and observed that Bright was "5 feet 9 inches and a half" in height. Round his belly, he was "6 feet 11 inches," and round the chest under the arms "5 feet 6 inches." More than a year before his death, Bright weighed forty-one stone and ten pounds or 584 pounds. But Coe suspected that by the time of his death, he may well have been above 616 pounds. In 1754, Bright's corpulence appeared in *A New and Complete Dictionary of the Arts and Sciences* as "the most extraordinary instance of corpulency perhaps ever known." Here, no doubt was left as to Bright's dimensions as it was pointed out that Mr. Bright's waistcoat could with great ease be buttoned round seven men of ordinary size.[51]

In mid-eighteenth-century Britain, Bright's extraordinary body instantiated a special case of the correlation between the spectacle of excessive fatness, the increased mortality of the corpulent body and its inertia. During his life, Bright had been "the gazing-stock and admiration of all people, as he walked along the street."[52] But his very death was turned into something of a show. Many attended the making of his massive coffin. Details of the coffin's dimensions were then publicized in the *London Magazine*, where it was also emphasized that "a way was cut thro' the wall and staircase, to let the corpse down into the shop."[53] When time came to celebrate the funeral, people "not only of the town but of the country for several miles round about" gathered to see how such "a corpse could be got to the ground." Coe himself lured readers with the voyeuristic tension accompanying Bright's interment and concluded his article by recalling that the coffin

> was drawn to the church on a low wheel'd carriage by ten or twelve men, and was let down into the grave by an engine fixed up in the church for that purpose.[54]

The same rhetoric of exaggeration characterizing the account of Bright's death found a particularly fertile field of expression in the description of the deaths of those who were affected by preternatural corpulency. As in the case of the "young *Englishman* of *Lincoln*" who died in 1724 "in the 28th year of his age," narratives of corpulence frequently ended with the sudden and premature death of the main character.[55] As a particular kind of literary *genre*, such narratives were codified at the point of intersection between the obituary and the curious report. In a letter to Mark Catesby published in the *Philosophical Transactions* of 1746, for instance, Thomas Knowlton reported that as one of the brothers of Halifax, Yorkshire, who weighed, respectively, thirty-four and thirty-five stone (respectively, 476 and 490 pounds), "was mounting an Horse, the poor Creature's Back broke under him, and he died on the spot."[56] Similarly, in the obituaries for the year 1754, the *Gentleman's Magazine* recorded that Mr. Jacob Powell, of Stebbing in Essex, who, together with Bright, was taken to be one of the largest men on record, weighed nearly "40 stone, or 560 pounds," and had "sixteen men to carry him to his grave."[57] Sometimes, as in the case of "the great Mr. Benjamin Bower, so called from his enormous size" who died in December 1763, part the wall of the room where he died had "to be taken down to get the corpse out."[58] In such reports, the cadavers of corpulent people were characterized by their extraordinary materiality. They were weighty, cumbersome, bulky, and firmly anchored to the ground in a way that was proportional to their mass.

Such correlation between the inertial aspects and sheer materiality of the corpulent body, and death, may be read against the image of corpulence physicians such as Cheyne and Short had helped to create, an image that was largely articulated in the vocabulary of decomposition and death. The very adjectives Cheyne used to describe his formerly overgrown body drew on the semantics of decomposition: "putrefying" and "cadaverous," his corpulent body was no longer a living human body, and Cheyne famously called it a "crazy carcase." For his part, as we have seen, Short described corpulence as the accumulation of "useless and pernicious Matter" leading to the untimely putrefaction of the living body.[59] The view that excessive fatness constituted a prelude to premature death was yet again spelled out in Coe's account of Bright's extraordinary corpulence, where it was observed that those who knew Bright were generally fond of him but also sorrowfully "looked upon him for several years as a man who could not live long."[60]

The Slenderness of the Miller

The deadly consequences affecting the characters populating eighteenth-century narratives of corpulence may have well informed the destiny of Thomas Wood, the miller from Billericay, whose growth to over-embodiment and ill health we saw at the beginning of this paper. Like some of the protagonists of the stories of corpulence reported in dictionaries and periodicals, Wood was depicted as a countryside glutton. As a voracious eater of meat, conspicuous consumer of butter, and avid drinker of ale, he seemed to have, as it were, pushed the characteristics of the "thorough-bred Englishman" to their ultimate and most lethal consequences. And yet, in the same way as Cheyne's, Wood's story ended up being an edifying one. In August 1764, Mr. Powley, "a worthy clergyman in the neighbourhood" was moved by Wood's ill state of health, recommended him to follow "an exact regimen," and suggested "*The Life of Cornaro*" as a book that was likely "to suggest to him a salutary course of living."[61]

First brought out in the second half of the sixteenth century, Luigi Cornaro's writings on the sober life of made a powerful case for the correlation between sobriety and longevity, and continued to be published, discussed, and quoted throughout the eighteenth century.[62] Drawing on personal experience, Cornaro's *Discorsi della vita sobria* (1591) narrated how, having spent his youth in debauchery and excesses, when "not above 35 or 40 Years Old" Cornaro found himself sick and ailing, decided to convert to sobriety, and was rewarded by a healthy and long existence. The main tenet informing Cornaro's work was that sobriety constituted a major relief to moral and physical evils. Although in his *Discorsi* he concentrated on food, Cornaro was aware that proper management of the other non-naturals also played an important part in the pursuit of health.[63] Cornaro's work convinced Wood that intemperance was the main cause of his illnesses and complaints, and made him resolved to follow Cornaro's own path. As he began to reduce his consumption of ale and animal food, he started to feel better. He then gave up all malt liquor, began to drink only water, and ate only the lighter meats. As he still suffered from rheumatism and occasional fits of the gout, he took for some time cold baths twice or three times a week and then began the exercise of the dumb-bell. From 25 October 1765 to 9 May 1766 he did not drink anything at all. In the summer of 1767, he gave up cheese and animal flesh, ate mainly a pudding made of sea-biscuit, and changed his sleeping patterns, going to bed no later than eight o'clock and waking up before two in the morning. Thanks to this strict course of abstinence, Wood recovered. As his health was reestablished, his spirits were again lively, his sleep was no longer disturbed by frightful dreams, and he felt stronger than ever. In short, he was metamorphosed "from a monster to a person of a moderate size; from the condition of an unhealthy, decrepit, old man, to perfect health, and to the vigour and activity of youth."[64]

The narrative of Wood's conversion to low regimen was articulated along the lines of Cornaro's and Cheyne's ones. As well as in the case of these latter, it unfolded as the story of the undertaking of a path of personal redemption leading from misery to happiness, as well as from corpulence to thinness, and from illness to health. As well as in Cornaro's and Cheyne's stories of moderation, moreover, it became exemplary. In fact, not only did Wood's embracement of low regimen and dramatic loss of weight save him from unbearable illness and precocious death, it also turned him into a healing authority and legitimated his role as a source of advise to others. As Wood's case was publicized, correspondents started to contact him in search of advice. Wood, for his part, replied to their requests and provided guidance on the preservation of health.[65] At the end of his course of conversion to sobriety, a portrait of the "abstemious miller" furthermore testified to his new physical state (figure 10.1). Here, Wood was depicted as a lean man dressed in gentlemanly jacket, and standing against a background where, at a distance, there lay some mills, the mark of his profession. By presenting Wood as a thin man, the portrait provided the evidence of the success of his course of dieting. As a representation of the happy outcome of Wood's conversion to moderation, it may have also offered a source of encouragement to those who found that the path towards leanness and health was not an easy one. In this sense, the portrait articulated visually what Cheyne's account of his corpulence had provided verbally, namely, the promise that even in the worst cases of corpulence, there was hope: all one had to do was to undertake a proper diet. Looking at the portrait, patients may have linked Wood's thin frame with the promise of health, youth, and vigor, which Wood claimed to have achieved along with weight loss. The portrait may have then contributed to legitimate Wood's credibility at the intersection of the correlation between leanness, health, and the promise of status.[66]

Conclusion

In eighteenth-century Britain, corpulence fell at the center of the tensions and contradictions of a society divided between the calls for moderation

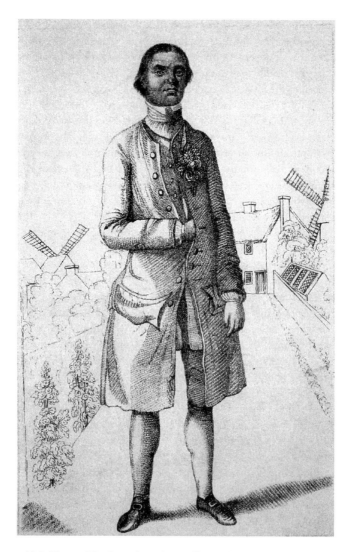

Figure 10.1 Thomas Wood, an abstemious miller, aged 53. Reproduction of a stipple engraving by R. Cooper after J. Ogberne, 1773 (Courtesy of Wellcome Library, London).

formulated within the culture of politeness and the interests and passions inscribed in the ethics of trade and consumption.[67] In this context, the physical impairment of the corpulent body epitomized the risks associated with excessive consumption. This essay has investigated how representations of corpulence were functional to the legitimation of a view of normalized embodiment that was associated with notions of physical, moral, and intellectual integrity. On this basis, it has read the motif of the marvelous deaths of corpulent people against the calls for temperance substantiating the status and authority of the self-controlled. As we have seen, eighteenth-century representations of corpulence played a part in the prescriptive literature on self-help that was addressed to the lay. Here, the corpulent body came to substantiate the fears and anxieties that informed the relationship between excessive consumption, mental instability, and untimely death. At the same time, narratives of corpulence also presented a special case of the interplay between prescriptive literature and bodily practice, between the shaping of an ideal of embodiment and individual forms of engagement with the norm encoded by such ideal. In the same way as Wood, a number of corpulent people responded to the warnings about the consequences of over-embodiment. The stories that thereby ensued provide a special insight into something as personal and as intimate as one's relationship with one's own body, the forms of uneasiness, discomfort, and dissatisfaction (as well as pleasure) generated by it, and the social pressures that were exercised on individuals to take steps to modify it. In doing so, they also shed light on the symbolic order of corpulence by providing a stage in which stories of recovery from excessive fatness tackled widely shared anxieties about the unsettling and potentially disruptive forces of consumer society. Bringing together the instantiation of ideals of self-control, a successful parable of redemption, and the codification of a socially exemplary role, Wood's portrait may then be regarded as a visual token of the part played by the abdomen (or the lack of it) in the articulation of the relationship between eighteenth-century bodies and selves. It tells us that eating like a gentleman encoded the promise of becoming one.

Notes

1. For comments and suggestions at various stages during the development of this essay, I would like to thank Daniel Beauregard, Cristina Chimisso, Serafina Cuomo, Silvia de Renzi, Patricia Fara, Marina Frasca-Spada, Colin Jones, George Rousseau, Valerie Taylor, the editors of this volume, and especially Joseph Berkovitz, Simon Schaffer, and Emma Spary. Roy Porter provided

insights into an early version of this paper. I have benefited from discussions in seminars and conferences at Cambridge University, Warwick University, and the University of Edinburgh. I would also like to thank Miriam Gutierrez-Perez for her help with the visual material and the Wellcome Trust for financial support.

2. George Baker, "The Case of Mr. Thomas Wood, a Miller, of Billericay, in the Country of Essex [. . .]. Read at the College on September 9, 1767," *Medical Transactions* (London: Baker and Dodsley, 1772), 259–274, esp. 261–263.

3. Thomas Short, *A Discourse Concerning the Causes and Effects of Corpulency together with the Method for his Prevention and Cure* (London: Roberts, 1727), iii–iv. On consumerism in the eighteenth century, see the classic Neil McKendrick, John Brewer, John H. Plumb, eds., *The Birth of a Consumer Society: The Commercialization of Eighteenth-Century England* (London: Europa Publications, 1982). See also Sara Pennell, "Consumption and Consumerism in Early Modern England," *The Historical Journal*, 42:2 (1999), 549–564.

4. Short, *Discourse*, 10.

5. Short, *Discourse*, v.

6. *Remarks on Cheyne's Essay of Health and Long Life* (Dublin: Watts, 1725), third edition, 7.

7. George Cheyne, *An Essay of Health and Long Life* (London: Strahan and Leake, 1724).

8. See Anita Guerrini, "Case History as Spiritual Autobiography: George Cheyne's 'Case of the Author,'" *Eighteenth Century Life*, 19:2 (1995), 18–27; David E. Shuttleton, "Methodism and Dr. George Cheyne's 'More Enlightening Principles,'" in *Medicine in the Enlightenment,* Roy Porter, ed. (Amsterdam-Atlanta: Rodopi, 1995), 316–335; George S. Rousseau, "Mysticism and Milleniarism: 'Immortal Dr. Cheyne,'" in *Millenarianism and Messianism in English Literature and Thought, 1650–1800 Clark Library Lectures 1981–1982,* Richard H. Popkin, ed. (Leiden: E.J. Brill, 1988), 81–126; and Brian J. Gibbons, "Mysticism and Mechanism: the Religious Context of George Cheyne's Representation of the Body and its Ills," *British Journal for Eighteenth-Century Studies*, 21:1 (1998), 1–23; Anita Guerrini, *Obesity and Depression in the Enlightenment: The Life and Times of George Cheyne* (Norman: University of Oklahoma Press, 2000); and Steven Shapin, "Trusting George Cheyne: Scientific Expertise, Common Sense, and Moral Authority in Early Eighteenth-Century Dietetic Medicine," *Bulletin of the History of Medicine,* 77:2 (2003), 263–297.

9. Short, *Discourse*, 9–25.

10. Short, *Discourse*, 68–79.

11. See Edward T. Renbourn, "The Natural History of Insensible Perspiration: A Forgotten Doctrine of Health and Disease," *Medical History,* 4 (1960), 135–152 and Jerome J. Bylebyl, "Nutrition, Quantification and Circulation," *Bulletin of the History of Medicine,* 51:3 (1977), 369–385. Having undertaken a long course of self-experimentation based on weight-watching in order to inquire into the correlation between bodily evacuation and health, the physician Santorio

Santorio (1561–1636) became the champion of the measurement and regulation of insensible perspiration. Santorio tenets linking health with insensible perspiration were still largely shared by those who wrote on corpulence in the eighteenth century. On eighteenth-century appropriations and elaborations of Santorio doctrine and practice, see Lucia Dacome "Living with the Chair: Private Excreta, Collective Health and Medical Authority in the Eighteenth-Century," *History of Science*, 39:4 (2001), 467–500.

12. On the non-naturals, see Lelland J. Rather, "The 'Six Things Non-Natural': A Note on the Origins and Fate of a Doctrine and a Phrase," *Clio Medica, 3* (1968), 337–347; Peter H. Niebyl, "The Non–Naturals," *Bulletin of the History of Medicine*, 45:5 (1971), 486–492; Antoinette Emch–Dériaz, "The Non-Naturals Made Easy," in *The Popularization of Medicine, 1650–1850,* Roy Porter, ed. (London: Routledge, 1992), 134–159; Heikki Mikkeli, *Hygiene in the Early Modern Medical Tradition* (Helsinki: Academia Scientiarum Finnica, 1999).

13. Short, *Discourse*, 68.

14. John Fothergill, "Case of an *Angina Pectoris*, with Remarks," *Medical Observations and Inquiries* (London: Cadell, 1776), vol. 5, 233–251, esp. 248–251.

15. Malcolm Flemyng, *A Discourse on the Nature, Causes and Cure of Corpulency Illustrated by a Remarkable Case, Read before the Royal Society, November 1757* (London: Davis and Reymers, 1760).

16. Ibid., 4–7.

17. Ibid., 10–15.

18. Ibid., 2.

19. Ibid., 20–21.

20. Ibid., 24–25.

21. "Case of a Preternatural Fatness, by Dr. Wade, Physician at Lisbon. *Read* November 7, 1763," in *Medical Observations and Inquiries* (London: Johnston, 1767), vol. 3, 69–84, esp. 83.

22. Flemyng, *Discourse*, 26–28.

23. See George Cheyne, *The English Malady: or, a Treatise of Nervous Diseases of all Kinds* (London: Strahan, 1733), 325 ff. On Cheyne's crisis, see Rousseau, "Mysticism and Millenarianism," 92–96 and Guerrini, *Obesity and Depression*, ch 1.

24. Antonio Cocchi, "Consulto primo: Eccessiva grassezza," in *Consulti medici, Opere di Antonio Cocchi* (Milan: Società tipografica dei Classici italiani, 1824), vol. 3, 1–4, esp. 3.

25. On the overlapping between medical and moral discourse in early modern England, see Keith Thomas, "Health and Morality in Early Modern England," in *Morality and Health,* Allan M. Brandt and Paul Rozin, eds. (New York: Routledge, 1997), 15–34; and Steven Shapin, "How to Eat Like a Gentleman: Dietetics and Ethics in Early Modern England," in *Right Living: An Anglo-American Tradition of Self-Help Medicine and Hygiene*, Charles E. Rosenberg ed. (Baltimore: Johns Hopkins University Press, 2003), 21–58.

26. Guerrini, "Case History."

27. See Cheyne, *The English Malady*, 325–326, 342, and 344.

28. George Cheyne, *The Letters of Doctor George Cheyne to Samuel Richardson (1733–1743)* (Columbia: University of Missouri, 1943), 76–77.

29. Ibid., 77.

30. Cheyne, *The English Malady*, 362.

31. In his analysis of the nightmare of 1753, for instance, the physician John Bond presented several cases of intemperate and corpulent individuals who were troubled by terrible nightmares. See John Bond, *An Essay on the Incubus, or Night–Mare* (London: Wilson and Durham, 1753), 55 and 64–65.

32. Cheyne, *The English Malady*, 261.

33. On the nervous body and nervous disorder in eighteenth-century Britain, see George S. Rousseau, "Nerves, Spirits, and Fibres: Towards Defining the Origins of Sensibility," in *Studies in the Eighteenth Century,* R. F. Brissenden and J. C. Eade, eds. (Toronto: University of Toronto Press, 1976), vol. 3: 137–157, and G. J. Barker-Benfield, *The Culture of Sensibility: Sex and Society in Eighteenth-Century Britain* (Chicago: University of Chicago Press, 1996), ch 1.

34. See, e.g., Roy Porter, "The Rage of Party: A Glorious Revolution in English Psychiatry," *Medical History,* 27:1 (1983), 35–50; and idem, "Introduction," in *George Cheyne: The English Malady (1733)* (London: Routledge, 1991), ix–li.

35. On anxieties of over-consumption in eighteenth-century Britain, see Roy Porter, "Consumption: Disease of the Consumer Society?" in *Consumption and the World of Goods,* John Brewer and Roy Porter, eds. (London: Routledge, 1993), 58–81.

36. Joseph Addison et al., *The Spectator* [1711–1714] (Oxford: Clarendon Press, 1965), vol. 2, 264.

37. Giovanni Andrea Gallini, *A Treatise on the Art of Dancing* (London: for the author, 1762), 154.

38. Ephraim Chambers, *Cyclopaedia: Or, an Universal Dictionary of Arts and Sciences* (London: James and John Knapton et al., 1728), 2 vols.

39. Philip Dormer Stanhope, *The Letters of Philip Dormer Stanhope, 4th Earl of Chersterfield* B. Dobrée, ed. (London: Eyre and Spottiwoode Publishers, 1932), vol. 2, 494–495. Cf. Gibbons, "Mysticism and Mechanism," 22.

40. See Akihito Suzuki, "Anti-Lockean Enlightenment? Mind and Body in Early Eighteenth-Century English Medicine," in *Medicine in the Enlightenment,* Roy Porter, ed. (Amsterdam: Rodopi, 1995), 336–359 esp. 349–351. See also James Raven, "Defending Conduct and Property: The London Press and the Luxury Debate," in *Early Modern Conceptions of Property,* John Brewer and Susan Staves, eds. (London: Routledge, 1995), 301–319.

41. On the role of dietetic advice in the moral discourse of early modern gentlemanly society, see Shapin, "How to Eat Like a Gentleman."

42. See John Mullan, *Sentiment and Sociability: The Language of Feeling in the Eighteenth Century* (Oxford: Clarendon Press, 1988) 216 ff. and Barker-Benfield, *The Culture of Sensibility.*

43. See Michèle Cohen, *Fashioning Masculinity: National Identity and Language in the Eighteenth Century* (London: Routledge, 1996) and idem, "Manliness, Effeminacy and the French: Gender and the Construction of National Character in Eighteenth-Century England," in *English Masculinities, 1660–1800,* Tim Hitchcock and Michèle Cohen, eds. (London: Longman, 1999), 44–61.

44. See Stephen Mennell, *All Manners of Food: Eating and Taste in England and France from the Middle Ages to the Present* (Urbana: University of Illinois Press, 1996), 92 and 96–98.

45. *The Young Gentleman and Lady Instructed in such Principles of Politeness, Prudence, and Virtue* (London: Wicksteed, 1747), vol. 2, 173–174.

46. *The Tryal of the Lady Allurea Luxury* (London: Noble, 1757), 6, 12–13 and 19.

47. Short, *Discourse,* 9–10.

48. Johann Georg Keysler, *Travels through Germany, Bohemia, Hungary, Switzerland, Italy and Lorrain,* translated from the second edition of the German (London: Linde and Field, 1756–1757), second edition, vol. 1, 189.

49. T. Coe, "A Letter from Dr. T. Coe, Physician at Chelmsford, in Essex to Dr. Cromwell Mortimer, Secr. R. S. concerning Mr. Bright, the Fat Man at Malden in Essex," *Philosophical Transactions of the Royal Society of London,* 47 (1751–1752), 188–193.

50. *The London Magazine: Or Gentleman's Monthly Intelligencer* (London: Baldwin, 1751), 82.

51. *A New and Complete Dictionary of Arts and Sciences* (London: Owen, 1744–1755), vol. 1, 758, entry on "Corpulency."

52. Coe, "A Letter," 189.

53. *The London Magazine,* 82.

54. Coe, "A Letter," 193.

55. See Keysler, *Travels,* 89.

56. Thomas Knowlton, "Extracts of Two Letters from Mr. Tho. Knowlton to Mr. Mark Catesby, F. R. S., concerning the Situation of the Ancient Town Delgovicia; and of two Men of an Extraordinary Bulk and Weight," *Philosophical Transactions of the Royal Society of London,* 44 (1746–1747), 102.

57. "List of Deaths for the Year 1754," *The Gentleman's Magazine* (London: Henry & Cave, 1754), 24, 483.

58. William Wadd, *Cursory Remarks on Corpulence; or Obesity Considered as a Disease* (London: Callow, 1816), 101.

59. Short, *Discourse,* v.

60. Coe, "A Letter," 192.

61. Baker, "The Case of Mr. Thomas Wood," 263.

62. Joseph Addison and George Cheyne were among those who discussed Cornaro in their writings. See Addison, *The Spectator,* vol. 2, 266–267 and George Cheyne, *The Natural Method of Cureing the Diseases of the Body, and the Disorders of the Mind depending on the Body* (London: Strahan et al., 1742), 296–298.

63. Luigi Cornaro, *Sure and Certain Methods of Attaining a Long and Healthful Life* (London: Midwinter, 1727), fourth edition, 14–15.
64. Baker, "The Case of Mr. Thomas Wood," 263–267.
65. George Baker, "A Sequel to the Case of Mr. Thomas Wood, of Billericay, in the County of Essex," in *Medical Transactions* (London: Dodsley *et al.*, 1785), vol. 3, 313.
66. For a discussion of the role of portraiture in the eighteenth-century medical world, see Ludmilla Jordanova, "Portraits, People and Things: Richard Mead and Medical Identity," *History of Science*, 41:3 (2003), 293–313.
67. See John Brewer, "The Most Polite Age and the Most Vicious: Attitudes towards Culture as a Commodity, 1660–1800," in *The Consumption of Culture: Image, Object, Text,* Ann Bermingham and John Brewer, eds. (London: Routledge, 1995), 341–361.

Chapter 11 ∾

"THE BELLY OF PARIS"

THE DECLINE OF THE FAT MAN IN FIN-DE-SIÈCLE FRANCE[1]

Christopher E. Forth

In early 1898, the journalist Séverine interviewed the renowned French novelist Émile Zola in his home shortly after he had published his essay "J'Accuse," an event that helped transform the Dreyfus Affair into a national crisis. Describing the rather Spartan interior of Zola's study, she detected a note of asceticism in her surroundings that seemed to conflict with her older impressions of the novelist, impressions that Séverine obviously thought her audience would share. "Zola, an ascetic?" she asked. "Really? Yes. Don't be too quick to smile or gasp." Zola's reputation as a successful novelist with a passion for fine food was quite well known, as was the rather considerable girth that he had acquired along the way. In fact, next to Sarah Bernhardt, Zola was the most frequently caricatured of French celebrities, so when some of his critics nastily dubbed him (after his novel of the same name) "the belly of Paris," everyone knew what they meant. Contrary to these conventional images of Zola, Séverine noted a profound change in the novelist that seemed to explain the heroic gesture he had just made. "And one should believe it when I say that this new Zola...reveals himself, asserts himself in such a way that I never noticed before.... He is not pleasing to look at; he is not ugly either; in any case, he is neither pudgy nor brutish. In the end he is simply well-shaped, like one of those hunting dogs of [the military academy at] Saint-Germain, of a superior race."[2]

This attention to the body of the "new Zola" seems trivial when one considers the gravity of the situation. In defense of a Jewish army officer unjustly found guilty in 1894 of selling military secrets to the Germans, the novelist had willingly exposed himself to libel charges by accusing highly placed army officers of a shameful breach of justice. Zola's scandalous gesture forced a public reconsideration of the case of Alfred Dreyfus and effectively divided large segments of the nation into warring factions, and thrust him even further into the limelight. Many observers believed this move had even transformed Zola himself. The writer Octave Mirbeau, for instance, perceived a most startling transformation in the man: "since these events, Zola is less nervous, less febrile than usual, he is more in possession of himself—body, mind, and soul . . . . He is ready to sacrifice his liberty, to give his life for the triumph of his cause, which is that of humanity."[3] As his pro-Dreyfus defenders saw it, the defense of republican ideals against the reactionary forces of religion and the military was no simple matter of political conviction; rather, taking up such a position was offered as proof of virile manhood grounded in a healthy body. Séverine's comments thus conform to a desire to view Zola as a hero whose body spoke volumes about his soul. Where Mirbeau found proof of Zola's heroism in his renewed vigor and determination, Séverine happily observed that the "new Zola" was no longer fat, but "simply well-shaped."

This chapter considers the relationship of Zola's body to the emerging cult of slenderness and muscularity that targeted the fat belly as one of the conspicuous signs of sensual excess and lack of self-control. The decline of the fat man or, more specifically, the emerging idea that manhood and obesity were mutually exclusive qualities, must be understood within the tangle of a series of cultural anxieties, from age-old medical warnings about the emasculating potential of the sedentary lifestyle to a renewed emphasis on bodily strength and vigor at the dawn of the twentieth century. Despite the dubious nature of the organ itself, a large belly had once nevertheless served as a symbol of male bourgeois power, a sign that he could afford to indulge in what so many others could only dream of. By the end of the century, however, boasting a large belly could no longer be seen as an unproblematic claim to manhood.

Gender and Willpower

When conceptualized as a defect of lifestyle rather than a congenital trait, fat is presented as a problem chiefly surmountable through acts of willpower (such as exercise and dietary reform), a faculty that has been considered intrinsically masculine for much of the modern period. During the nineteenth century physicians often emphasized the amorphousness of female psychology, alleging an inherent instability that rendered women especially prone to nervousness and more subject to the demands of the flesh. This is not to say that women were not often implored to perform feats of self-denial that might attest to their solid moral standing—indeed, numerous examples of female self-abnegation in the nineteenth century illustrate this fact. Rather, these gendered medical assumptions in a sense provided women with a moral safety net when they erred: after all, lapses of the female will ultimately testified to what most men considered the "natural" weakness of women, which meant that nervous and weak-willed women were still safely within the parameters of their sex. The fate of the so-called "fasting girls" in the hands of nineteenth-century physicians illustrates this point. By diagnosing them as anorectics doctors were able to explain the female refusal of food by reference to an irrational compulsion rather than conscious design, thereby transforming what might have been viewed as an act of will into a simple subordination to a fixed idea.[4] There is thus a gender dimension to the issues of fat and weight loss. When not reduced to a hereditary or glandular problem, fat people attested to a failure of the will, suggesting their inability to overcome the demands of the flesh: "What compounds the difficulty of treatment," noted one physician, "is that nearly all fat people suffer from a veritable intellectual apathy; among them the force of will has diminished considerably. . . ."[5] For all of the scorn heaped upon her, a weak-willed woman still qualified as feminine (despite her straying away from feminine conventions of beauty), while a weak-willed man was no man at all, at least not in any normative sense.

What was called "educating the will" at the turn of the century was in many respects a continuation of the long cultural process whereby a sense of discrete individuality was being carved out by members of the bourgeoisie, allowing them at once to distance themselves from their own bodily functions while displacing anxiety about those functions onto other social groups. Throughout modern history, dietetics and the management of appetite have provided critical means of constructing such an identity. Stephen Mennell claims that a veritable "civilizing of appetite" had been underway at least since the mid eighteenth century when instances of gluttony were increasingly described as throwbacks to earlier manners. With the rising bourgeoisie aping the aristocracy at every step, Mennell argues, new practices of social distinction were installed at the level of refined eating habits rather than in the quantity of food consumed. One effect of these new practices was a growing contempt for gluttony and the physical excess it sometimes wrought. This seems to have been the case with King Louis XVI, whose excesses at the table were noted with contempt, whereas less than a century before the gluttony of Louis XIV was considered more or less acceptable. Such themes came to a head on the eve of the French Revolution, where references to the fatness of the "pig-king" were often coupled with revelations about his sexual impotence, providing early evidence of a growing distance between obesity and emerging ideas of manhood.[6]

A more pronounced shift toward thinner bodies took place around the 1890s and coincided with what many considered to be an acute crisis of masculine identity, a growing anxiety about gender roles that stemmed in part from a humiliating defeat at the hands of Prussia in 1870 and from the inability of the French to revitalize their stagnating birthrate. The fact of depopulation frustrated a desire for revenge against the newly formed and surprisingly fecund German empire by restricting the number of French troops that could be called upon in the inevitable rematch between the two countries. This natalist discourse constituted what Robert Nye has called the period's "master pathology" and was the common denominator of many other concerns, from the apparent rise of criminals and sexual "deviants" to the emergence of the independent New Woman and a modest feminist movement.[7] Against this rising tide of effeminacy and weakness, the campaign to foster "real" men was carried out in places like high schools, where physical education was used to supplement what many saw as an overly cerebral pedagogy, and in sporting clubs, where the sedentary bourgeoisie could work their bodies so as to stave off neurasthenia and other disorders. "Educating the will" was a phrase on everyone's lips, and often implied a reform of the body as a means of combating nervous disorders and rebuilding character. Insofar as most medical texts conceived of the will in more or less materialist terms—that is, as being itself an epiphenomenon of somatic processes—few regarded the exercise of volition as a simple case of mind over matter. Rather, the will was an inhibiting force that kept the self together by inhibiting the flow of passionate drives that would otherwise overwhelm the person. To the extent that a strong will was seen as being necessarily grounded in a healthy physicality, educating the will meant an ability to wield the body against itself or, more specifically, against those unruly aspects of corporeality so frequently regarded as "flesh." As many health reformers noted, this privileging of the ordered body over the unruly flesh had an important antecedent in Rousseau, who noted in *Émile* that "The weaker the body, the more it commands; the stronger it is, the more it obeys. All the sensual passions lodge in effeminated bodies."[8]

The triumph of appetite over self-control was inscribed in the fat man's belly, and signified the connection between modernity's material abundance and sensual pleasures, and the physical decline of men. As the next section demonstrates, the effeminate qualities attributed to the fat man bore a more than passing resemblance to the neurasthenic, the epitome of failed manhood at the fin de siècle. Insofar as both were marked by sexual impotence, muscular weakness, and diseases of the will, the fat man and the gaunt neurasthenic were far removed from the normative masculine standards of the day. While neither of these male figures were pathologized to the same extent as criminals, sexual deviants, homosexuals, and the insane, they were constructed out of the same discursive materials: each stood outside of the vaguely defined sphere of heroic male volition.

"A Good Cock is Never Fat"

Although fat people had often provided fodder for caricaturists throughout the modern period, one does not encounter many self-help manuals devoted to weight loss before the 1890s, after which obesity became a "disease" that threatened to diminish the manly force of men and the feminine charms of women. Three arguments allowed physicians to successfully gender the fat man as feminine in the eyes of contemporaries, all of which sketched sharp contrasts to what was considered normative masculine behavior. First, physicians drew close connections between genital activity and digestive processes, and commonly suggested that fat men were sexually inadequate. Second, in an attempt to dispel the perceived equivalence between excessive body weight and manly strength, physicians emphasized repeatedly that a large body often concealed an inner weakness, both in terms of the energy burned off and the body's capacity for physical force. Third, they invoked widespread anxieties about pathologies of male volition to suggest that fat men lacked willpower and initiative.

The connection between digestion and gender identity is surely one of the least explored aspects of the cultural history of the body. Although during the premodern period the dominance of humoral physiology made it possible for Western medicine to draw close connections between digestion and the moral complexion of the person, such liaisons were frequently noted well into the twentieth century. Insofar as they envisioned the body as an inner economy where the excessive expenditure of energy in one area threatened to diminish it in other parts, nineteenth-century physicians posited a relationship between digestion and genital activity that has often been overlooked in histories of sexuality. Under normal circumstances the functions of the stomach do not provoke a loss of equilibrium, noted an 1852 text on impotence, though extremely obese people sometimes find it functionally difficult to copulate and in order to be successful must resort to sexual positions normally reserved for libertines. Yet in cases of overeating, this physician observed, the stomach draws upon forces from throughout the body to compensate for this overexcitation. "Everyone knows that after a large meal, especially if one has imbibed spiritous liqueurs, the genital forces are far from responding to the ardors of desire."[9] So widespread was this belief that even Brillat-Savarin counseled his readers against undertaking sexual activity or even intellectual pursuits in the aftermath of a good meal.[10]

Such concerns with digestion and sexuality were easily transferred to the issue of obesity. When it came to matters of nutrition and digestion one could not hope for a more authoritative guide than Dr. Charles Bouchard, whose theory of intestinal autointoxication resonated across the western world. Bouchard's take on obesity was nevertheless somewhat surprising insofar as he insisted that neither overeating nor lack of exercise could be isolated as dominant causes of the disorder. On the contrary, in his writings genital factors played an especially prominent role. Not only are women twice as disposed to obesity as men, Bouchard explained, but more than three quarters of obese women become obese after pregnancy, that is after "one of the acts of the genital life." An inverse development takes place among men, he noted, upon whom "genital activity has a slenderizing effect; on the contrary chastity or castration engender obesity." Hence, in Bouchard's mind, the urgency that obesity merited, for "obesity is really a disease because it leads to impotence and sterility."[11] The *Dictionnaire encyclopédique des sciences médicales* came to a similar conclusion about the relationship between virility and obesity: "Among obese men the sexual instinct is in general barely developed; some are absolutely impotent." Like some of his colleagues, the author had recourse to an old French proverb to illustrate his point: "a good cock, they say, is never fat."[12] Another physician even observed the complete absence of spermatozoa in the semen of certain fat men, thus ruling out any possibility of conception.[13] Not only did body weight become a more or less direct expression of one's capacity to procreate, but fat men came off as less virile than thin men, either by choice or by accident. Amid the welter of natalist discourses and anxieties about depopulation, fat men visibly embodied their helplessness in the face of a national crisis.

This opinion was by no means unanimous, however. Physicians like Adrien Proust and Albert Mathieu found evidence that sexual excess could just as easily lead to obesity as to slenderness.[14] On the other hand, their description of the classic obese weakling was explicitly gendered: "Weak, anemic, and plethoric fat people," they wrote, "are pale, fatigued, lifeless. . . . they are apathetic, drowsy, without energy and without courage." Significantly, this form of obesity was to be found most often among children and young people, and especially among girls.[15] Along with Bouchard, Proust and Mathieu also recognized a direct relationship between obesity and nervous disorders that suggested the femininity of overweight people. Bouchard too had noticed that hysteria was frequently accompanied by instances of excessive obesity: "Given the predominant role that the nervous system plays in all nutritional changes," he wrote, "one should count on a close relationship between certain nervous disorders and obesity."[16] Such observations convinced many physicians of the need to treat the nerves as an indirect means of curing obesity and other digestive problems, and often recommended such conventional therapies as hydrotherapy.[17]

Allied with the inability to engender children was the charge that fat men lacked the capacity for physical force. Traditional popular beliefs were perhaps the most formidable obstacle for the physicians to overcome in the pathologization of obesity, especially in those cases where fat had once seemed synonymous with strength and well-being. Medical opinion militated explicitly against the notion that a large frame signified strength, suggesting instead that what had been ordinarily considered a sign of vitality and fertility was in fact evidence of weakness and even impotence. "Many men who seem vigorous exist only in their stomachs," explained the author of *La santé virile par l'hygiène*: "the little real energy they have is concentrated there . . . they are certainly not as strong as they seem."[18] Another physician suggested close attention to the words typically used to describe fat men: "Let's ask these 'strong'—read 'bloated'—individuals, whom the vulgar believe enjoy perfect health, to perform some physical labor and our opinion will be *faite de coup*."[19] The joys of frivolity and excess found in the "grotesque body" no longer played a central role in a bourgeois culture where bodily strength was subordinated to productivity and the work ethic. No doubt part of the problem had to do with appearance, and Peter Stearns has noted cases in which aesthetics played a central role in the growing French disgust with obesity. Yet when it came to men it was physical force rather than health or beauty that was the primary consideration. It is not that obese men were simply unhealthy, but that they lacked the strength and productive power that was frequently expected of "true" men.[20]

A similar tendency found in medical studies of hysteria and neurasthenia marked studies of obesity: by emphasizing the predominance of women among those afflicted with the malady (not to mention the "feminizing" nature of the illness), doctors implicitly situated male patients in a largely female diagnostic category. Some physicians were no doubt aware of the implications of such diagnoses and took steps to masculinize either the disease or the cure. This was certainly the case with Jean-Martin Charcot, who insisted that the existence of hysterical men did not necessarily imply the wholesale feminization of such patients, many of whom he described as working class and quite virile in every other respect.[21] Insofar as diet provided testimony to one's strength of will, fat men could redeem themselves through the strict adherence to a daily regimen and submission to a variety of other weight loss techniques. If weakness of the will had resulted in obesity, then surely a triumph of volition would lead to its cure.

Willpower was therefore a crucial aspect of the kind of bodily control that signified masculine identity, and was seen as woefully lacking in most fat people. In the medical literature on obesity one finds repeated references to the lack of will and "intellectual apathy" manifested by the obese, qualities that posed significant obstacles to treatment. Nevertheless, Proust and Mathieu invoked the importance of will and perseverance as part of a manly triumph over the seductive (and thus "feminine") allure of gustatory delights. "In order to stop gaining weight and to shed one's pounds," they wrote, "one must first of all possess great force of character. One must resist the temptations of the table, resist seduction and the bad habits one has acquired."[22] This fantasy about the manly encounter with seductive food had a precedent in a more general cultural tendency to treat the dining experience as a male bonding ritual. It was not until late in the century that it was considered appropriate to take women to restaurants and, as Jean-Paul Aron has demonstrated, the meal itself was often cast as a woman to be taken or as an enemy to be overcome. The masculine credentials that were once confirmed through the gourmand's symbolic conquests could be similarly affirmed through the gastronomical chastity of *l'homme à régime*.[23]

A range of obesity treatments were available to the French during this period, from thyroid pills, massage, and exercise to a wide selection of dietary regimes. In fact, by 1912 obese people were offered at least twenty different weight-loss diets from several countries. A number of French spas had been identified as featuring waters whose laxative properties were considered especially conducive for weight loss; yet the undisputed capital of obesity treatment was the sanitarium at Brides (Savoie), where taking the waters was complemented by a severe regime that reportedly produced the most favorable results.[24] A medical consultant at Brides, Dr. Laissus, explained the various therapeutic measures practiced at the spa, which ranged from hot and warm baths in running water to massage, dietary restrictions, and the so-called "light bath" [*bain de lumière*]. In the latter technique the patient was hermetically sealed in a box whose interior is lined with up to eighty electric light bulbs. With only his head emerging from a hole in the top, the patient's body was subjected to temperatures of between 55 and 60 degree Celsius for up to 20 minutes, after which he or she was removed from the box and wrapped in blankets before being ushered off to the shower. Through such practices, Laissus promised, most patients could expect to lose between twelve and twenty pounds in about three weeks.[25]

The cure that Laissus illustrated through a series of notable case studies suggested an interplay between doctor and patient that, despite its insistence on total submission to medical authority, nevertheless congratulated the male patient's ability to follow orders fully. Female patients, it was suggested, might require greater intervention. Although this affirmation of the male patient did not exactly confirm free agency, it did attest to the exercise of the will in a manner that would allow for the conquest of obesity and the recovery of manhood. It is therefore striking that in his two case studies of male curists Laissus selected men who could not have been considered utter weaklings before arriving at Brides. For example, Mr C... was a big eater and drinker who had steadily gained weight after performing his military service. Yet it was because he was "full of confidence and animated by a great desire to make a serious cure" that he was able to lose more than 27 kilograms in less than two months. In order to explain this success, Laissus observed, "it is enough to show that he had willpower and that the doctor had much vigor [*fermeté*]." A similar scenario was illustrated in the case of Mr D..., who, despite being strong and muscular, "confessed readily that he had an enormous appetite and that he could not moderate it." Central to this patient's success was his apparent "force of character" which allowed him to keep to a strict dietary regimen even after leaving the spa. When he returned the following season he had become considerably more slender, so much so that the doctor hardly recognized him.[26]

The adolescent Miss B... was a very different case. At more than 125 kilograms this unfortunate fifteen-year-old did not demonstrate much force of character, but was rather "a formless mass nearly incapable of moving."

214 ~ Christopher E. Forth

Believing that his firm instructions had made an impression on this girl, Laissus was later surprised to find steadfast opposition to his insistence that she reform her eating habits. "I realized that I would have difficulty with this capricious child," lamented the doctor, "and that I would need to double my energy and surveillance in order to triumph over this invincible apathy." After investing a great deal of personal attention in this case Laissus eventually triumphed over his patient, who adhered to the prescribed dietary and exercise regimen with only occasional lapses.[27] Contrary to the male patients, whose willpower seemed to complement the firmness of the physician, Miss B...'s participation in her own cure was barely acknowledged, affirming at once the perceived weakness of female volition and the physician's commendable ability to impose his own will over such recalcitrant patients.

While medical literature was not always explicit about the association between obesity and male weakness, in the early twentieth century proponents of physical culture did not mince words in their wholesale assault upon the fat man. Edmond Desbonnet, the period's best known proponent of physical culture, promised a cure to obesity, stomach ailments, and neurasthenia in his chain of bodybuilding centers. Heralding a veritable sporting renaissance around 1910, the physical culture movement self-consciously fostered "a virile education" that would reverse the international image of the Frenchman as being intelligent but "without virility and without initiative."[28] In such circles physique was a sheer matter of willpower and proper lifestyle, and even among those with a hereditary predisposition to obesity, for whom "the aptitude to fatten is developed by the hygienic faults of the subject.... It is less the inevitable result of a temperament than the unhealthy administration of that temperament."[29] Harkening back to Greek models of the ideal male body, physical culturists emphasized wide chests and slender waists that attested to strength as well as beauty, and called attention to the abdominal muscles as being central to a manly bearing. For the sake of the "regeneration of the race," one of the explicit aims of Desbonnet's magazine, *La Santé par les sports*, it was imperative that the public cease to confuse physical bulk and muscular force, so that by becoming more discerning in their choice of husbands women might avoid procreating with a "ridiculous and horrible" fat man.[30] Although during the prewar years the rhetoric of bodily force surely triumphed over the reality of an iron-pumping population, the weakened and perhaps impotent fat man was quickly becoming an object of ridicule. "A fat belly is synonymous with physical degradation,"[31] noted one physical culturist, while another put the matter quite baldly: "To be obese is to be disgraceful."[32] As the bodybuilding entrepreneur Richard Andrieu claimed, men whose overcivilized habits had distanced them from their warrior heritage could regain their manhood by joining a new kind of hunt. If their ancestors had stayed in shape by hunting the now extinct European buffalo known as the auroch, Andrieu proposed that the hunt be turned inward. "If we can no longer hunt aurochs, let's hunt . . . fatty tissue whose cells are nowhere near close to disappearing."[33]

Zola's Body

In light of Zola's well-known appetite and the gathering contempt for male obesity, it is safe to say that designating Zola the "belly of Paris" was no innocent metaphor. Indeed, the novelist had been since the 1870s a frequent guest at the celebrated banquets of the literary brothers Jules and Edmond Goncourt, and on more than one occasion surprised his hosts with his culinary discernment and formidable appetite. In 1876 Jules de Goncourt observed "a Zola I never knew before, a Zola who was a glutton, a gourmand, and a gourmet, a Zola spending all his money on food, running to food merchants and grocers of great renown, gorging himself on the best." Even famous gastronomes like the Goncourts were taken aback by Zola's obsession with food: "I fully understand the caprice of the stomach's imagination that compels one, every now and then, to have a fine, delicate, and original dinner, but to do so every day strikes me as intolerable."[34]

The novelist's immense appetite and refined tastes formed just one part of a well-known study of Zola carried out by Édouard Toulouse, a physician who ambitiously planned a multi-volume series exploring the bodies and minds of famous intellectuals. Taking such a celebrated figure as a subject ensured that Toulouse's study would not be consigned to the commercial oblivion that awaited more specialized medical texts. On the contrary, his book seems to have attracted a readership among those who were at once familiar with the novelist's writings and interested in matters of health.[35] Some scholars have interpreted Toulouse's study as providing a negative appraisal of Zola's health by concluding that the novelist ranked among the "superior degenerates" who often comprised great culture heroes.[36] Yet the issue of Zola's obesity provided an important counterpoint to whatever "feminizing" effects such a diagnosis may have entailed, and thus renders the effect of Toulouse's book ambiguous at best.

As Toulouse revealed in his case history of the novelist, Zola's obesity began at a fairly early age and increased as he grew older and more successful. In time he began to experience physical difficulties that compelled him to rethink his daily regimen: "He was winded by the least physical effort." When Zola decided to start dieting in 1887 he weighed 192 pounds and his belly measured 1.14 meters around.[37] By the time of the Affair he had dropped nearly twenty pounds, but still manifested a certain roundness reminiscent of his old self. In his analyses Toulouse paid special attention to the novelist's nervous character, which in many circles would have suggested a psychological disposition more commonly found among women. Nevertheless Toulouse countered the potentially negative effects of his appraisal by emphasizing qualities that would be easily construed as evidence of manliness. Zola was "Robust, energetic, tenacious, combative, composed and very reasonable despite his nervous troubles and some morbid thoughts."[38] Toulouse was particularly impressed by Zola's willpower, his "tenacity, his persistence in effort. We find this quality in everything he does. If a difficulty arises when he is working, he does not stop, he does not get up in order to divert his mind; on the contrary he remains at his desk, working intently on the obstacle and only breathing easy once he is free of it." This capacity to devote himself single-mindedly to his goal was the motor force behind Zola's professional success, and it "appeared also in his private life, for example, in his struggle against obesity. He is the man of combat who is impassioned and sustained by combat."[39]

Ironically, Zola himself had often expressed doubts about his capacity for self-mastery, and once confided to Goncourt that his own work habits owed more to nervous compulsion than inner strength: "you should not think that I have willpower, I am by nature the weakest being and the least capable of training. In me the will is replaced by *l'idée fixe,–l'idée fixe* which makes me ill if I do not submit to its obsession."[40] On the one hand this self-revelation accords well with Toulouse's general finding that Zola was at heart "truly a neuropath" who displayed traits of "nervous disequilibrium, [and] a really morbid exaggerated emotivity."[41] On the other hand, Toulouse made every effort to salvage the novelist's sense of manly self-control that could have been forfeited by dwelling on nervous disorders, and underscored Zola's struggle against obesity as one aspect of his essentially robust nature that made him a "man of combat" despite his condition as a "superior degenerate." It is perhaps for this reason that Zola remained quite pleased by the findings of Toulouse, and thanked the doctor for presenting an analysis that showed such "great care for the truth while maintaining balance and a great deal of tact." Zola was especially pleased that revelations of his daily struggle for artistic creation might finally put to rest the old myths about him being a beast of burden who labored only for money: "Thank you for having studied and labeled my dirty laundry. I believe that I have benefited from it."[42]

Heroic weight-loss through strict dieting was for Toulouse evidence of a strong will in action, a belief echoed by other contemporaries. In his 1903 memoirs of the Société des gens de lettres, of which Zola was president four times, the novelist Albert Cim eulogized the "iron will" wielded by the writer, a quality embodied in his notable weight loss. This was a transformation that "only the most energetic will could impose," declared Cim. "Haven't we gone so far as to claim that if, as big, heavy, and obese as he was for 30 years, he became thin and slender at fifty, it was only *because he wanted it*, because he applied himself, tenaciously, to make himself diet?"[43] Such celebrations of Zola's willpower were also made by John Grand-Carteret, an amateur cultural critic who had written several books on caricature and the graphic arts at the height of the Dreyfus Affair. Dwelling on the difference between the fat Zola and the thin Zola, Grand-Carteret applauded the novelist's decision to abandon his "disgraceful proportions" by exercising and controlling his appetite. Like Séverine, he too saw Zola's role in the Affair as a heroic struggle against injustice and the forces of tradition, and noted that the novelist's timing could not have been better: "before hurling himself head on into the struggle, Zola wanted first to obtain a victory over himself." Grand-Carteret saw in this physical reform something for others to emulate, a veritable conquest of the flesh that epitomized the manly will in action: "Whoever wants to go to war against human cowardice should first triumph over his own troubles. It was with this goal in mind ... that Zola proclaimed, through his outward appearance, the rejuvenation and transformation of his person."[44]

Grand-Carteret thus echoed a sentiment shared by many Dreyfusards and conveyed clearly the period's association of the fat man with effeminacy. The struggle against military lies and religious superstition required a manly stance best exemplified by Zola, whose conquest of his own body stood as a beacon to those who also struggled for the light of Truth against the darkness of the flesh.

Notes

1. For a fuller discussion of the male body in France, see my *The Dreyfus Affair and the Crisis of French Manhood* (Baltimore: Johns Hopkins University Press, 2004).
2. Séverine, *Vers la lumière* (Paris: Stock, 1900), 47–50. On images of Zola in popular culture, see Pierre-Olivier Perl, "Les caricatures de Zola: Du naturalisme à l'affaire Dreyfus," *Historical Reflections/Réflexions Historiques,* 24 (Spring 1998), 137–154.

3. Octave Mirbeau, "Un matin, chez Émile Zola," *Livre d'hommage des lettres françaises à Émile Zola* (Paris: Société libre d'Édition des Gens de Lettres, 1898), 73.

4. Joan Jacobs Brumberg, *Fasting Girls: The Emergence of Anorexia Nervosa as a Modern Disease* (Cambridge: Harvard University Press, 1988).

5. Dr. G. Rouhet, "De l'obésité," *La Culture physique* (April 1910), 246.

6. Stephen Mennell, "On the Civilizing of Appetite," in *The Body: Social Process and Cultural Theory*, Mike Featherstone, Mike Hepworth, and Bryan S. Turner, eds. (London: Sage, 1991), 126–156.

7. Robert A. Nye, *Crime, Madness, and Politics in Modern France* (Princeton: Princeton University Press, 1984), 140.

8. Jean-Jacques Rousseau, *Émile, or On Education*, Allan Bloom, trans. (New York: Basic Books, 1979), 54.

9. Dr. Rauland, *Le Livre des époux: Guide pour la guérison de l'impuissance* (Paris: 1852), 96–97.

10. Jean Anthelme Brillat-Savarin, *The Physiology of Taste*, M.F.K. Fisher, trans. (New York: Knopf, 1972), 205.

11. Charles Bouchard, *Leçons sur les maladies par ralentissement de la nutrition* (Paris: Librairie F. Savy, 1890), 118–120, 127.

12. E. Demange, "Obésité," *Dictionnaire encyclopédique des sciences médicales,* 14 (1880), 14.

13. Dr. Dheur, *Comment on se défend contre l'obésité* (Paris: Société d'éditions scientifiques, n.d.), 24.

14. Adrien Proust and A. Mathieu, *L'Hygiène de l'obèse* (Paris: Masson, 1897), 60.

15. Ibid., 20.

16. Bouchard, quoted in Ibid., 90.

17. See also Dr. M. Leven, *La névrose: Étude clinique et thérapeutique* (Paris: G. Masson, 1887).

18. E. Detois, *La santé virile par l'hygiène* (Aurillac: Roux, 1901), 8.

19. Dr. H. van de Velde, *L'Alimentation des gens bien portants et des malades* (Paris, 1899), 11.

20. Peter N. Stearns, *Fat History: Bodies and Beauty in the Modern West* (New York: NYU Press, 1997), 153–167.

21. Mark S. Micale, "Hysteria Male/Hysteria Female: Reflections on Comparative Gender Construction in Nineteenth-Century France and Britain," in *Science and Sensibility: Gender and Scientific Enquiry, 1780–1945*, Marina Benjamin, ed. (Oxford: Blackwell, 1991), 200–239.

22. Proust and Mathieu, *L'Hygiène de l'obèse*, 207.

23. Jean-Paul Aron, *Le Mangeur du XIXe siècle* (Paris: Éditions Robert Laffont, 1973).

24. E. Demange, "Obésité," 33.

25. Docteur Laissus fils, *Considérations sur la cure de l'obésité* (Paris: A. Maloine, 1909), 10–11.

26. Proust and Mathieu criticized the thermal milieus, claiming that the "advantage of these cures is that one obtains among the patients a docility that they would no longer have at home. Their drawback is bringing about a rapid thinning through intense methods which cause fatigue. Obese people treated in this manner show a great tendency, once they return home and resume their bad habits, to regain quickly all they had lost." Proust and Mathieu, *L'Hygiène de l'obèse*, 339.

27. Laissus, *Considérations,* 12-29.

28. Jean Daçay, "Le Renaissance athlétique en France," *La Culture physique* (15 September 1910), 526.

29. Docteur Ruffier, *Le traîtement de l'obésité par la culture physique* (Paris: Librairie de "Portez-vous bien!," 1912), 8.

30. Edmond Desbonnet, "Ne confondons pas grosseur et force," *La Santé par les sports* (15 May 1912), 337–338.

31. Dr. J. B. Wauquier, "L'Obésité: Gros ventre est synonyme de déchéance physique," *La Santé par les sports* (8 March 1914), 4.

32. Anonymous, "Comme quoi il est prouvé que la Beauté est un gage de Santé," *La Santé par les sports* (8 April 1913), 6.

33. Richard Andrieu, "Étude sur l'initiation à l'athléticisme par la culture physique," *La Culture physique*, 3:39 (15 August 1906), 637.

34. Edmond and Jules de Goncourt, 15 October 1876, *Journal: Mémoires de la vie littéraire, 1864–1878* (Paris: Fasquelle, 1956), vol. 2, 1149–1150.

35. The inaugural issue of *Paris-santé illustré,* a small product-oriented magazine published by the Pharmacie Pigalle (34, Boulevard de Clichy), featured a review of Toulouse's work as a cover story. Against literary doubts about the usefulness of such an enterprise, the author stressed the scientific potential for better understanding the man behind the works. Dr. Jehan, "Émile Zola, par le Dr. Toulouse," *Paris-santé illustré,* 1 (June 1897), 2.

36. Daniel Pick, *Faces of Degeneration: A European Disorder, c. 1848–c. 1918* (Cambridge: Cambridge University Press, 1989).

37. Dr. Édouard Toulouse, *Enquête médico-psychologique sur les rapports de la supériorité intellectuelle avec névropathie* (Paris: Société d'Éditions scientifiques, 1896), 119.

38. Ibid., 266–267.

39. Ibid., 262.

40. Edmond and Jules de Goncourt, 3 June 1872, *Journal*, II: 898.

41. Toulouse, *Enquête*, 166.

42. Zola to Toulouse, 15 October 1896, in *Correspondance*, 358.

43. Albert Cim, *Le dîner des gens de lettres: Souvenirs littéraires* (Paris: Flammarion, 1903), 73–74.

44. John Grand-Carteret, *Zola en images: 280 illustrations* (Paris: Librairie Félix Juven, 1908), 22–23.

Chapter 12 ✏

HOW FAT DETECTIVES THINK

Sander L. Gilman

If there is a moment in Western history when fat seems to become a positive quality in shaping the image of the "fat man," it is at the close of the nineteenth century. It is here, particularly in the crime fiction of this period, where the body of the fat detective seems to aid his mental processes, his body size and shape seeming to account for his different way of thinking. In his essay on the eating habits of philosopher-scientists throughout the past, Steven Shapin reveals that, at least in the Western world, a powerful myth as early as Marsilio Ficino's renaissance book on the health of the scholar assumes that such men should have a "lean and hungry look."[1] That all of his examples are men is not incidental. Our collective fantasy of the appropriate body of the male thinker stands at the center of Shapin's work. I want to ask the corollary question: What happens to the image of the "thinking male" when that male body is fat, even obese? Shapin's point, of course, is that Sir Isaac Newton, that proverbial thinker who is reputed to have forgotten whether he had eaten his chicken or not, actually died hugely bloated. Equally true is the representation of the body of Erasmus Darwin (1731–1802), who was so fat that he had to cut a circle out of his dining table to accommodate his paunch. At that very same table sat the members of the Birmingham Lunar Society, the intellectual leaders of his day, including James Priestly (the discoverer of oxygen) and James Watt (the creator of the steam engine).[2] What Shapin addresses is that there is great disparity between the way we imagine how bodies should look and function, and our mythmaking about them. In complicated ways, the fat detective is the antithesis of the lean philosopher and his fat analogue.

The Science of Thinking with Your Gut

To understand the notion of the fat detective, it is necessary to examine the perceptions regarding the faculties of thinking and judgment in relation to the body during the long turn of the century from 1880 to 1914. During the course of the nineteenth century, the relationship between the brain and the nervous system came to be relatively well established. The notion of "thought," which had been a component of the "soul," was transmuted with the introduction of a medical materialism by scientists such as Johannes Müller, into a model of thinking by way of the body. The nervous system was seen as the place where thought and therefore judgment took place. The central discoveries were in the realm of the nature of the nerves themselves and one of the most important developments through the course of the nineteenth century was the discovery that nerves consisted of two types of fiber. One fiber carried electrical impulses and the other, in the terms of the model of electricity dominant in representing the nervous system during this period, served as insulation. The substance surrounding the nerve was a fat, which by mid century came to be called "myelin." It was understood as absolutely necessary to the correct function of the nervous system in that it increased the speed of the transmission of nerve impulses.[3] One can think of this model of the nerve as insulation wrapped around energy: the inert shielding the active, or thought clothed in fat. It was seen as the sign of evolutionary development that enabled human beings to become human. And that leap was defined in their new ability to think, but, most specifically, to make judgments.

Historically, fat has a central role in constituting the neurological body. It was Robert Remak who, in 1836, demonstrated that the "nerve" has differentiated "parts," identified as the myelinated and unmyelinated fibers.[4] He thus discovered that white-matter tracts are really attached to cell bodies. This took place as Justus von Liebig at Giessen University was uncovering how fat was formed in the animal body and how this was connected to the animal's nutrition. Liebig as a chemist spent his career studying the energy-producing function of food through careful measurement. He saw carbon-containing fats as a type of fuel that was absolutely necessary for the maintenance of the healthy body. He labeled carbohydrates and fats as "respiratory foods." From this came his view that when such foods were eaten to an excessive amount, fat accumulated on the body. Diet was for Liebig the cause and control of morbid obesity, but fat was recognized as essential for the proper functioning of the body. This work, initially published in 1840, paralleled and influenced the work of those interested in the functioning of the nervous system.[5] For if fat was necessary for the well-being of the entire body, should it not also be for the function of the nerves?

While Remak never actually used the word myelin, he recognized the difference between fat and nerve tissue, building upon Albrecht Haller's eighteenth-century notion of the irritability of nerve tissue. It is not simple coincidence that paralleled the discovery of the "fat" of the nerves as the key to their function to the discovery of the meaning of fat in the metabolic process. There had been older views that collapsed the image of body fat with the fat imagined about the nerves following Haller's view of the irritability of the nerves. In 1811, Thomas Jameson had written that obesity "also diminishes the irritability of the system, since fat people are remarked for good humor, and for bearing cold better that those who are lean, on account of the defensive coat of fat surrounding their nerves."[6] Here there is a basic assumption of the nature of fat men and their fat nerves, which is made universal by Remak. All of our nerves are covered with fat that enables them to function. Yet the new neurology continues to carry hidden assumptions about masculinity and character. Based on Remak's observations in the 1830s, new theories of human development and the way we ascertain it evolved, but they carried with them older ideas of the meaning of fat.

Louis Ranvier (1872), continuing Remak's work, showed there were nodes in the myelin and that these "adipose cells" [*endoneurium*] are part of the connective tissue of the nerves.[7] Unlike Remak, who used a microscope to make his distinction between the two types of fiber, Ranvier used a new silver impregnation stain, which provided the first detailed "look" at the nature of the myelin sheath and the "node of Ranvier" in the nerve. While this was an obvious anatomical structure when it was stained, it was not so to the unaided eye. The ability to "see" fat made it real. "Seeing" fat in the body was as important to the neurologists as acknowledging its presence. A complete nerve was a nerve with a myelin sheath, and the discovery of demyelenating diseases, such as multiple sclerosis that afflicted major personages from K. F. W. Marx at the beginning of the nineteenth century to Jean-Martin Charcot at its close, demonstrated the pathological effect of the loss of "fat."[8] Nerves worked only with the presence of the sheath of fat and they ceased to work once it was lost. If the loss could be seen, as in the inability for muscle to operate, could not the loss also impact on those qualities that defined the human being even more directly, on thought and the thought processes?

After the job of identifying and making myelin visible for inspection, it was Paul Emil Flechsig who returned to the earlier premise of Remak and in 1900 theorized how it developed.[9] (Yes, it is *that* Flechsig, Daniel Paul Schreber's doctor, and the subject of his most intense fantasies. The vocabulary of Flechsig's scientific studies of the brain and the nerves find their way in grotesque and complex ways into Schreber's text.[10]) Flechsig built on the localization work of Freud's teacher, Theodor Meynert, who first related regional structural differences in the cerebral cortex to the specific functions. Flechsig was able to identify groups of fibers and the thirty-six specific and constant regions of the cortex with which they are associated. Most importantly, he showed how these cortical areas developed in a chronological sequence. Fibers in various parts of the nervous system acquire myelin sheaths at different stages of development. Thus, a study not of where "fat" appears but when "fat" appears provided a clue to an archeology of the human nervous system. Fat was the key to the history of human judgment. It provided the benchmarks by which one could distinguish between "primitive" and "higher" stages of development. Myelin was the sign of the potential for human intelligence. With its appearance, according to Flechsig's theory, there was a leap in the possibility for thought.

Flechsig's theoretical work mapping neural development began in 1893 and was based on the discovery of myelinization in the subcortical white matter of the fetus and infant. He observed that there seemed to be three zones and periods of development of the nerves based on the nature of the myelin. First, there were the motor and sensory areas that matured earlier (primordial zones); then, the intermediate zones; and finally, the regions of late development, the terminal zones. Flechsig notes that his project of myelogenetic localization seemed to be "falling back to the phrenology of Gall." Like the eighteenth-century phrenologist Franz Gall, there was an attempt to see in the structure of the brain and nervous system reflections on the higher or lower "nature" of human responses. He postulated a developmental scheme that would have seen "fat" (now understood as myelin) as the means by which the nerve functioned and thus made thought possible. It was a measure for the course of the development of the nervous system from the most primitive, uninsulated nerves through to the highest cortical function. To extrapolate, fat detectives think with their guts, but only because of the heavy myelinization of their nervous system.

It was with another neurologist of the time, Sigmund Freud, that the idea of myelin became closely connected to the ability to produce judgments. It is clear that in Flechsig's model, the increased intelligence ascribed to the presence of myelin implied the ability to judge, but Freud makes this explicit. Freud's early, unpublished project for a scientific psychology of

1895 proposes a neurological model of the body, and this is really never lost in his way of conceiving the biological "space" for the psyche. It postulates a basic or primitive neural network that underlies all consciousness. Freud makes a distinction between the permeable and the impermeable neurons. The former offering no resistance and are the transmitters of perception, and the latter the place of memory and are "loaded with resistance."[11] Freud makes an analogous distinction (in the same essay) on the difference between remembering and judging (1:330–331). Perception has implanted memory on the impermeable neurons, and judgment occurs when there is a disparity between new perception and stored perceptions. Thus, for Freud, judgment is "not a primary function but presupposes the cathexis from the ego of the disparate non-comparable portions of the perception" (1:332). Judgment is an unconscious process, which is, as Freud notes, a "method of proceeding from the perceptual situation that is given in reality to the situation that is wished-for" (1:332). All judgment resides in the nerve's ability to retain mimetic images of actual perceptions and to recall them on an unconscious level. It is judging through the body's memory.

Fat thinks; fat judges. Or at least, the fat about the nerves provides the most elemental level of response to one's world. This positive evaluation of fat is no different when we turn to the therapeutics of the period and look at those places where fat comes to be understood as curative. S. Weir Mitchell in his *Fat and Blood and How to Make Them* (1877), ties the lack of "visible" body fat to the notion of an insufficiency of the nerves.[12] Hysteria can result when the body becomes too thin: "I think the first thing which strikes an American in England is the number of inordinately fat people, and especially fat women . . . this excess of flesh we usually associate in idea with slothfulness" (15). In fact, he proceeds to state, such fat is a prophylaxis against disease: "This must make . . . some difference in their relation liability to certain forms of disease" (15). It is primarily women who suffer from this loss of fat and the resulting nervousness: "a large group of women, especially said to have nervous exhaustion, or who are described as having spinal irritation. . . . They have a tender spine, and soon or later enact the whole varied drama of hysteria" (25-26). They are "lacking in color and which had not lost flesh" (27). But even men can suffer from such a debility of the nerves, specifically through traumatic experiences: "Nor is this less true of men, and I have many a time seen soldiers who had ridden boldly with Sheridan or fought gallantly with Grant, become, under the influence of painful nerve wounds, as irritable and hysterically emotional as the veriest girl," undergoing "moral degradation" (28). Fat men and women are mentally healthy; thin men and women suffer. The result, of course, is the "rest cure," made popular in our own day in the readings of Charlotte Perkins Gilman's 1892 tale, "The Yellow Wallpaper," which is the account of her own treatment by Mitchell.[13] But the neurological basis of Mitchell's understanding of the definition of fat has not been explored, nor has the notion that fat impacts on a specific type of thinking, the intuitive. For S. Weir Mitchell, a certain amount of fat was necessary to protect the nervous system and thus the psyche from distress. He argued that "blood thins with the decrease of tissues and enriches as they increase" (15). And the more blood, the more psychic energy. It is a sign of "nutritive prosperity" (16). Such prosperity is signaled by the social station of the individual. Thus, he proposes that the "upper classes gain weight in the summer" (and intelligence) while the working classes lose it. But it is also determined by the individual's gender. All in all, fat men are healthier than fat women. Body fat is thus the visible equivalent to the myelin about the nerves. Fat makes the body healthy since it prevents the exposure of the nerves. It is thus the sign of the possibility of higher thought (as in the fat sheath around the nerves) and the preservation of mental health (bodily fat).

Fat Male Sleuths and Their Nerves

This model of the thinking and judging body, as it is found from 1891 to the mid twentieth century, is embodied in the fat sleuth. His body is a thinking and judging body, unlike the "fat" body of the female of the time, which is a reproductive body. S. Weir Mitchell differentiates between the soldierly and reproductive functions of the healthy, fat body of men and women. The male body thinks with its visible fat. It is empathetic and responsive. His body is a healthy body because of its fat. The fat detective only functions in his role as an intuitive solver of problems when he responds to his "gut" feelings. His body thinks and judges. It is a basic form of rationality. Thus, as we will see, the passivity of Tubby Schaumann and Mycroft Holmes becomes a means, in their own narratives, of remembering the forgotten, of sensing that which cannot be experienced, which shapes their ability to discover hidden or forgotten truths. It seems to be primitive (like a sloth or walrus), but it is indeed the hallmark of the most sophisticated and highly developed male body. It is the body that thinks. Here our contemporary notion of the "enteric nervous system that is pharmacologically more complex than the sympathetic or parasympathetic systems, involving many neuropeptide and other transmitters (such as 5-hydroxytryptamine [a.k.a. serotonin]) often described as a collection of 'little brains,'"[14] can be evoked. The body itself is understood as the place of thinking. The parallel nature of the nineteenth-century understanding of fat and thinking is that the cultural assumptions that shape the language of neurology simultaneously shape the language of popular fiction. It is a language that sees the need for "fat" as part of a cultural discourse of appropriate, if slightly quirky, masculinity.

In 1891, Wilhelm Raabe, best known as one of the foremost regional colorists in late nineteenth-century German letters, published his novel *Stopfkuchen*, subtitled "A Murder and Sea" tale.[15] Translated into English as "Tubby Schaumann," a rough approximation of the nickname of the protagonist, it is the exemplary and, perhaps, the first account of the mental process of the fat detective. Here we have an amateur sleuth whose primary quality seems to be his huge body and his insatiable appetite. Heinrich "Stopfkuchen" Schaumann's bulk and his fleshly desires make it seemingly impossible to leave the world of the small village where he was raised. He lives for cakes and pies; his primary position is lying prone under the hedges looking for people who come down the paths. He is the prototypical fat man, "so lazy and so fat and so decent and so loveable."[16] His body is "seen" as different. Indeed, his name, Schaumann, means one who sees or is seen.

The antithetical body in this murder mystery is that of his youthful friend, Edward, whose narrative frames the novel. He returns from making a new life in South Africa in order to visit his hometown. There, he discovers his old friend Schaumann had married the daughter of Quakatz, the owner of the isolated and infamous Red Bank Farm. Decades before, the farmer Kienbaum was found dead and Quakatz was immediately accused of the murder as he had often quarreled with the deceased. Quakatz was not prosecuted for the crime due to lack of evidence, but his guilt was evident to everyone in the town. Nevertheless, he had spent all of his waking hours trying to prove his innocence. Into this home, and infamy, came the young Tubby Schaumann who married Quakatz's vivacious, red-haired daughter. "How a man with Tubby Schaumann's physical constitution managed to have her fall in love with him so quickly I don't know, but he did" (186). Told through the perspective of someone who arrived after the fact, the novel then goes on to reveal how Schaumann uncovered the identity of the real murderer.

In the process of unraveling the mystery, Tubby's fat body is his most powerful ally. He is invisible in his bulk and tenacious in his powers of observation. He is the scientist-observer as the late-nineteenth-century detective story used to great effect. In this case he is an amateur paleontologist, whose discovery of a mammoth skeleton makes his reputation in scientific circles. But his contemporaries see him in much the same terms which he sees his discovery—as a huge, unwieldy, primitive object. This double vision frames his scientific gaze. Tubby's body is a primitive body, which should infer a primitive consciousness.[17] His school biology teacher had compared him to the bradypus: "Look at him, all of you, Schaumann, the sloth. There he sits again on the dullard's bench, like the bradypus, the sloth. Has hair the color of withered leaves and with four molars. Crawls slowly up onto another class—I mean, climbs up a tree and stays there until he has eaten the last leaf" (215). Even his friend sees his preoccupation with food as a sign that he should be "let to crawl sloth-like into his tree" (225). But this sloth-like demeanor has "cold-bloodedness which had something uncanny about it" (225). But, of course, the fat body of the detective here is not the body of the sloth. What appears to be slothfulness is, in fact, introspection. Tubby's hobby, the collecting of fossils, is a closer clue to his relationship to the "primitive" body of the sloth. He is the observer whose passivity masks the rational mind at work. He is pure intellect encased in an immobile body.

Schaumann proves, at least to himself, that he had solved the crime when, in good detective style, he deduces the murderer at the grave of his accused father-in-law. Evoking the means by which Hamlet captured the conscience of the king, Tubby watches the postman Störzer as he listens to the preacher's eulogy at Quakatz's grave. Tubby Schaumann knows that Störzer is the murderer by observing him silently; his trick is to place his bulk in one place and look at the world, whether at the landscape of Quakatz's Red Bank Farm or the world of the murderer. He sees Störzer's discomfort in confronting the corpse and perceives his guilt. He knows because of his bulk, and his bulk seems almost an extension of the farm. Schaumann later unveils the crime to Edward, revealing to him that Störzer, whose friend and disciple Edward was, had committed the crime. Störzer himself had died just before Edward's return. But the perpetrator is unknown to everyone else.

The gut truth of the fat detective is not to be found in the world of the intellect, but in his body. Tubby's doctor warns him to avoid the "strain of the mind." This is ironic, as the life of the mind is and has been Tubby's hallmark. But the doctor believes that too much mental activity might be harmful. At the pub, Tubby is invited formally to expose Störzer to the public prosecutor so as to clear the name of his father in law: "I'd love to, if it were possible and my doctor hadn't forbidden it," laughed Schaumann. "Oh, if you had any idea, Schellbaum, how emphatically that man Oberwasser has forbidden me intellectual stimulus of any kind, you would leave me lying under my hedge as in other and better days" (301). He leaves with his friend having solved the murder and without claiming the laurels of the detective, but with the truth revealed to all who would overhear.

The fat detective in Raabe's novel is able to solve the case of Kienbaum's murder over the course of decades simply because of the passive, sedentary nature of his body. His body, which appears to be bloated and obese, is the perfect vehicle for the sort of emotional—not intellectual—exploration of the inner souls of those about him. He is not an "intellectual" but a keen observer. His ability to place the real murder into circumstances where, like Cracker, he reveals his crime, is the reflex of the fat which forms his body and which reflects the empathetic nature of his soul. He does not track him down, but waits until he comes to him and confesses. This is another form of intelligence, an intelligence seemingly contradicted by the visible form of Tubby's "slothful" body. Schaumann is more than corpulent; he is fat incarnate. His fat is not only the sign of the successful farmer, as one of his friends notes; it is also a sign of the type of archeology of the soul, which the detective undertakes. Tubby's girth seems to be an impediment to his role as a scientist; indeed, it becomes the sign of his success as a farmer, a paleontologist, and a sleuth.

The clear antithesis of Tubby Schaumann is the most important detective of the 1890s, Arthur Conan Doyle's Sherlock Holmes.[18] Created in 1887, whip-thin, addicted to cocaine rather than food, always ready to head off on a chase at the drop of a clue, Holmes remains the exemplary rational detective.[19] (Joshua Duke in 1885 suggested that the new drug "Cuca" could be used as an aid for dieting. Perhaps Holmes knew how to keep his body so thin?[20]) His regular feats of observation stun his rather dull-witted companion Dr. John Watson, but all rely on the ability causally to link "facts" following the model of analytic thinking he learned in medical school.[21] Again it is the scientist, but here the scientist as activist, who makes the perfect intellectual detective. He often sinks into a contemplative stupor, aided by his tobacco and cocaine. But this detective also goes out into the world gathering facts. Holmes roams the length of Europe—all the way to Tibet—for knowledge. His is the explorer's body, Sir Henry Morton Stanley's body, as well as that of the detective.

But there is another Holmes in these tales. Holmes's older and wiser brother, Mycroft, is introduced in *The Strand Magazine*'s publication of "The Case of the Greek Interpreter" (1892).[22] Like Tubby Schaumann, this sleuth is huge and sedentary. "Mycroft Holmes was a much larger and stouter man than Sherlock. His body was absolutely corpulent, but his face, though massive, had preserved something of the sharpness of expression which was so remarkable in that of his brother."[23] Mycroft's intelligence glimmering in his eyes (the mirrors of the soul) seems overburdened by his primitive body. There is something quite archaic about it; he has "a broad fat hand, like the flipper of a seal" (295). He is not quite a sloth but close enough.

Mycroft is the better brother, as his younger sibling grudgingly admits. Holmes states that "... he was my superior in observation and deduction. If the art of the detective began and ended in the reasoning from an armchair, my brother would be the greatest criminal agent that ever lived" (293). What makes Holmes the better is that he is willing to use his powers in the world. Mycroft, like Tubby Schaumann, in the end is merely an amateur sleuth, not really a consulting detective, unlike the pompous fat detective whom Sherlock Holmes bests in *The Sign of the Four* (1890). And the amateur nature of his undertaking is seemingly tied to his lack of desire to pursue truth to its bitter ends: "What is to me a means of livelihood is to him the merest hobby of a dilettante" (294). Here the quality of the amateur, in Tubby's case the amateur paleontologist as detective, is central. These are not the professional detectives whose world is the world of action, but the amateur whose interest includes other models of the world besides that of rational detection. This is the model that eventually evolves into a string of fat detectives, culminating in *Cracker.* Such detectives of the 1890s and the turn of the century are imagined as thinking differently. Unlike Sherlock Holmes, they appear to think through their bodies; yet this is deceptive. Rather their bodies provide an image of obesity that masks their sharp powers of observation and deduction.

Other versions of the fat amateur sleuth followed Raabe and Conan Doyle. In 1911, G. K. Chesterton began the publication of his Father Brown tales.[24] Here the question of belief and the body of the fat amateur detective are again linked. The priest's body is represented as chubby; his response to the murders he investigates is rational rather than intuitive. Indeed, Chesterton saw the Father Brown stories as a means of furthering his Anglo-Catholicism, seen in England as a form of the irrational. The squat body of Father Brown represents the innate seeking for truth beyond logic. He is the embodiment of the idea of thought and faith being aspects of one truth. It is a truth to be found by those who are able to see it, not necessarily by those ordained by the state to seek it.

By 1934 and the publication of Rex Stout's first Nero Wolfe mysteries, the tradition of the fat detective as a counter type had been well established.[25] In 1929, there was Duddington Pell Chalmers, the obese detective hero of John T. McIntyre's *The Museum Murder,* as well as Gerald Verner's

Superintendent Budd, the stout detective, "who is fat, lazy, graceful on his feet," "prone to shut his eyes while thinking," and "not susceptible to feminine beauty."[26] Like Mycroft Holmes and Father Brown, who is celibate by definition, Nero Wolfe's body is not a sexualized one. Yet, this feminizing quality of the male body masks a life of passion. In the course of the Nero Wolfe mysteries we learn of his earlier romantic attachments, all of which took place before his bulk both inhibited and freed him from the power of physical passion.

In Rex Stout's first novel, *Fer-de-Lance* (1934), the hard-boiled associate of Wolfe, Archie Goodwin, notes the almost archaic form of Wolfe's body as similar to the early-twentieth-century fantasies of Neolithic man: "Wolfe lifted his head. I mention that, because his head was so big that lifting it struck you as being quite a job. It was probably really bigger than it looked, for the rest of him was so huge that any head on top of it but his own would have escaped your notice entirely."[27] Wolfe's fat is the fat which protects: "I said to him something I had said before more than once, that beer slowed up a man's head and with him running like a brook, six quarts a day, I never would understand how he could make his brain work so fast and deep that no other men in the country could touch him. He replied, also as he had before, that it wasn't his brain that worked, it was his lower nerve centers...."[28] Wolfe, unlike Archie, thinks with his guts, and invoking the popular beliefs of his day regarding fat, states, "I am too sensitive to strangers, that is why I keep these layers over my nerves."[29] His fat isolates his nerves: "I carry this fat to insulate my feelings. They got too strong for me once or twice and I had that idea. If I had stayed lean and kept moving around I would have been dead long ago."[30] One of the best commentator's on the Wolfe novels observed that "upholders of order are our romantic heroes, and Wolfe qualifies under that category. His daily schedule is as much an insistence on order as a tribute to it: similarly, Wolfe's fat, his gruffness, and his seclusion betray his struggle to insulate himself from emotions, to harness them, to grant them a place, but a smaller one than they claim. Reason then is a goal; it is also a process, a struggle. The Wolfe novels value it as both."[31] The archaic body struggles with its basic emotional nature. And fat is the weapon that enables Wolfe to succeed as a detective.

The very act of thinking for Wolfe is thinking with his body: "Wolfe looked up again, and his big thick lips pushed out a little, tight together, just a small movement, and back again, and then out and back again. How I loved to watch him doing that! That was about the only time I ever got excited, when Wolfe's lips were moving like that... I knew what was going on, something was happening so fast inside of him and so much ground was being covered."[32] The pursed lips are the organ of eating but also the organ of thought. Here the parallel to Tubby Schaumann and other fat detectives is clear. The body has its own life and its own rules. It compliments or contradicts the rational mind and provides the means by which fat detectives set themselves off from all other scientific observers.

When, in 1942, Wolfe decides to diet, the result is a shambles. In the novella "Not Quite Dead Enough," Rex Stout's own major commitment to the war effort is emulated by his character, who also decides to get into shape. The thin man within him desires to reappear. Wolfe was thin before he gained weight so as to protect his nerves because of the unpleasantness with a certain woman in Montenegro. But the effect of a thin Wolfe is ludicrous, as Archie comments: "He didn't look smaller, he merely looked deflated. The pants were his own, an old pair of blue serge. The shoes were strangers, rough army style. The sweater was mine, a heavy maroon number that I had bought once for a camping trip, and in spite of his reduction of circumference it was stretched so tight that his yellow shirt showed though the holes."[33] Wolfe simply looks ridiculous. He moves, he acts, and he believes that he is thin, but it is only a simulacrum of thinness. Running up and down the stairs, short of breath, he is simply the fat man within the thinner one. Most importantly, according to Archie, Wolfe's intelligence has lost its edge. His fat self conquers when he is confronted with a fascinating case that demands his attention. He leans back "comfortably in his chair, his arms folded, with his eyes closed, and I had a suspicion that he was about two-thirds asleep. He had finished two bottles of beer, after going without for over a month, and he was back in the only chair in the world he liked, and his insane project of going outdoors and walking fast twice a day was only a hideous memory."[34] Wolfe returns to that state of obese equilibrium in which thought and body seem to be one. When he later tries to lose weight as part of a case in which he has to disguise himself in the novel *In the Best of Families* (1950), he seems shrunken and ill-proportioned: "with more skin supplied for his face than was needed, it had taken up the slack in his pleats and wrinkles, and that may have accounted for his sporting a pointed brown beard, since it must be hard to shave pleats."[35] The natural Wolfe is not the thin man of his youth, but the fat boy of his old age.

The fat detective Nero Wolfe took to the screen in *Meet Nero Wolfe* (1936) with Edward Arnold as the protagonist. Arnold was one of the very few clearly portly leading men of the age who could do Nero Wolfe and in the same season play romantic leads, as he did in *Come and Get it* (1936). The popularity of Nero Wolfe continued with a rather long series of spin-offs of fat detectives in the mass media, beginning with Dashiell Hammett's Brad Runyon, which aired on ABC radio (1946–1950). The announcer opened the show with the following observation: "He's walking into that drug-store...he's stepping onto the scales...(SNICK! CLICK!) Weight: 237 pounds.... Fortune: Danger! Whoooo is it? The...Fat Man!" The oversized actor J. Scott Smart, who actually outweighed his character by thirty pounds, played him on radio. World-weary, Runyon was a cross between Wolfe and Sam Spade. The first episode, written by Hammett, was *The Black Angel*, broadcast on 26 November 1946. The body of the fat detective on the radio could only be evoked by the image in the listener's mind. As such, his bulk became part of the fantasy of the obese body as heard rather than seen. Rex Stout's Nero Wolfe himself became part of the invisible world of the fat detective on the radio. In 1982, the Canadian Broadcasting Corporation tried their hand at bringing back old-time radio with thirteen one-hour episodes of Nero Wolfe, all based on novellas or short stories written by Stout. The svelte Mavor Moore played the bulky Nero Wolfe, but all that the listener heard was the voice of the fat detective.

A more visible world of the fat detective played itself out on television.[36] William Conrad, whose voice was well-known from his role as the lanky sheriff on radio's version of *Gunsmoke*, went on to play Frank Cannon in *Cannon*, as a tough, expensive, overweight private detective; a sort of hybrid between Sam Spade and Nero Wolfe.[37] Directed by George McCowan, it began a highly successful run in 1971, which concluded only in 1976. According to the plot, the key to Cannon's character lies in the fact that his wife and infant son die in an automobile accident after which he placed all his energy and considerable weight into his new profession of private detective. In 1981, NBC aired a TV series based on novellas and short stories by Rex Stout, which starred Conrad as Nero Wolfe. Then, in 1987, Conrad continued a version of the Nero Wolfe character in *Jake and the Fatman*, in which his role as J. L. "Fatman" McCabe was much more seden-tary. He was transformed into a slovenly former Hawaiian-cop-turned-Honolulu district attorney. From the "Fatman" to "Cracker," the space of the fat detective comes again to be one filled with the emotional, elemen-tal, intuitive, and empathetic. And yet all of these qualities are shown to be a form of judgment, oftentimes more compelling than "pure" rationality. And all of this began on a German farm with Tubby Schaumann's careful observations of the world about him as the key to solving the murder that haunted his world.

No modern fat detective has been more purposely immobile than Raymond Burr as Ironside. Burr, already quite portly in his successful

Perry Mason television series, became this new role with a made-for-TV movie in 1967. While as Perry Mason, Burr played Nero Wolfe to his detective, Paul Drake, in *Ironside* (1967–1975) he undertook the role of Robert Ironside, chief of detectives at the San Francisco police department. Shot by a gunman, Ironside was paralyzed from the waist down and wheelchair bound in the initial movie. Ever large, Burr returned in 1993 for a last time with a made-for-TV-film. Ironside's limitations seem to be that of the thinking detective. As a private detective, Ironside is able to function because his staff serves as his "legs." He is also transported in a specially fitted van to pursue the villains. The coupling of the portly actor and his sedentary role provides a further rationale for the immobility of the fat detective.

Certainly, the most notable figure in the contemporary representation of the "fat detective" is to be found on ABC's long running television drama, *NYPD Blue*. He is Detective Andy Sipowicz, played by Dennis Franz. Since premiering in 1993, the show has centered itself about this character. Cocreators Steven Bocho and David Milch, along with executive producers Mark Tinker and Michael Robin, continued Franz's character from one who had appeared in Bocho and Milch's earlier success, *Hill Street Blues*. Franz had played Lt. Norman Buntz on the show from 1985 to 1987. But Buntz was merely a "tough cop." In Sipowicz, the darkness and complexity of the figure was clearly related to his sense of self as a detective. Sipowicz is portrayed as a recovered alcoholic, the father of a son he had neglected (and who is killed in the course of the show), a man of open emotions and clear prejudices. He is a muscular man gone to fat. It is because of, rather than in spite of, these "flaws," that he is able to be empathetic with his colleagues and generally to have insight into his own character. The flaws in his character, represented by his overweight body, make him into a better detective. Franz had acted in two short-lived detective series (*Beverly Hills Buntz* [1987] and *NYPD Mounted* [1991]) in which the complexity of the "fat" character was lacking. It was in *NYPD Blue* that he is at last able to develop his role as a detective, self-consciously using his fat body as the outward projection of his flawed character. Bocho and Milch use this quite self-consciously in the series. The body-size of the character was literally exposed in a nude scene—one of the first on commercial television—in which Franz was filmed from the rear. In addition to this overt pointing to the size of the character, an ongoing theme of the early seasons was a new, official mandate for all overweight police officers to lose weight, and the subsequent diets and exercise that they undertook to do so. All but Sipowicz. Dennis Franz's body became the key for the figure of the fat detective. His mode of approach is that of the hard-boiled detective, the muscular detective gone to seed, but his fat body is also seen as an external sign of his empathetic nature.[38]

The image of the giant, hulking, primitive body, which responds seemingly intuitively to a stimulus more basic than rational thought, remains a powerful cultural commonplace. It is only the appearance of the fat detective that leads us to assume his "primitive" state. In a cartoon drawn by Scott Adams, the creator of *Dilbert*, a baby dinosaur comments to Dogbert: "my Dad says that good is what you know in your heart. He says evil is a bad gut feeling." Dogbert replies "Well, of course, your dad's brain is so tiny that his other organs have to pitch in like that." The baby dinosaur replies: "Maybe I shouldn't learn about life from a guy who counts with his toes." And Dogbert concludes: "And thinks with his guts."[39] This is the way that fat detectives seem to think—but, of course, we know better.

Notes

1. Steven Shapin, "The Philosopher and the Chicken: On the Dietetics of Disembodied Knowledge," in *Science Incarnate: Historical Embodiments of Natural Knowledge*, Christopher Lawrence and Steven Shapin, eds. (Chicago: University of Chicago Press, 1998), 21–50.
2. Jenny Uglow, *The Lunar Men: Five Friends Whose Curiosity Changed the World* (New York: Farrar, Straus and Giroux, 2002).
3. On the history of myelin see especially the second edition of Edwin Clark and C. D. O'Malley, *The Human Brain and Spinal Cord* (San Francisco: Norman, 1996).
4. Clarke and O'Malley, *Human Brain*, 46–52.
5. Timothy O. Lipman, "Vitalism and Reductionism in Justus von Liebig's Physiological Thought," *Isis,* 58 (1967), 167–185 and K. Y. Guggenheim, "Johannes Müller and Justus Liebig on Nutrition," *Koroth,* 8 (1985), 66–76.
6. Thomas Jameson, *Essays on the Changes of the Human Body, at its Different Ages* (London: Longman, Hurst, Bees, Orme and Brown, 1811), 91.
7. Clarke and O'Malley, *Human Brain*, 78–80.
8. George E. Berrios and J. I. Quemada, "Multiple Sclerosis," in *A History of Clinical Psychiatry*, George E. Berrios and Roy Porter, eds. (New York: NYU Press, 1995), 174–192.
9. Clarke and O'Malley, *Human Brain*, 547–553.
10. Eric L. Santner, *My Own Private Germany: Daniel Paul Schreber's Secret History of Modernity* (Princeton: Princeton University Press, 1996), 70–77.
11. Sigmund Freud, *Standard Edition of the Complete Psychological Works of Sigmund Freud*, J. Strachey, A. Freud, A. Strachey, and A. Tyson ed. and trans., 24 vols. (London: Hogarth, 1955–1974), vol. 1, 299–300.

12. S. Weir Mitchell, *Fat and Blood and How to Make Them* (Philadelphia: Lippincott, 1877).

13. Martha J. Cutter, "The Writer as Doctor: New Models of Medical Discourse in Charlotte Perkins Gilman's Later Fiction," *Literature & Medicine,* 20 (2001), 151–182.

14. D. Rang, *Pharmacology* (London: Churchill Livingstone, 1995), 105.

15. Gerhart von Graevenitz, "Der Dicke im schlafenden Krieg: Zu einer Figur der europäischen Moderne bei Wilhelm Raabe," *Jahrbuch der Raabe-Gesellschaft* (1990), 1–21.

16. Wilhelm Raabe, *Novels*, ed. Volkmar Sander, trans. Barker Fairly (New York: Continuum, 1983), 174. Hereafter pages are cited in the text.

17. Hubert Ohl, "Eduards Heimkehr oder Le Vaillant und des Riesenfaultier: Zu Wilhelm Raabes *Stopfkuchen*," *Jahrbuch der Deutschen Schiller-Gesellschaft,* 8 (1964), 247–279.

18. D. F. Rauber, "Sherlock Holmes and Nero Wolfe: The Role of the 'Great Detective' in Intellectual History," *Journal of Popular Culture,* 6 (1972), 483–495.

19. James D. Smead, "The Landscape of Modernity: Rationality and the Detective," *Digging into Popular Culture: Theories and Methodolgies in Archeology, Anthropology and Other Fields*, Ray B. Browne and Pat Browne, eds. (Bowling Green, OH: Popular, 1991), 165–171.

20. Joshua Duke, *Banting in India with Some Remarks on Diet and Things in General* (Calcutta: Thacker, Spink and Co., 1885), 55.

21. Ronald R. Thomas, "Minding the Body Politic: The Romance of Science and the Revision of History in Victorian Detective Fiction," *Victorian Literature and Culture,* 19 (1991), 233–254.

22. Thomas M. Sobottke, "Speculations on the Further Career of Mycroft Holmes," *The Baker Street Journal,* 2 (1990), 75–77.

23. *The Original Illustrated Sherlock Holmes* (New York: Castle, n.d.), 294. This is a facsimile edition of the serial publication of the Holmes stories. Hereafter pages are cited in the text.

24. On Father Brown and Sherlock Holmes see Walter Raubicheck, "Father Brown and the 'Performance' of Crime," *The Chesterton Review,* 19 (1993), 39–45.

25. Frederick Isaac, "Enter the Fat Man: Rex Stout's *Fer-de-Lance*," in *In the Beginning: First Novels in Mystery Series*, Mary Jean DeMarr, ed. (Bowling Green, OH: Popular, 1995), 59–68.

26. John Mc Aleer, *Rex Stout: A Biography* (Boston: Little, Brown, and Co., 1977), 552.

27. Rex Stout, *Fer-De-Lance* (1934; New York: Bantam, 1984), 2.

28. Ibid.

29. Ibid., 164.

30. Rex Stout, *Over my Dead Body* (1939; New York: Bantam Books, 1994), 119.

31. David R. Anderson, *Rex Stout* (New York: Frederick Ungar Publishing Co., 1984), 23.

32. Stout, *Fer-De-Lance*, 4–5.

33. Rex Stout, *Not Quite Dead Enough* (New York: Bantam Books, 1992), 13.

34. Ibid., 81.

35. Rex Stout, *In the Best of Families* (New York: Bantam, 1993), 142. See also Neil Brooks, "Not Just a Family Affair: Questioning Critical and Generic Orthodoxies through the Nero Wolfe Mysteries," *Clues*, 20 (1999), 121–138.

36. Jerry Mosher, "Setting Free the Bears: Refiguring Fat Men on Television," *Bodies out of Bonds: Fatness and Transgression*, Jana Evans Braziel and Kathleen LeBesco, eds. (Berkeley: University of California Press, 2001), 166–193.

37. Tom Gunning, "Tracing the Individual Body: Photography, Detectives, and Early Cinema," *Cinema and the Invention of Modern Life*, Leo Charney, and Vanessa R. Schwartz, eds. (Berkeley: University of California Press, 1995), 15–45.

38. One can note that there is a fat female detective in Barbara Neely's "Blanche" series from the 1980s. She is a black detective of large proportions.

39. Scott Adams, *Bring Me the Head of Willy the Mailboy!* (Kansas City: Andrews and McMeel, 1995), 82.

Chapter 13 ✐

FAT IN AMERICA

Peter N. Stearns

American fat plays no small role in the contemporary world if only because it is unusually voluminous and evident. It serves as a national symbol and symbol. And while the American-ness can be overdone, there is a distinctive national experience that is both fascinating and cautionary.

To be sure, the history of fat in the United States follows many contours familiar in other Western, industrial countries. Fat began to be identified as a health and aesthetic issue at the very end of the nineteenth century, on bases shared with Western Europe. American concern may have lagged just slightly—the mid 1890s serve as a good beginning date for the United States—but there was substantial overlap not only in timing but also in basic causation. Most obviously, the United States participated in the results of new medical discovery and the more basic shift from concerns about contagious to degenerative diseases, as primary factors in mortality. The nation also saw an upsurge in the abundance and regular availability of food, just as work habits became more sedentary for many groups, while transportation improvements gradually reduced the need to walk. The result framed a new debate about fat that has continued to the present— and again, in broad outline, this fits a larger pattern.[1]

At least three distinctive twists make the national version of the standard story more interesting. Most obviously, as efforts to denigrate fat continued, Americans began to put on more weight—gradually around the middle of the twentieth century, much more rapidly since the 1980s. By this point, American obesity became a global issue, in its own right and sometimes as part of a larger critique of American policies and culture. As a French magazine recently put it, and not too kindly: "The United States is simply one big eating machine."[2] The unusually rapid rise of American obesity begs for explanation, and the history of American fat helps provide it. The second distinctive twist relates to the first: elements of the American approach to fat control differed from those used elsewhere, and seem to have been particularly counterproductive. As increasing obesity becomes a global issue, there may be some worthwhile lessons here that go beyond American shores, though they also have potential bearing on the national future. Finally, debates within the United States about the nature of obesity as a problem—whether fat, or attacks on fat, constitute the graver issue—while not unprecedented, have been particularly keen, obviously complicating national response to recent trends.

★　★　★

There are few indications of intense, widespread concern about fat in the United States before the 1890s. Fashions varied somewhat during the nineteenth century, and there was emphasis on the importance of slenderness in young adult women. One folk test involved a suitor's ability to touch hands around the waist of his beloved. It was perfectly legitimate, however, in the same middle-class circles, to use restraining garments to achieve the desired results: corsets, though criticized by doctors for distorting female organs, were widely used in the same age group.[3] There was also a considerable history of moralistic concern about purity and restraint in nutrition, including a presumed relationship between overindulgence in foods and in sex.[4] At the same time, plumpness in middle age was not only acknowledged, but also appreciated. The feminist leader Elizabeth Cady Stanton was praised for her mature figure, seen as a badge of motherhood and a sign of balanced character; feminist leaders who were more slender were reproved, with more than a hint of the traditional linkage between thinness and discontent.[5] Even younger women could draw comment for thinness. The French actress Sarah Bernhardt, during her first visit to the United States in the 1880s, was judged unattractive because she was too angular.[6] Plumpness was praised for more than aesthetic reasons. In men even more than women, it served as a sign of prosperity and, in an age appropriately worried about wasting diseases like tuberculosis, good health. A certain degree of weight was associated with good judgment and avoidance of extremes. In the 1860s, reflecting social tolerance if not approval, a Fat Man's Club was formed in Connecticut; it would last until 1907, when it disbanded because an altered culture made its watchword unacceptable. An extremely rotund president, William Howard Taft, encountered some banter about his weight in the early twentieth century—and he did lose a bit as part of his campaign strategy, while remaining very heavy—but comments were mild compared to those directed at a much less corpulent president, Bill Clinton, at the end of the century, when fat had become a badge of dishonor.[7]

Granting limited evidence, there is no particular sign that Americans had any particular incidence of fat, compared to other Western societies and to later national patterns. Students at the military academy of West Point, admittedly a perhaps atypical group, were quite slender, and there is no indication of average weight gain until after the 1920s.[8] For many, strenuous physical labor and, in the growing cities, lots of walking served to limit weight. While cases of obesity must have existed, they drew little public comment. Doctors were more likely to focus on particular symptoms, like gout, than on overeating as a general category. Overall, in fact, lack of adequate weight drew more medical and aesthetic comment than the reverse. Other-than-plump babies were a sign of ill health and bad parenting. Newspaper advertisements touted products designed to help young adults put on weight.

It is true that the national self-image included satisfaction at the abundance of food. Some scholars have argued that this was a general characteristic among people of European origin in the Americas, as they encountered fewer problems with food shortage than had been characteristic of peasant Europe—because of the different ratio between people and rich agricultural lands. Possibly self-congratulation on abundance helped counter other feelings of inferiority toward the old world.[9] Whatever the overall experience of the New World, American delight with plenty, noted by many scholars, definitely included food.[10] Rich recipes figured largely in nineteenth-century women's magazines. While replicating many features of conventional harvest festivals, the national holiday of Thanksgiving, as it spread from the 1860s onward, included strong emphasis on massive amounts of food surrounding the traditional turkey. Eating contests were a staple feature of many county fairs. All of this suggests a somewhat distinctive culture that had few further consequences in the nineteenth century itself, but which, maintained later amid more sedentary patterns, undoubtedly contributed to the unusual American weight trends.[11]

A special version of the commitment to plenty developed among many immigrant groups during the early twentieth century. Adjusting to a strange environment, often experiencing urban conditions for the first time, many immigrants delighted in food abundance. It provided comfort and a justification for the risky project of leaving familiar conditions. Weight gains among many ethnic groups, like Greek or Italian Americans, compared to their nonimmigrant counterparts, became common.[12]

Foreign observers also noted, from the early nineteenth century onward, an unusual national propensity to eat rapidly. Many young urban American men, including many immigrants, lived in boarding houses, where rapid eating among other things helped assure an adequate share at table. The "boarding house reach" entered the national vocabulary, designating people who greedily spooned into serving plates across their tablemates to make sure they got enough. The demands of industrial work also encouraged rapid eating. Again, in the nineteenth century itself this had no distinctive results in terms of body mass, but it constituted another set of national conventions that proved less suitable to the conditions of a more sedentary society later on.[13]

★   ★   ★

As noted, the modern history of fat in the United States begins around the middle of the 1890s, when fat began to be obsessively discussed, in middle-class circles, and vigorously reproved. Quite suddenly, slenderness became newly popular. Some established stage stars found their popularity eroding, and some went on crash diets in response. Sarah Bernhardt, on a second visit, was lionized as a considerable beauty. Women's fashions stressed thinness. The new "Gibson girl" look, popularized by artist Charles Gibson in *Life* magazine, featured a very slender young woman (with a similarly slender young man in the background). Soon after 1900, the United States participated in the great corset debate. While results were inconclusive, and support garments continued to be widely sold, there is no question that fashion for many women, as clothing became less stiff and constrained and might even include exercise garb, now included the ability to look thin without artificial aid.[14]

New attention from medical and insurance circles compounded the fashion trend, and applied more clearly to men as well as women. It's relevant to note that American doctors were a bit more hesitant than their leading European counterparts in admitting health issues associated with overweight. This reflected the fact that, around 1900, the United States had fewer medical research centers; all the pertinent research, at least until the 1920s, emanated from abroad. A number of practitioners wrote scornfully of their patients' interest in losing weight, which they found annoying;

considerable gender bias against women crept into some of the remarks.[15] This medical hesitancy could have contributed to a gap between fashion rhetoric about weight and actual individual commitments. (This was definitely the case concerning children, as we will see later on; and even in the early twenty-first century a number of critics called American doctors to task for being too timid with their patients in stressing weight issues.) Gradually, however, doctors did climb on board, at least officially; by the 1920s weight checks became a standard (and often dreaded) component of routine physical examinations in doctors' offices.[16] American insurance companies displayed none of the complexities of their medical colleagues. By 1900 insurance companies were issuing clear actuarial tables claiming a strong relationship between low weight and long life expectancy. In a nation increasingly committed to the purchase of life insurance policies, this information had considerable potential impact. In a familiar pattern, through succeeding decades insurance companies not only publicized their figures with growing zeal but also displayed a heightened rigor, such that desirable weights, adjusted to height, tended to go down steadily for both women and men. This trend toward rigor interestingly paralleled fashion trends where, except during the 1930s and 1950s, increasingly slender waists were emphasized. (The same applied to the most widely advertised models and film stars—thus, waist sizes for Miss America decreased fairly steadily, in relation to height, from the inception of the contest in the early 1920s.)[17] Insurance tables, fashion, and the media world operated in implicit harmony, fairly consistently raising the bar for acceptability.

This was the context in which weight issues received increasing discussion among middle-class Americans, from 1900 onward. This was the context in which interest in diet standards and devices steadily intensified, creating a major product industry. Newspaper advertisements for diet aids began to proliferate early in the twentieth century, quickly outstripping recipes for weight gain by the too-thin. To be sure, a new enthusiasm also developed for body-building among men; it was important not to be too scrawny, and a variety of systems were touted for moving from "98-pound weakling" to muscle-rippling beach hunk. But here too, leaders cautioned strongly against fat, one even rather nastily wondering, in 1920, whether fitness-enthusiast former president Teddy Roosevelt had died because he never managed to take off excess pounds.[18]

As they took root and fairly steadily expanded, diet enthusiasms in the United States followed patterns familiar in many parts of the Western world, and indeed there was considerable sharing of fads at least across the Atlantic, and with Australia and New Zealand as well. An American cachet was added to certain diet products sold in France, for instance, just as French fashions had particular resonance in New York and Chicago. In the United States, again as elsewhere, pressures were particularly keen for women, where the fashion industry sponsored draconian, youth-oriented standards, as among the flappers of the 1920s.[19] But there was a quieter male concern too, evident in the pages of new men's magazines like *Esquire*. Diet discussions subsided a bit during the 1930s, when concern about depression-induced malnutrition trumped attention to fat and over-weight. But they resumed with a vengeance in the 1950s, when they became a staple among women's magazines and in bookstores. Special diets, special products, and even weight-fighting organizations gained growing prominence.[20]

Three aspects of American diet enthusiasm stand out for their distinc-tiveness during the first six decades of the twentieth century and even beyond, though not all lend themselves to easy interpretation. First, clearly by the 1950s, but with some outcroppings as early as the 1920s, American diet promoters often seized on cases of truly spectacular weight losses, among both women and men. *The Ladies Home Journal*, for example, fea-tured a series of stories in the 1950s about people who had dropped 150 or more pounds. The success was compounded by the dramatic life results that accompanied such a personal achievement: love blossomed, jobs beck-oned, and all was right with the world. To be sure, occasional follow-ups noted falls from grace, as some fatties returned to older habits. But the emphasis on huge triumphs of the will was interesting, and it has resumed in the early twenty-first century with advertising programs from sources like the Subway sandwich chain trumpeting similar achievements through a combination of willpower and particular products. The growing rigor of slenderness ideals may have promoted this search for miracles.[21]

Critics have wondered if this American penchant for the miraculous was not counterproductive. Huge success claims could be discouraging for run-of-the-mill dieters, who simply could not win such results. A hope for miracles might distract from realistic daily commitments.

A second distinctive product of American diet enthusiasm was the group approach. Beginning in the 1930s with Alcoholics Anonymous, Americans began to place considerable trust in groups of strangers, united by a personal problem, who could support each other in remediation.[22] From the 1950s onward a number of groups formed, like Overeaters Anonymous, which used group confession as a tool in weight loss pro-grams. Many supplemented the use of collective shame and approval (I am an overeater, proclaimed to a room full of strangers; I have kept 30 pounds off for six months, to warm applause from the same strangers) with particular diet cookbooks or other products. But the use of shaming techniques, in a culture that in other respects resisted shame, was intriguing.[23] It blossomed particularly among women. It also proved exportable to a degree, as branches were established in Europe as elsewhere. But nowhere did the true confessions approach flourish as readily as in the United States; the French, for example, even more committed to slenderness, disliked discussing their eating transgressions in public.[24]

Self-help groups around weight issues related to the third and most significant American characteristic in the fight against fat: an early and deep-seated tendency to equate overeating and a fat appearance with moral deficiency. As *Living Age* magazine proclaimed in 1914: "Fat is now regarded as an indiscretion and almost as a crime." Plays might have titles like *Nobody Loves a Fat Man* (1907), and jokes about fat proliferated. During World War I, "Anybody healthy, normal individual, who is now getting fat is unpatriotic," according to popular magazines.[25] While the migration of the word *slob* (originally a Welsh word for gooey mud) began in Britain, it picked up steam in the United States. Moral opprobrium against fat people, particularly women, continued between the wars, where they were accused of sloth and simple lack of willpower,—"lazy and undisciplined," as one doctor put it, punishable of course by their sexual unattractiveness. Extreme adjectives that could be applied to the fat, with terms like "monstrous deformity" insultingly expressed not only in print, but to individuals (again particularly women) in doctors' offices. New twists were added by the 1950s, when the fat were widely assumed to be psychologically disturbed, doubtless because of inadequate childhoods. In characteristic psychobabble: "Circumstances leading to a high-weight mark usually stem from a fatal character flaw and other psychological manifestations." Women's and adolescent magazines filled with stories of people whose fears and anxieties propelled them to overeat. "Girls get fat because they're emotionally disturbed."[26]

The American penchant for moral judgments about fat was not of course unique. Elements occurred in other cultures as they faced the new ease of overweight that accompanied advanced industrial societies. But the penchant was unusually great. French doctors by the 1970s were at pains to reassure patients that their problems had nothing to do with personal fault, while widely criticizing the American approach.[27]

Distinctiveness, in turn, calls for assessments both of special causes and special results. As to cause: Americans clearly have a cultural penchant for turning health issues into moral crusades; they would do the same with smoking during the 1970s and 1980s. Compared to most other Western societies, the United States remained highly religious, which helps explain the ease of moralism. In the case of fat, two other prompts may have been involved. First, the fight against fat began at a time when Americans were increasingly indulging in consumer society. The delight in new products was widespread, but it also occasioned some guilt: was indulgence compatible with personal worth? Having a target for self-control, like dieting, helped express but also reconcile moral concerns about consumer affluence. Many articles directly equated dieting with a combat against a "soft" society. The association with ethical consumerism was directly expressed by some experts even early in the twentieth century—thus economist Simon Patten who praised the new ease of living but also insisted that it be accompanied by personal discipline in areas like eating.[28] A second moral spur, specifically applied to women, involved the decline of motherhood. Many Americans, headed by the middle class, participated eagerly in the falling birth rate of the early twentieth century. But the trend had its discomforts, particularly as women simultaneously began to express their sexual appetites more openly and as sex, by definition, was increasingly designed for pleasure, not procreation. Dieting was a way, again, to express virtue and self-control even in a changing sexual climate. And the results of dieting, rendering the maternal body image less popular, may have confirmed the association. In a moralistic culture, in other words, the association of fat with personal fault was compounded by the possibility of demonstrating virtue amid new contemporary moral uncertainties.[29]

The results of the moral crusade element of the battle against fat were several. Most obviously, it encouraged open prejudices against fat people. Employment discrimination against the overweight began to come to light by the 1970s, particularly in jobs like flight attendance that were disproportionately female and associated with physical attractiveness. But bias against fat showed vigorously off the job as well, for example in teenage culture, which could be vicious against the overweight—particularly among white girls. And it affected men, with the physical culture literature ridiculing the ineffectiveness of fat men.

Moralism had at least two other consequences, clearly counterproductive. In the first place, moralism tended to associate campaigns against overweight with the dominant white, middle-class culture. This in turn contributed to the desire of some minority groups, most vocally African Americans, to dissociate themselves from these goals—if only because they were so often the targets of this same moralism.[30] Second, even for white middle-class people themselves, the moral stakes attached to slenderness could add, ironically, to compulsions to eat. A woman tries a diet; she registers no improvement or even falls back a bit (a statistically common occurrence in all contemporary societies); she berates herself as a moral failure and eats to console. As one commentator put it, "Dieting while growing fatter is an inverted spiritual exercise: every time you break your resolution you eat even more, for consultation and in defiance." The linkage is convoluted, but it has been reported in a number of individual cases and may apply more widely.[31]

In sum, mainstream American standards converted to hostility to fat over a century ago. The process had some distinctive features, certain of which undoubtedly have complicated the goals involved. For the United States displayed a final unusual quality, even amid the din of the diet industry: amid deep commitments to slenderness and majority involvement with dieting (either about to diet, dieting, or just finished) by the 1970s, Americans began to put on weight.

★   ★   ★

There were various straws in the wind. Between 1939 and 1971, women's dress sizes were recalibrated for larger dimensions (a size 12 allowed for a one-inch expansion in waist). Seats in some stadia had to be widened. Between 1950 and 1978, caloric intake, by some estimates, went up six percent. Insurance company weight reports brought the message home. Between 1941 and 1963, men's average weight increased by eight pounds, in early to mid-adulthood, while women's weight went up at a slightly slower rate (though women remained more likely than men to be overweight). A 1979 study found an average weight increase of five pounds for both genders. Another estimate suggested a two-pound average weight gain during the 1970s alone. Height was also increasing, of course, thanks to better nutrition and less childhood illness, which modifies some of these findings, but the weight increase was more substantial. Several studies pinpointed weight gains when height was held constant. Nothing revolutionary, but an apparently inexorable trend.[32]

These steady gains are the more interesting compared to some European standards. Data complicate claims to precise comparison, but during much of the same period French weight seems to have declined modestly, again height held constant.[33] And of course the weight gains occurred against a backdrop of cultural pressure for slenderness and dieting: ideals and reality were increasingly diverging in the United States.

What was going on? Several factors contributed to the new weight trends. We have seen that older eating patterns and expectations complicated the realization of slenderness ideals in a society increasingly sedentary. Much of this period coincided with rapid expansion of desk-bound white collar jobs and also suburbanization with its deterrents to walking. Traditional pleasures in food abundance and fast eating could have new effects in this context. To a lesser extent, some of the counterproductive features of the diet craze, including excessive moralism and expectations of miraculous results, might have served a role as well.

Three additional factors came into play. First, the United States was blessed by unusually productive agriculture and an unusually powerful commercial food industry. These features could combine with the expectation of food plenty and fast eating. Most notably, from the 1880s onward American companies generated a growing array of snacks, first touted as contributions to health or work efficiency (through the energizing effects of sugar) but increasingly sold as just plain fun. Commercially baked crackers were the first entrants, along with sugary sodas initially intended to reduce the consumption of alcohol. By the interwar period snacks expanded to include cookies, chips, and packaged ice cream, and soda production proliferated. American grocery stores began their revealing reconfiguration to include huge rows of snack items. The 1920s also saw the origins of fast-food restaurants in the United States, with their standard fare of hamburgers and fried potatoes. With the formation of McDonalds in the 1950s, targeting family dining, the impact of fast foods accelerated. Unusual forms of food availability, in other words, combined with larger eating traditions to contribute to steady weight gains.[34]

Factor two was related: an interesting hesitation to impose slenderness standards on children. Here American habits contrasted with those of at least several European countries, where assumptions that children needed discipline in their eating were common. Despite sincere commitment to fighting fat in adults, Americans continued to value plump children as a sign of health and good parenting. Childrearing manuals relatively rarely raised the possibility of fat as a childhood problem until the 1970s, despite some medical concern from the 1940s onward. In contrast, malnutrition among children gained much attention, heightened by Depression-era concerns and then by the growing publicity given to phenomena such as anorexia nervosa. Experts long warned that even plump children might suffer from inadequate nutrition. For boys, the popularity of football, where overweight could be a positive advantage, may have added to the widespread tolerance of childhood fat. Obviously, this does not mean that no parent or doctor addressed children's overweight, but the phenomenon was not widely discussed.[35] One of the reasons adult Americans so often proclaimed the need to diet is that they reached adulthood with an active heritage from a childhood of some overindulgence. A 1952 pediatric text pinpointed the issue: "It is interesting that parents worry so little about fat children and so much about thin ones."[36] Even as doctors warned increasingly about childhood obesity, parental habits proved hard to change, including the impulse to use food to reward children and demonstrate that parents were sources of pleasure.

Finally, American weight gains were dramatically affected by open disagreements about fat and beauty standards. More culturally diverse than many modern societies, the United States embraced a number of large or growing groups who openly if implicitly, dissented from the official middle-class ideals and who were also in less frequent contact with doctors and medical literature. African Americans, most obviously, retained aesthetic standards that sanctioned big women, and to a lesser extent big men. From the 1940s onward, the pages of *Ebony* magazine, aimed at the black middle class, were revealing. Dieting advice was sparse, while clothes advertisements (when they did not use white models) featured women noticeably larger than the mainstream American average. Michelle Zeno, for example, carried 193 pounds on her 5 feet 10 inches when she became an *Ebony* model, noting simply: "I come from large people." A number of articles explicitly rejected dieting pressure. Ms. Zeno again: "You have to feel beautiful, just as beautiful as the next person." The magazine also frequently featured comments from men praising amplitude and associating substantial girth with sexiness. "Truth be told, my ideal woman is a size 20." "The only things a thin woman can do for me is to introduce me to a woman of size." These were not just the foibles of an individual publication. Polls during the 1980s and 1990s found African-American adolescent girls far more likely to be content with their bodies than their white counterparts, despite the fact (or to an extent because) they were noticeably bulkier on average.[37]

And there was no question, during the third quarter of the twentieth century and beyond: African Americans were heavier than their white counterparts, and they gained weight more rapidly during this specific period. Weight gains among African-American women were twice as substantial as those among whites, while African-American men more than quadrupled the gains of white men.

Other subcultures contributed as well. The growing Latino population maintained an active culture of heavy eating, and cities like San Antonio, Texas, with large Latino groups committed to high-calorie cuisine, were among the heaviest in the United States.

American weight patterns exhibited some of the social differentiations common in industrial countries: some traditional rural areas were heavier than the national average (Mississippi and West Virginia routinely tipped the scales at the top), and the working class was heavier than the middle class. But these patterns were exacerbated by subcultures with particular eating and aesthetic standards, subcultures that pushed heaviness in some deliberate defiance to middle-class American norms. Here was the final explanatory factor in the larger combination that produced noticeable weight gains in the diet-conscious decades.

★   ★   ★

By the 1980s, the clash between diet trends and reality added another component to the American mix: a strong backlash against slenderness standards. Civil rights legislation from the 1960s gave a number of individuals legal encouragement to file suit against employers who discriminated against them on grounds of weight. Several cases were won against airlines, police departments and other agencies. This contributed to a larger advocacy climate for the overweight, arguing against prejudice on the part of the general society. Into this mix came a strong feminist current, which generated a number of books and articles contending that slenderness campaigns were a plot to trap women into exhausting beauty regimens. Beauty advocates were obvious villains in this line of argument, but so were medical authorities. Some feminists simply rejected the idea that overweight had adverse health implications. A variety of groups formed around praise for fat bodies as beautiful, valid, and sexy.[38]

This was a small though vocal movement. Its impact was hard to calculate, but it certainly complicated the warnings about obesity in ways that could be confusing (or possibly liberating) for some. Advocacy groups for the overweight were more vocal in the United States than for example in France, which both reflected and encouraged less agreement on basic standards. The new opinion current, along with actual weight trends, surely contributed to some softening of media presentations of overweight by the 1990s. While models and real stars continued to shine by their slenderness, a number of television shows features hefty performers (including a number of African Americans). Whether all of this contributed to actual weight trends was uncertain, but it unquestionably made for vigorous debate.

★   ★   ★

The final chapter to date in the fat history of the United States began in the 1980s and has continued to the present day: an unprecedentedly rapid increase in weight gains and in percentages of obesity. This is the point at which American weight patterns began to win widespread international comment and criticism, as the nation unquestionably led the world in excess poundage.

The average American adult gained eight pounds between 1985 and 1995, and the momentum continued, with white Americans actually leading African Americans in rates of change (though still not in absolute levels). By 2002 the average individual American gained 20 pounds between his or her twenties and fifties, twice the rate of the 1970s. The percentage of obese and overweight rose to 62 percent, up from 48 percent in 1980; rates of outright obesity doubled. Growth in levels of childhood obesity soared even more rapidly, to about 19 percent by 2003; some claims pointed to a tripling here, over two decades.[39]

What was going on? Previous trends, including eating habits and attitudes to children, were still in play, and perhaps a greater permissiveness on weight issues contributed as well. Changes in the food industry played a considerable role, and some observers found them predominant. Restaurant meal size increased considerably. With food cheap, restaurants found that people responded more eagerly to larger meals than to reductions in prices. New kinds of corn syrups, introduced in the early 1980s, added to the caloric content of sodas. Marketing of snacks and other caloric foods became steadily more aggressive. The huge surge in coffee houses, offering cream-laden options, was another contribution to weight gains.[40]

Adding to this factor were undeniable changes in domestic habits. With more married women and mothers working, attention to home cooking declined. More people took their meals in restaurants or from prepackaged foods, and this reduced care in monitoring portion size and often contributed to increased haste as well. Fewer meals were taken in families, with socializing and group controls monitoring eating behavior; more family members took food on the run, and this included many busy adolescents. More children were left to their own devices after school, as both parents worked; this too reduced supervision of snack eating. Parental guilt, at leaving children alone, could express itself in provision of comforting but high-calorie foods.[41]

Compounding all of this of course were further moves toward sedentary lifestyles. Not only extensive television watching, but also the new commitment to computers (and for children, computer games) reduced exercise for many, adults and children alike.

Many of these trends were common in the industrial world, and indeed obesity rates began to mount quite generally in the global middle class and among the class's children. But the United States saw some trends, like aggressive food marketing, mount particularly rapidly; restaurant meal size was a case in point. And the trends built on preexisting national patterns, which again differentiated the American case from many other countries.

A final factor may have entered in as well, helping to explain, for example, the new vulnerability to the lures of the food industry. Many Americans began working longer hours during the 1980s and 1990s, pressed at once by constrictions on real wages and by the excitement of the 1990s economic boom. By the 1990s, Americans enjoyed less formal vacation time than their counterparts in all other industrial societies, now including Japan. Work pressure obviously contributed to changes in domestic eating habits. But it added inducements of its own: working more strenuously, many Americans took meals at their desks, and sought comfort foods that would provide quick satisfaction as other, more elaborate recreational outlets, including more leisurely dining, were unavailable. This element in causation is difficult to prove definitively, though it does help explain America's particularly rapid ascent into turn-of-the-century fat. It was at the least revealing that most places of work began to install food outlets in each building, to facilitate the quick bite. Americans were becoming uncomfortable with work, or leisure, that did not have a food source within easy reach, a change which both reflected and encouraged the new weight trends.[42]

And of course, as an interesting imponderable, the 1970s and 1980s constituted the point at which large numbers of Americans stopped smoking, or never started, a huge national change that proceeded much more rapidly than in most other countries. Clearly a customary solace, for example at work, was being removed for all but the 25 percent who persisted, and possibly other eating needs were encouraged as well—if only because, proud of their self-control in one area, many felt authorized to relax it in another.

By the early twenty-first century, the impact of growing weight gains began to penetrate the national consciousness, even amid some continued agitation for greater tolerance for fat. Diet enthusiasms multiplied, including some revivals of older approaches that had initially been shunted aside. As a popular cartoon held, carbohydrates replaced the devil in the chic American lexicon of evils. National warnings about the problem gained greater attention, though of course the results of this new attention remained unclear.

★   ★   ★

This essay has emphasized some distinctive American features among common trends and contexts in advanced industrial societies over the past century. The United States participated in the common phenomenon of more abundant food, more sedentary work and life styles. A few special traditions, a few distinctive twists including quite recent ones, embellish this basic challenge in recent United States history. It is important, however, not to overdo the comparative distinctions. By the early twenty-first century, it was becoming clear that recent weight gains in the United States had simply anticipated and exceeded larger global trends, with increased obesity reports from India and China, as well as places like France. Gibes at American gluttony may still be warranted, as eating habits may symbolically link with an aggressive foreign policy, but problems are not American alone.

And in this regard, aspects of the American historical experience also provide some potential lessons, for the nation itself as it faces a new round of concern about weight, and possibly for other countries as well. It is fairly clear, in the American context but possibly more widely, that guilt trips really do not work effectively. Making people feel personally deficient as they face weight problems does not motivate remediation very widely, and often leads to compounding behaviors. As some countries face a newer weight problem—France is an example again—there is a strong temptation to develop new levels of blame, trying to scare people into thinness by invoking both personal guilt and a failure to live up to a proud national image. The American experience suggests that this is a bad idea and should be reconsidered.

A clear product of the accusatory approach, again becoming more visible in places like France, is that its unfairness conflicts with other contemporary cultural norms that argue against discrimination against any group, including the heavy. The result is a series of conflicting reports, conferences, even formal scholarship, as to whether fat or campaigns against fat represent the real problem. Here too, it would be helpful to move beyond recent history, to a slenderness rhetoric that is less intolerant and therefore a set of responses that is less confusing.

Recent discussions, in the United States and of course globally, do suggest the possibility of moving to a new stage in the contemporary approach to fat. The argument is, simply, that the contemporary pressures toward excess weight need to be seen as social, and not just or even primarily as individual issues. Solutions, therefore, must be sought that go beyond individual self-control as well. Some American companies, faced with the medical cost implications of current weight trends, have been reorganizing spaces to encourage walking, even placing elevators so that use of stairs may seem more efficient. International proposals for special taxation on promotions for certain kinds of foods, mostly snacks, are interesting as well. We may be moving past the purely individualistic approach to fat issues, which so easily lends itself to moralism and blame.

Even this, however, will be contentious. When the World Health Organization floated its tax idea, many Republican leaders promptly replied that eating was in fact a purely individual concern, a matter for self-control and nothing more. This stance mirrored their take on other social issues, such as teenage pregnancy, where "just say no" campaigns predominate over some of the collective approaches common elsewhere, and it also reflected extreme sensitivity to regulations that might adversely affect business, along with a general reluctance to credit international recommendations of any sort. A certain American distinctiveness would not vanish.

Still, the scope of this distinctiveness should not be overdrawn. Elements of the national experience do provide useful examples. Time will tell whether American exceptionalism persists with regard to fat, or whether the United States will turn out to have been first among equals in a complex global transition to changes in eating habits and styles of life.

Notes

1. Peter N. Stearns, *Fat History: Bodies and Beauty in the Modern West* (rev. ed., New York: NYU Press, 2002); Hillel Schwartz, *Never Satisfied: A Cultural History of Diets, Fantasies and Fat* (New York: Free Press, 1983).
2. *Nouvel Observateur* (July 2000).
3. Lois Banner, *American Beauty* (Chicago: University of Chicago Press, 1983).
4. Stephen Nissenbaum, *Sex, Diet and Debility in Jacksonian America* (Westport, CT: Greenwood, 1980). The early moral efforts to purify nutrition, associated with people like Sylvester Graham and Kellogg, were not directed specifically to fat, though they provided some precedents for later applications.
5. Banner, *American Beauty*.
6. Lois Banner, *In Full Flower: Ageing Women, Power and Sexuality* (New York: Knopf, 1992); see also idem, *American Beauty*.
7. Hillel Schwartz, *Never Satisfied* (New York: Smithmark Publishers, 1995).
8. Timothy Cuff, "The Body Mass Index Values of Mid Nineteenth-Century West Point Cadets," *Historical Methods*, 26 (1993), 171–181; John Komlos and Peter Coclanis, "Nutrition and Economic Development in Post-Reconstruction South Carolina," *Social Science History*, 19 (1995); M. F. Najj and M. Rowland, *Anthropometric Reference Data and Prevalence of Overweight, 1976–1980*, National Center for Health Statistic, Vital and Health Statistic Series, report no. DHH5/PUB/PHS-87-1688 (Hyattsville MD, 1987); M. F. Nazz and R. J. Kuczmarski, *Anthropometric Data and Prevalence of Overweight*

for Hispanics: 1982–1984, National Center for Health Statistics,Vital and Health Statistics Series, report no. DHH5PUB/PHS-87-1689 (Hyattsville, MD: 1989).

9. John C. Super, *Food, Conquest and Colonization in Sixteenth-Century Spanish America* (Albuquerque: University of New Mexico Press, 1988), 84–85.

10. David Potter, *People of Plenty: Economic Abundance and American Character* (Chicago: University of Chicago Press, 1954), 191–193.

11. Leon Baritz, *The Good Life: The Meaning of Success for the American Middle-Class* (New York: Knopf, 1982); Reay Tannahill, *Food in History* (New York: Penguin, 1973).

12. Donna Gabaccia, *We Are What We Eat: Ethnic Food and the Making of Americans* (Cambridge: Harvard University Press, 1998).

13. Waverley Root and Richard de Rochemont, *Eating in America* (New York: William Morrow and Co., 1976), 124–125; Constantin Volney, *View of the Soul and Climate of the United States of America* (London: J. Johnson,1803), 323. See also Richard Cummings, *The American and His Food* (Chicago: University of Chicago Press, 1940).

14. Schwartz, *Never Satisfied*; Jill Fields, "Fighting the Corsetless Evil," *Journal of Social History* 30 (1996).

15. James McLester, "Principles Involved in the Treatment of Obesity," *Journal of the American Medical Association,* 82 (1924), 2103; Lulu Graves, "Coping with Overweight," *Modern Hospital,* 32 (1929), 63, 64.

16. Schwartz, *Never Satisfied.*

17. Stearns, *Fat History,* ch. 2; Viviana Zelizer, *Morals and Markets: The Development of Life Insurance in the United States* (New York: Columbia University Press, 1979). For precedents, see Nissenbaum, *Sex, Diet and Debility.*

18. James Whorton, *Crusaders for Fitness: The History of American Health Reformers* (Princeton: Princeton University Press, 1982).

19. M. Pumphrey, "The Flapper, The Housewife and the Making of Modernity," *Cultural Studies,* 2 (1987); Kathy Peiss, *Hope in a Jar: The Making of American Beauty Culture* (New York: Metropolitan Books, 1998); Estelle B. Freedman, "The New Woman: Changing Views of Women in the 1920s," *Journal of American History,* 16 (1974), 372–393.

20. Naomi Wolf, *The Beauty Myth: How Images of Beauty are Used Against Women* (New York: Anchor Books, 1991); Joan Jacobs Brumberg, *Fasting Girls: The Emergence of Anorexia as a Modern Disease* (Cambridge: Harvard University Press, 1988).

21. Roberta Pollack Seid, *Never Too Thin: Why Women are at War with their Bodies* (New York: Prentice Hall, 1989); see *Ladies Home Journal,* January 1924 and 1953, passim.

22. Klaus Makela, ed, *Alcoholics Anonymous as a Mutual-Help Movement* (Madison, WI: University of Wisconsin Press, 1996).

23. On the decline of shame in American culture, John Demos, "Shame and Guilt in Early New England," in *Emotion and Social Change,* Carol Z. Stearns and

Peter N. Stearns, eds. (New York: Holmes and Meier, 1988), 69–86; see also Peter N. Stearns, *American Cool: Constructing a Twentieth-Century Emotional Style* (New York: NYU Press, 1994). Of course some shaming persisted anyway, but its specific use in the self-help groups is an intriguing and distinctive throwback. Part of the explanation involves sensitivity to one's image with others in an other-directed society.

24. Annick Peinge, "Nous maigrons ensemble," *Le temps des femmes* (1988), 14–16; *Le Monde*, 28 June 1995.

25. Edith Lowry, *The Woman of Forty* (Chicago: Forbes and Co., 1919); "On Growing Fat," *Atlantic Monthly*, 99 (1907), 431; *The Nation* 101 (1918), 355–357.

26. Murray Segal, *Think Thin* (New York, 1971), 28 and 103; Theodore Rubin, *The Thin Book* (New York: Trident Press, 1966), 11, 46, 54; Sidney Petrie, *The Lazy Lady's Easy Diet* (West Nyack, NY: Parker Publishing Co., 1969); Frank J. Wilson, *Glamour, Glucose and Glands* (New York: Vantage Press, 1956). See also Richard Stein and Carol Nemeroff, "Moral Overtones of Food: Judgments of Others Based on What They Eat," *Personality and Social Psychology Bulletin*, 21 (1995), 480–490.

27. Gilbert Dreyfus, *Pourquoi l'on grossit et comment mincir* (Paris: Stock, 1977). Dreyfus had made similar comments in earlier editions going back to the 1950s.

28. Simon Patten, *New Basis of Civilization* (1910; reprint Cambridge: Harvard University Press, 1969); idem, "Overnutrition and its Social Consequences," *Annals*, 10 (1897), 44–46; Daniel Fox, *The Discovery of Abundance: Simon N. Patten and the Transformation of Social Theory* (New York: American Historical Association, 1976).

29. Peter N. Stearns, *Battleground of Desire: The Struggle for Self-Control in American History* (New York: NYU Press, 1999).

30. Maya Brown, "Dying to the Thin" (article ms., *Western Psychiatric Institute*, Pittsburgh, PA); S. K. Kumanyika, F. F. Wilson, and M. Guildford-Davenport, "Weight-related Attitudes and Behaviors of Black Women," *Journal of the American Dietetic Association*, 93 (1993), 416–422.

31. Richard Klein, "Big Country: The Roots of American Obesity," *New Republic* (19 September 1994), 351.

32. David Williamson, "Descriptive Epidemiology of Body Weight and Weight Change in U.S. Adults," *Annals of Internal Medicine* (1953), 646–649; "Trends in Average Weights, Insured Men and Women," *Statistical Bulletin of the Metropolitan Life Insurance Company* (1966), 1–3; "Trends in Average Weights and Heights of Men: An Insurance Experience," *Statistical Bulletin of the Metropolitan Life Insurance Company* (1970); 6–7; *Society of Actuaries and Association of Life Insurance Medical Directors of America, Build Study* 1979 (New York, 1980); Edward Lew, "Mortality and Weight: Insured Lives and the American Cancer Society Studies," *Annals of Internal Medicine* (1989), 1024–1029.

33. A. Charraud and H. Valdeliévre, "Le Taille et le poids du francais," *Economie et Statistique,* 132 (1981), 22–38; Dominique Laurier et al., "Prevalence of Obesity: A comparative Survey," *International Journal of Obesity,* 16 (1992), 568; Stearns, *Fat History,* chart, 212.

34. Harvey Levenstein, *Revolution at the Table: The Transformation of the American Diet* (New York: Oxford University Press, 1988), 44–60 and passim.

35. Gladys Schultz, "Our Underfed Children," *Ladies Home Journal* (March 1951), 44–45; L. E. Holt, "The Reluctant Eater," *Good Housekeeping* (November 1956), 132; Charles Aldrich, *Cultivating the Child's Appetite* (New York, 1931); Marion Farmer, "Between Meals," *Nation's School* (January 1934), 256; Frank Richardson, "Your Underweight Child," *Good Housekeeping* (January 1930), 35; Josephine Kenyon, "Thin Child," *Good Housekeeping* (October 1933), 98; Lettie Gay, "Feeding the Under-Weight Child," *Parents' Magazine* (March 1936), 40.

36. James Hughes, *Pediatrics in General Practice* (New York, 1952), 144.

37. "Big Can Be Beautiful," *Ebony* (October 1978); "When Bigger is Better," *Ebony* (July 1994); "Women Fight Back," *Ebony* (March 1990), 27–31.

38. Wolf, *The Beauty Myth*; Seid, *Never Too Thin*; Rosalyn Meadows and Lillie Weiss, *Women's Conflicts about Eating and Sexuality* (Binghamton, NY: Haworth Press, 1993); Marcia Millman, *Such a Pretty Face: Being Fat in America* (New York: Norton, 1980).

39. Robert Kuczmarski et al., "Increasing Prevalence of Overweight Among US Adults," *Journal of the American Medical Association,* 272 (20 July 1994), 205–211.

40. Greg Critser, *Fatland: How Americans Became the Fattest People in the World* (New York: Houghton-Mifflin, 2003). The question of which comes first, food lures or new individual motives, applies earlier to American snacking and now to portion size. A bit of both is a common sense conclusion: the lures do not explain the whole behavior.

41. Peter N. Stearns, *Anxious Parents: The History of Modern American Childrearing* (New York: NYU Press, 2003).

42. See Stearns, *Fat History,* preface to the new edition; Gary Cross, *An All-Consuming Century: Why Commercialism Won in Modern America,* (New York: Columbia University Press, 2000) and *Time and Money: The Making of Consumer Culture* (New York: Routledge, 1993).

Index